AF360906

Recent Advances and Clinical Outcomes of Kidney Transplantation

Recent Advances and Clinical Outcomes of Kidney Transplantation

Special Issue Editors

Charat Thongprayoon
Wisit Cheungpasitporn
Napat Leeaphorn

MDPI • Basel • Beijing • Wuhan • Barcelona • Belgrade • Manchester • Tokyo • Cluj • Tianjin

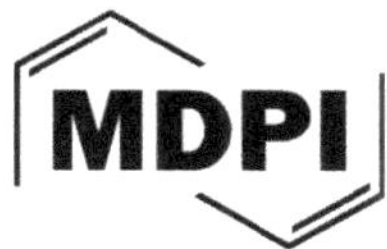

Special Issue Editors

Charat Thongprayoon
Division of Nephrology and Hypertension
USA

Wisit Cheungpasitporn
University of Mississippi Medical Center
USA

Napat Leeaphorn
Saint Luke's Health System
USA

Editorial Office
MDPI
St. Alban-Anlage 66
4052 Basel, Switzerland

This is a reprint of articles from the Special Issue published online in the open access journal *Journal of Clinical Medicine* (ISSN 2077-0383) (available at: https://www.mdpi.com/journal/jcm/special_issues/outcomes_kidney_transplantation).

For citation purposes, cite each article independently as indicated on the article page online and as indicated below:

LastName, A.A.; LastName, B.B.; LastName, C.C. Article Title. *Journal Name* **Year**, *Article Number*, Page Range.

Volume 2
ISBN 978-3-03936-407-7 (Pbk)
ISBN 978-3-03936-408-4 (PDF)

Volume 1-2
ISBN 978-3-03936-409-1 (Pbk)
ISBN 978-3-03936-410-7 (PDF)

Contents

About the Special Issue Editors

Charat Thongprayoon, M.D.; Division of Nephrology and Hypertension, Department of Medicine, Mayo Clinic, Rochester, MN, USA. Email: charat.thongprayoon@gmail.com. Dr. Charat Thongprayoon, M.D., is affiliated with Mayo Clinic Hospital Rochester. His research interests include nephrology, electrolytes, acute kidney injury, renal replacement therapy, epidemiology, and outcome studies.

Wisit Cheungpasitporn, M.D.; Division of Nephrology, Department of Medicine, University of Mississippi Medical Center, Mississippi, USA. Email: wcheungpasitporn@gmail.com. Dr. Wisit Cheungpasitporn is board-certified in both Nephrology and Internal Medicine. He completed his nephrology fellowship training at Mayo Clinic, Rochester, Minnesota. Dr. Cheungpasitporn also completed his additional training at Mayo and has become an expert on kidney transplantation. He completed his postdoctoral diploma in the clinical and translational science (CCaTS) program in 2015. Dr. Cheungpasitporn received the 2016 Donald C. Balfour Research Award, given in recognition of outstanding research as a junior scientist whose primary training is in a clinical field at Mayo Clinic, Rochester, Minnesota, as well as the 2016 William H. J. Summerskill Award, given in recognition of outstanding achievement in research for a clinical fellow at Mayo Clinic, Rochester, Minnesota. Dr. Cheungpasitporn has been part of Division of Nephrology at UMMC since August 2017.

Napat Leeaphorn, M.D., is a nephrology specialist in Kansas City, MO. He currently practices at Saint Luke's Kidney Transplant Specialists. Dr. Leeaphorn is board-certified in Internal Medicine and Nephrology.

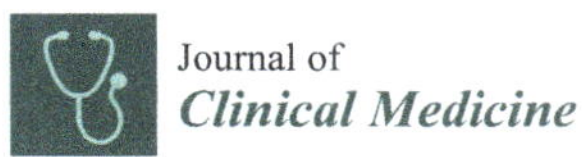 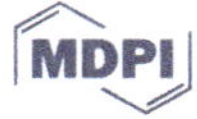

Journal of
Clinical Medicine

Article

Chronic Use of Proton-Pump Inhibitors and Iron Status in Renal Transplant Recipients

Rianne M. Douwes [1,*], António W. Gomes-Neto [1], Michele F. Eisenga [1], Joanna Sophia J. Vinke [1], Martin H. de Borst [1], Else van den Berg [1], Stefan P. Berger [1], Daan J. Touw [2], Eelko Hak [3], Hans Blokzijl [4], Gerjan Navis [1] and Stephan J.L. Bakker [1]

[1]   Department of Internal Medicine, Division of Nephrology, University Medical Center Groningen, University of Groningen, 9700 RB Groningen, The Netherlands
[2]   Department of Clinical Pharmacy and Pharmacology, University Medical Center Groningen, University of Groningen, 9700 RB Groningen, The Netherlands
[3]   Unit PharmacoTherapy, -Epidemiology and –Economics, Groningen Research Institute of Pharmacy, University of Groningen, 9713 AV Groningen, The Netherlands
[4]   Department of Gastroenterology and Hepatology, University Medical Center Groningen, University of Groningen, 9700 RB Groningen, The Netherlands
*   Correspondence: r.m.douwes@umcg.nl; Tel.: +31-050-3612-277

Received: 14 August 2019; Accepted: 28 August 2019; Published: 3 September 2019

Abstract: Proton-pump inhibitor (PPI) use may influence intestinal iron absorption. Low iron status and iron deficiency (ID) are frequent medical problems in renal transplant recipients (RTR). We hypothesized that chronic PPI use is associated with lower iron status and ID in RTR. Serum iron, ferritin, transferrin saturation (TSAT), and hemoglobin were measured in 646 stable outpatient RTR with a functioning allograft for $\geq$ 1 year from the "TransplantLines Food and Nutrition Biobank and Cohort Study" (NCT02811835). Median time since transplantation was 5.3 (1.8–12.0) years, mean age was 53 $\pm$ 13 years, and 56.2% used PPI. In multivariable linear regression analyses, PPI use was inversely associated with serum iron (β = −1.61, p = 0.001), natural log transformed serum ferritin (β = −0.31, p < 0.001), TSAT (β = −2.85, p = 0.001), and hemoglobin levels (β = −0.35, p = 0.007), independent of potential confounders. Moreover, PPI use was independently associated with increased risk of ID (Odds Ratio (OR): 1.57; 95% Confidence Interval (CI) 1.07–2.31, p = 0.02). Additionally, the odds ratio in RTR taking a high PPI dose as compared to RTR taking no PPIs (OR 2.30; 95% CI 1.46–3.62, p < 0.001) was higher than in RTR taking a low PPI dose (OR:1.78; 95% CI 1.21–2.62, p = 0.004). We demonstrated that PPI use is associated with lower iron status and ID, suggesting impaired intestinal absorption of iron. Moreover, we found a stronger association with ID in RTR taking high PPI dosages. Use of PPIs should, therefore, be considered as a modifiable cause of ID in RTR.

Keywords: proton-pump inhibitors; iron; iron deficiency; renal transplantation

---

1. Introduction

Iron deficiency (ID) is very common in renal transplant recipients (RTR), with reported prevalence of 20% to 30% more than 12 months after transplantation [1–3]. ID is an important contributor to post-transplant anemia, which affects approximately 20% to 49% of RTR within the first year after transplantation and is associated with adverse health outcomes [1,4–6]. Besides clinical symptoms associated with ID, such as fatigue, dyspnea, and decreased exercise tolerance, iron deficiency anemia (IDA) has been associated with an increased risk of graft failure and mortality in RTR [4,6,7]. Moreover, iron deficiency, independent of anemia, has been shown to be a risk factor for mortality in RTR [3].

Identifying modifiable risk factors of post-transplant ID may improve transplant outcomes and quality of life in RTR. In this regard, drug-induced factors should not be ignored. Recently, several observational studies have demonstrated that chronic proton-pump inhibitor (PPI) use may negatively affect iron status and is associated with ID in the general population [8–11]. It is postulated that PPIs interfere with the absorption of iron in the duodenum, where non-heme iron is primarily absorbed in its ferrous form (Fe^{2+}) after the reduction from its less absorbable ferric form (Fe^{3+}), which is facilitated by gastric acid and membrane reductases localized at the apical membrane of the enterocytes [12,13]. This hypothesis is supported by a study from Ajmera et al., who found a reduced response to oral supplementation of ferrous sulfate in iron deficient patients taking omeprazole [14]. In a large population-based case-control study, an increased risk of ID was found among patients receiving PPI therapy for at least one year and even among intermittent long-term PPI users compared to PPI non-users [8]. These findings are in line with previous results from another large cohort study in the United States, which demonstrated a higher risk of ID among chronic users of both PPIs and H2-receptor antagonists (H2RAs), which diminished after treatment discontinuation [9].

PPIs are frequently prescribed after renal transplantation to prevent gastrointestinal complications from immunosuppressants, and may therefore possibly contribute to the high burden of post-transplant ID in RTR. It is currently unknown whether chronic PPI use adversely affects iron status in RTR and studies investigating this hypothesis are lacking. In the present study, we aimed to investigate the association of PPI use with iron status in a large single-center cohort of stable outpatient RTR.

2. Methods

2.1. Study Design

For this cross-sectional cohort study, we used data from a previously well-described cohort of 707 stable RTR registered at clinicaltrials.gov as "TransplantLines Food and Nutrition Biobank and Cohort Study", NCT02811835 [15]. In brief, all adult RTR with a functioning graft for at least 1 year without known or apparent systemic illnesses (i.e., malignancies, opportunistic infections) who visited the outpatient clinic of the University Medical Center Groningen (UMCG) between November 2008 and March 2011 were invited to participate. Written consent was obtained from 707 of the initially 817 invited RTR. Study measurements were performed during a single study visit at the outpatient clinic.

2.2. Exposure Definition

RTR using any PPI on a daily basis during a period of at least 3 months before the study visit were defined as chronic PPI users. For statistical analyses we excluded RTR with missing data on PPI dosage (n = 1), with on-demand PPI use (n = 3), with missing data on iron status parameters (n = 7), or using iron supplements or EPO stimulating agents (n = 50), leaving 646 RTR eligible for analysis.

2.3. Study Approval

The study protocol was approved by the institutional review board (METC 2008/186, approved on 17 September 2008) of the UMCG and all study procedures were performed in accordance with the Declaration of Helsinki and the Declaration of Istanbul.

2.4. Clinical Measurements and Iron Status Parameters

Information on medical history, including reported history of gastritis or peptic ulcer disease, was obtained from electronic patient records as described previously [15]. Medication use, including the use of PPIs, diuretics, renin-angiotensin-aldosterone system (RAAS) inhibitors, antiplatelet drugs, anti-diabetic drugs, mycophenolate mofetil (MMF), calcineurin inhibitors (CNIs) and prednisolone, was recorded at baseline. Blood pressure was measured using a standard protocol, as described previously [16]. Information on alcohol use and smoking behavior was obtained using a questionnaire.

Blood samples were collected after an 8–12 h overnight fasting period. Serum creatinine was measured using an enzymatic, isotope dilution mass spectrometry traceable assay (P-Modular automated analyzer, Roche Diagnostics, Mannheim, Germany). Estimated glomerular filtration rate (eGFR) was calculated applying the serum creatinine-based chronic kidney disease epidemiology collaboration (CKD-EPI) equation. Concentrations of glucose, hemoglobin A1c (HbA1c), and high-sensitivity C-reactive protein (hs-CRP) were determined using standard laboratory methods. Serum iron was measured using photometry (Modular P800 system; Roche Diagnostics, Mannheim, Germany). Serum ferritin concentrations were determined using the electrochemiluminescence immunoassay (Modular analytics E170; Roche Diagnostics, Mannheim, Germany). Transferrin was measured using an immunoturbidimetric assay (Cobas-c analyzer, P-Modular system; Roche Diagnostics, Mannheim, Germany). Transferrin saturation (TSAT, %) was calculated as 100 × serum iron (μmol/L)/25 × transferrin (g/L). Iron deficiency was defined as transferrin saturation (TSAT) < 20% and ferritin < 300 μg/L, as described in literature previously and commonly used in patients with pro-inflammatory conditions, such as chronic heart failure and chronic kidney disease [3,17–19]. Proteinuria was defined as urinary protein excretion ≥ 0.5 g/24 h.

2.5. Assessment of Dietary Iron Intake

Total dietary iron intake (i.e., heme and non-heme iron) was assessed using a validated semi-quantitative food frequency questionnaire (FFQ), which was filled out at home [20,21]. Dietary data were converted into daily nutrient intake using the Dutch Food Composition Table of 2006 [22].

2.6. Statistical Analyses

Statistical analyses were performed using Statistical Package for the Social Sciences (SPSS), version 23.0 (IBM corp., Armonk, NY, USA). Data are presented as mean ± SD for normally distributed data, median with interquartile range (IQR) for skewed data, and number with percentage for nominal data. Differences between PPI users versus PPI non-users were tested using independent sample T-tests, Mann–Whitney U-tests, and Chi-square tests or Fishers exact test when appropriate.

To investigate the association of PPI use with serum iron, serum ferritin, TSAT, and hemoglobin levels, univariable and multivariable linear regression analyses were performed with adjustment for potential confounders of iron status including: age, sex, eGFR, proteinuria, time since transplantation, history of gastrointestinal disorders (i.e., reported history of gastritis or peptic ulcer disease before baseline), lifestyle parameters (BMI, smoking behavior, and alcohol use, dietary iron intake), inflammation (hs-CRP), MMF use, and other medication use (i.e., diuretics, RAAS-inhibitors, anti-platelet therapy, CNI use, and prednisolone use). Serum ferritin was natural log (ln) transformed to obtain a normal distribution. To investigate a dose-response relationship, we performed additional analyses in which RTR were divided into three groups based on daily PPI dose defined in omeprazole equivalents: no PPI, low PPI dose (≤20 mg omeprazole equivalents/day (Eq/d)), and high PPI dose (>20mg omeprazole Eq/d) [23]. Tests of linear trend were conducted by assigning the median of daily PPI dose equivalents in subgroups treated as a continuous variable. To investigate the association between PPI use and ID, we performed logistic regression analyses with adjustment for the same potential confounders used in multivariable linear regression analyses. In sensitivity analyses, H2RA users (n = 20) were excluded to assess the robustness of the association between PPI use and ID. Additionally, we performed sensitivity analyses using an alternative definition of ID as proposed in a position statement by the European Best Practice (ERBP) group and previously recommended in the United Kingdom-based National Institute for Health and Care Excellence (NICE) guideline (NG8) (TSAT < 20% and ferritin < 100 μg/L) [24,25]. A two-sided *p*-value < 0.05 was considered statistically significant in all analyses.

3. Results

3.1. Baseline Characteristics

Baseline characteristics are shown in Table 1. At baseline, RTR were 53 ± 13 years old and 382 (59.1%) were male. Mean BMI was 26.7 ± 4.8 kg/m^2, and 157 (24.3%) had diabetes. RTR were included at a median of 5.3 (1.8–12.0) years after transplantation. Mean eGFR was 53.5 ± 19.9 mL/min/1.73 m^2 and 135 (21.0%) had proteinuria. Mean serum iron and median ferritin concentrations were 15.2 ± 5.9 μmol/L and 115.5 (53.0–213.3) µg/L, respectively. Mean hemoglobin concentration was 13.3 ± 1.7 g/dL and mean TSAT was 25.1 ± 10.5%. Iron deficiency was present in 193 (29.9%) RTR. PPIs were used by a small majority of 363 (56.2%) RTR and omeprazole was the most often prescribed PPI (n = 317). Other PPIs used included esomeprazole (n = 28), pantoprazole (n = 15), and rabeprazole (n = 3). RTR who used PPIs were older than RTR who did not use PPIs, had a higher BMI, and had shorter time between transplantation and baseline measurements. Furthermore, diabetes was more prevalent in RTR using PPIs and PPI users had higher glucose and HbA1c levels, and lower levels of hemoglobin, iron, ferritin, and TSAT. Dietary iron intake was not significantly different between PPI users and PPI non-users. Additionally, CNIs and MMF, diuretics, anti-diabetic drugs, and antiplatelet drugs were more often used by PPI users compared to PPI non-users.

Table 1. Baseline characteristics of 646 renal transplant recipients.

Characteristics	Total Population	Non-PPI User	PPI User	*p*
Number of subjects, n (%)	646 (100)	283 (43.8)	363 (56.2)	n/a
Demographics				
Age, years	53 ± 13	51 ± 13	54 ± 12	0.001
Men, n (%)	382 (59.1)	170 (60.1)	212 (58.4)	0.7
BMI, kg/m^2	26.7 ± 4.8	26.0 ± 4.6	27.3 ± 4.8	<0.001
Diabetes Mellitus, n (%)	157 (24.3)	54 (19.1)	103 (28.4)	0.006
History of gastrointestinal disorders, n (%)	42 (6.5)	10 (3.5)	32 (8.8)	0.007
Time since transplantation, years	5.3 (1.8–12.0)	9.5 (4.1–15.0)	4.0 (1.1–8.0)	<0.001
Lifestyle parameters				
Current smoker, n (%)	79 (13.1)	33 (12.4)	46 (13.6)	0.7
Alcohol consumer, n (%)	409 (70.6)	186 (72.7)	223 (69.0)	0.3
Iron intake, mg/d	11.3 ± 2.9	11.2 ± 2.7	11.4 ± 3.0	0.5
Renal function parameters				
eGFR, mL/min/1.73 m^2	53.5 ± 19.9	56.2 ± 19.7	51.4 ± 19.8	0.002
Serum creatinine, µmol/L	122 (99–156)	117 (98–150)	126 (101–164)	0.03
Proteinuria (≥0.5 g/24 h), n (%)	135 (21.0)	60 (21.2)	75 (20.8)	0.9
Laboratory parameters				
Iron deficiency, n (%)	193 (29.9)	63 (22.3)	130 (35.8)	<0.001
Hb, g/dL	13.3 ± 1.7	13.6 ± 1.6	13.1 ± 1.8	<0.001
Iron, µmol/L	15.2 ± 5.9	16.4 ± 6.1	14.2 ± 5.6	<0.001
Ferritin, µg/L	115.5 (53.0–216.3)	136.0 (77.0–222.0)	93.0 (42.0–196.0)	<0.001
Transferrin saturation, %	25.1 ± 10.5	27.3 ± 10.1	23.3 ± 10.5	<0.001
Glucose, mmol/L	5.3 (4.8–6.0)	5.2 (4.7–5.8)	5.3 (4.9–6.2)	0.01
HbA1c, mmol/mol	40 (37–44)	39 (36 – 42)	41 (38 – 45)	<0.001
HsCRP, mg/L	1.6 (0.8–4.2)	1.6 (0.8–3.8)	1.6 (0.7–4.6)	0.8
Medication use				
Calcineurin inhibitors, n (%)	369 (57.1)	137 (48.4)	232 (63.9)	<0.001
Mycophenolate mofetil, n (%)	431 (66.7)	171 (60.4)	260 (71.6)	0.003
Prednisolone, n (%)	641 (99.2)	282 (99.6)	359 (98.9)	0.4
Diuretics, n (%)	253 (39.2)	87 (30.7)	166 (45.7)	<0.001
RAAS–inhibitors, n (%)	314 (48.6)	144 (50.9)	170 (46.8)	0.3
Antiplatelet drugs, n (%)	131 (20.3)	46 (16.3)	85 (23.4)	0.03
H2-receptor antagonists, n (%)	20 (3.1)	19 (6.7)	1 (0.3)	<0.001

Data are presented as mean ± SD, median with interquartile ranges (IQR) or number with percentages (%). Abbreviations: BMI, body mass index; eGFR, estimated glomerular filtration rate; Hb, hemoglobin; HbA1c, hemoglobin A1c; HsCRP, high-sensitivity C-reactive protein; PPI, proton-pump inhibitor; RAAS-inhibitors, renin-angiotensin-aldosterone system inhibitors.

3.2. Association of PPI Use with Iron Status Parameters

In univariable linear regression analyses, PPI use was associated with a 2.18 µmol/L lower serum iron (95% CI: −3.09 to −1.27, *p* < 0.001), −0.34 µg/L lower ln serum ferritin (95% CI: −0.49 to −0.18, *p* < 0.001), 3.9% lower TSAT (95% CI: −5.5 to −2.3, *p* < 0.001), and 0.52 g/dL lower hemoglobin levels (95% CI: −0.78 to −0.25, *p* < 0.001). The association between PPI use and lower iron status parameters remained independent of adjustment for potential confounders, as shown in Table 2.

Table 2. Association of PPI use with iron status parameters in 646 stable renal transplant recipients.

n = 646	Serum Iron, μmol/L			Ln Serum Ferritin, μg/L			Transferrin Saturation, %			Hemoglobin, g/dL		
	β	95% CI	p	β	95% CI	p	β	95% CI	p	β	95% CI	p
Crude	−2.18	−3.09; −1.27	<0.001	−0.34	−0.49; −0.18	<0.001	−3.92	−5.52; −2.32	<0.001	−0.52	−0.78; −0.25	<0.001
Model 1	−2.03	−2.94; −1.12	<0.001	−0.35	−0.50; −0.20	<0.001	−3.80	−5.40; −2.20	<0.001	−0.52	−0.78; −0.26	<0.001
Model 2	−1.61	−2.57; −0.65	0.001	−0.31	−0.48; −0.15	<0.001	−2.85	−4.55; −1.15	0.001	−0.35	−0.61; −0.10	0.007
Model 3	−1.67	−2.67; −0.66	0.001	−0.31	−0.48; −0.14	<0.001	−3.00	−4.80; −1.20	0.001	−0.41	−0.67; −0.14	0.003
Model 4	−1.54	−2.48; −0.60	0.001	−0.32	−0.48; −0.16	<0.001	−2.75	−4.43; −1.07	0.001	−0.35	−0.61; −0.09	0.007
Model 5	−1.62	−2.58; −0.66	0.001	−0.31	−0.47; −0.15	<0.001	−2.90	−4.60; −1.20	0.001	−0.35	−0.61; −0.01	0.007
Model 6	−1.37	−2.33; −0.41	0.005	−0.27	−0.43; −0.11	0.001	−2.33	−4.03; −0.63	0.007	−0.33	−0.58; −0.07	0.01

Model 1: PPI use adjusted for age and sex. Model 2: model 1 + adjustment for eGFR, proteinuria, time since transplantation, history of GI-disorders. Model 3: model 2 + adjustment for lifestyle parameters (BMI, smoking behavior, alcohol use, dietary iron intake). Model 4: model 2 + adjustment for inflammation (hs-CRP). Model 5: model 2 + adjustment for MMF use. Model 6: model 5 + adjustment for other medication use (diuretic use, RAAS-inhibition, antiplatelet therapy, CNI use, and prednisolone use). Abbreviations: CNI, calcineurin inhibitor; Ln, natural log transformed; MMF, mycophenolate mofetil; RAAS-inhibitors, renin-angiotensin-aldosterone system inhibitors.

3.3. Association of PPI Use with ID

In crude logistic regression analysis, PPI use was associated with ID (OR: 1.95; 95% CI 1.37–2.77, $p < 0.001$), as shown in Table 3. The association remained independent of adjustment for age, sex, eGFR, proteinuria, time since transplantation, and history of GI-disorders (OR: 1.57; 95% CI 1.07–2.31, $p = 0.02$). Further adjustment for lifestyle parameters, including dietary iron intake (OR: 1.57; 95%CI 1.04–2.38, $p = 0.03$) and inflammation (OR: 1.56; 95% CI 1.06–2.30, $p = 0.03$), did not materially affect the association. In model 5 we adjusted for MMF use, which is known for its myelosuppressive nature. In this model, PPI use remained independently associated with ID (OR: 1.57; 95% CI 1.07–2.31, $p = 0.02$). The association between PPI use and ID lost significance when we additionally adjusted for other medication use (OR: 1.43; 95% CI 0.96–2.12, $p = 0.08$). In further models, in which we adjusted separately for each type of medication, it appeared that mainly diuretic use contributed to the attenuation of the association (Table S3). Associations of all potential confounders with ID are provided in Table S4. These analyses demonstrated that besides PPI use, also female sex, proteinuria, time since transplantation, diuretics use, and CNI use were independently associated with ID.

Table 3. Logistic regression analyses investigating the association of PPI use with iron deficiency in 646 renal transplant recipients.

n = 646	Iron Deficiency		
	Odds Ratio	95% CI	*p*
Crude	1.95	1.37–2.77	<0.001
Model 1	1.94	1.36–2.78	<0.001
Model 2	1.57	1.07–2.31	0.02
Model 3	1.57	1.04–2.38	0.03
Model 4	1.56	1.06–2.30	0.03
Model 5	1.57	1.07–2.31	0.02
Model 6	1.43	0.96–2.12	0.08

Model 1: PPI use adjusted for age and sex. Model 2: model 1 + adjustment for eGFR, proteinuria, time since transplantation, history of GI-disorders. Model 3: model 2 + adjustment for lifestyle parameters (BMI, smoking behavior, alcohol use, dietary iron intake). Model 4: model 2 + adjustment for inflammation (hs-CRP). Model 5: model 2 + adjustment for MMF use. Model 6: model 5 + adjustment for other medication use (diuretic use, RAAS-inhibition, antiplatelet therapy, CNI use, and prednisolone use). Abbreviations: CNI, calcineurin inhibitor; MMF, mycophenolate mofetil; RAAS-inhibitors, renin-angiotensin-aldosterone system inhibitors.

3.4. Dose-Response Analyses

In this study, 237 RTR received a low PPI dose ($\leq$20 mg omeprazole Eq/d) and 126 RTR received a high PPI dose (>20 mg omeprazole Eq/d). As shown in Table 4 and Figure 1, the point estimate of the odds ratio in RTR taking a high PPI dose as compared to RTR taking no PPIs (OR 2.30; 95% CI 1.46–3.62, $p < 0.001$) was higher than in RTR taking a low PPI dose (OR:1.78; 95% CI 1.21–2.62, $p = 0.004$). After adjustment for potential confounders, PPI use remained associated with ID in patients taking a high PPI dose (OR: 1.73, 95% CI 1.05–2.86, $p = 0.03$), but not in RTR taking a low PPI dose (OR: 1.29, 95% CI 0.84–1.98, $p = 0.25$), as shown in Table 4.

Table 4. Subgroup analyses of the association of PPI use with iron deficiency in 646 stable renal transplant recipients.

	Categories of PPI Use						
	No PPI		Low PPI Dose		High PPI Dose		
Number of subjects	283		237		126		p trend
	Odds ratio (95% CI)	p value	Odds ratio (95% CI)	p value	Odds ratio (95% CI)	p value	
Iron deficiency							
Crude	1.00 (reference)	n/a	1.78 (1.21–2.62)	0.004	2.30 (1.46–3.62)	<0.001	<0.001
Model 1	1.00 (reference)	n/a	1.76 (1.19–2.62)	0.005	2.33 (1.47–3.69)	<0.001	<0.001
Model 2	1.00 (reference)	n/a	1.38 (0.90–2.10)	0.14	2.00 (1.23–3.25)	0.005	0.005
Model 3	1.00 (reference)	n/a	1.43 (0.91–2.24)	0.12	1.88 (1.11–3.16)	0.02	0.02
Model 4	1.00 (reference)	n/a	1.39 (0.91–2.13)	0.12	1.93 (1.18–3.15)	0.009	0.008
Model 5	1.00 (reference)	n/a	1.38 (0.91–2.10)	0.14	2.00 (1.23–3.26)	0.005	0.005
Model 6	1.00 (reference)	n/a	1.29 (0.84–1.98)	0.25	1.73 (1.05–2.86)	0.03	0.03

Model 1: PPI use adjusted for age and sex. Model 2: model 1 + adjustment for eGFR, proteinuria, time since transplantation, history of GI-disorders. Model 3: model 2 + adjustment for lifestyle parameters (BMI, smoking behavior, alcohol use, dietary iron intake). Model 4: model 2 + adjustment for inflammation (hs-CRP). Model 5: model 2 + adjustment for MMF use. Model 6: model 5 + adjustment for other medication use (diuretic use, RAAS-inhibition, antiplatelet therapy, CNI use, and prednisolone use). Abbreviations: CNI, calcineurin inhibitor; MMF, mycophenolate mofetil; RAAS-inhibitors, renin-angiotensin-aldosterone system inhibitors.

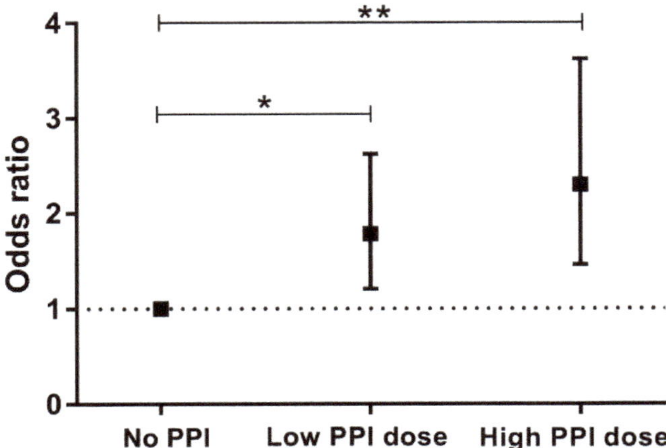

Figure 1. Crude association between PPI use and risk of iron deficiency stratified by subgroups of PPI use. No PPI, low PPI dose (≤20 mg omeprazole Eq/d), high PPI dose (>20 mg omeprazole Eq/d). Presented are odds ratio's with 95% confidence intervals. ** and * represent significant *p* values compared to No PPI subgroup.

3.5. Sensitivity Analyses for Risk of ID

In sensitivity analyses, H2RA users (n = 20) were excluded from analyses (Table S1). The association between PPI use and risk of ID remained materially unchanged when H2RA users were excluded (OR: 1.99, 95%CI 1.39–2.86, *p* < 0.001). Moreover, the association between PPI use and ID became slightly stronger when the alternative definition of ID (TSAT < 20% and ferritin < 100 µg/L) was used (OR: 2.90, 95% CI 1.94–4.35, *p* < 0.001), and remained significant independent of adjustment for potential confounders (Table S2).

3.6. Description of Excluded RTR Receiving Oral Iron Supplementation

Baseline differences between RTR with oral iron supplementation and without oral iron supplementation are described in the supplemental results and are demonstrated in Table S5.

4. Discussion

In this study, we demonstrate that PPI use is associated with lower iron status and ID in a large cohort of stable RTR. Remarkably, the association between PPI use and risk of ID remained independent of adjustment for important potential confounders, and appeared to be independent of dietary iron intake, a finding that has not been shown previously. Furthermore, we found that RTR using a high PPI dose have a higher risk of ID. These results indicate that PPI use possibly contributes to the high burden of post-transplantation ID in RTR.

During the past few years, several case reports have demonstrated a relationship between PPI use and the occurrence of IDA [11,26]. Recently, these findings have been strengthened by two large population based cohort studies demonstrating an increased risk of ID among subjects from the general population [8,9]. Lam et al. were the first to observe in a large population that chronic use of both PPIs and H2RAs was associated with an increased risk of ID (adjusted OR: 2.49 for PPI use and 1.58 for H2RA use) [9]. A recent study in a large U.K. population found that the risk of ID was 3.6 times higher in subjects using PPIs for at least one year continuously, i.e., with time gaps between PPI prescriptions of less than 30 days [8]. Consistent with our findings, both studies found a positive dose-response relationship, which suggests a potential causal effect of PPIs. However, compared to these studies, the adjusted odds ratios in our study were lower. This may in part be explained by a higher predisposition of ID in RTR compared to subjects from the general population. ID is highly prevalent after renal transplantation and the etiology is multifactorial. For example, high hepcidin and interleukin-6 levels as a result of inflammatory conditions after transplantation may lead to lower intestinal iron uptake due to the down regulation of the ferroportin transporter responsible for iron transport across the enterocyte [13,27,28]. Furthermore, insufficient iron stores at time of transplantation, per-operative blood loss, and inadequate intake of vegetables rich in iron may add to the risk of ID in RTR [29]. Another potential explanation for the lower odds ratio found in our study might be the relative high incidence of the CYP2C19*17 variant in Caucasian populations, which results in ultra-rapid metabolism of PPIs in the liver [30]. Therefore, the association between PPI use and ID might be more pronounced in populations with lower incidences of this CYP polymorphism, such as Asian populations in which the slow metabolizer phenotype is more common [31]. Interestingly, the present study shows that PPI therapy also appears to be an important risk factor of post-transplantation ID. Since this is a modifiable risk factor, we think this finding is worth discussing given that clinicians may not be aware of the additional risk that PPI use constitutes in RTR.

In contrast to our study, no association was found between PPI use and ID in a cohort study of patients with Zollinger–Ellison syndrome [32]. However, these results cannot simply be extrapolated to other populations and it is likely that the negative effect of PPIs on enteric iron absorption may be less pronounced in patients with gastric acid hypersecretion. In another study among 34 patients with primarily reflux esophagitis, there was also no clear evidence that chronic PPI therapy lead to decreased levels of serum iron and ferritin [33].

Several mechanisms by which PPI use may induce ID are proposed in literature. The main mechanism postulated is decreased intestinal absorption of dietary non-heme iron as a consequence of reduced gastric acid secretion by PPIs [34]. In contrast to the absorption of heme iron, dietary non-heme iron is highly dependent on gastric acid to enhance its absorption [13]. Non-heme iron remains soluble as long as the environment remains acidic and is reducing, of which the latter is necessary to form ferrous iron. It has been shown that in an environment with a pH above 2.5 absorption fails [35]. This theory is supported by a study from Hutchinison et al., who demonstrated that absorption of non-heme iron was lower in patients with hereditary hemochromatosis after the use of PPIs for seven days [34].

However, other factors by which PPIs could affect iron absorption are reported. For example, vitamin C is known to facilitate non-heme iron absorption, since it is a strong reducing agent. Secretion of vitamin C by gastric cells is dependent on intragastric pH and decreased bioavailability of vitamin C has been demonstrated in *Helicobacter pylori* positive and negative subjects after 28 days of omeprazole administration [36]. A low vitamin C intake may add to this, which may be a consequence of patients being over-correct in avoiding all citrus juices, while they actually only need to avoid pomelo containing juices to avoid interaction with CNI use [37]. This suggestion is corroborated by the fact that we recently found that vitamin C depletion is very common in RTR [38]. Moreover, interactions between the gut microbiome and iron bioavailability are reported in literature [39–41]. It is known that PPIs tremendously alter the composition of the gut microbiome, which may potentially affect intestinal iron absorption [42]. It is furthermore known that 50% of patients do not take their long-term therapy for chronic diseases as prescribed [43]. This is a further unknown factor that could interact with the results and could weaken the associations that we found.

To our knowledge, the influence of iron intake on the association between PPI use and ID has not been previously investigated. Lam and colleagues argued that possibly only subjects with low-normal iron levels or with a low dietary iron intake may become iron deficient [9]. In the present study, the association between PPI use and ID remained unchanged after adjustment for dietary iron intake, which shows that the association between PPI use and ID is not confounded by iron intake. Besides PPI use, we also found that female sex, proteinuria, time since transplantation, diuretics use, and CNI use were independently associated with ID. To date no evidence has been found linking diuretic use to ID [44]. However, it cannot be excluded that diuretics adversely affect iron status via decreased tubular reabsorption, resulting in increased urinary excretion of iron. The same accounts for proteinuria, which is a sign of either glomerular damage, tubular damage, or both. This may lead to increased protein filtration, decreased protein reabsorption, or both, which may result in increased urinary loss of transferrin-bound iron [45]. We also found that CNI use was independently associated with ID. In a previous study among liver transplant recipients, erythropoietin production and hematocrit levels were significantly reduced in CNI users, however the association with iron deficiency was not investigated [46].

Our study has some limitations. First, our study is cross-sectional in nature, and therefore we cannot assume causality. Next to that, we cannot exclude the possibility that the observed association between PPI use and decreased iron status parameters and ID are caused by residual confounding or indication bias. However, several analyses were performed to decrease this possibility. As described above, adjustment for iron intake and history of gastritis or peptic ulcer disease, conditions that can be the cause of a lower iron status, did not change the association between PPI use and ID. Moreover, in sensitivity analyses we excluded RTR using H2RAs and performed logistic regression analyses using an alternative definition of ID, which did not materially change the association. However, when we adjusted for medication use in model 6, the association between PPI use and ID lost significance, which could possibly mean two things. First, other medications may also negatively affect iron status, which attenuates the effect of PPIs on ID. Second, RTR using other medications may be more prone to ID compared to non-users. Furthermore, soluble transferrin receptor (sTfR) measurements were not available, and it should be realized that other than recording history of overt GI-disorders, patients were not thoroughly screened for presence of GI-disorders at the moment of sampling. Lastly, this is a single center study consisting of predominantly Caucasian RTR, which may limit generalizability of results to other populations.

Our study also has several strengths. It is the first study in its kind investigating the association of PPI use with iron status parameters and ID in a large cohort of stable RTR. The main strength is the well-characterized cohort of RTR, in which multiple iron status parameters and dietary iron intake were measured. Extensive data collection made it possible to correct for many possible confounding factors, including lifestyle parameters, inflammation, and medication use. Lastly, to define ID we used a definition previously used in chronic kidney disease and in RTR, including both functional and absolute iron deficiency situations [3,17,18].

5. Conclusions

In conclusion, we demonstrated that PPI use is associated with lower iron status and ID, indicating impaired intestinal absorption of iron potentially related to reduced gastric acid secretion. Moreover, we demonstrated that the association was stronger among RTR taking a high PPI dose. Taken together these results infer that PPI use is an important modifiable factor that potentially contributes to the high burden of post-transplantation ID after renal transplantation. Based on these results it should be advised to actively manage iron status in RTR using chronic PPI therapy. Reevaluation of treatment indication or switching to a less potent acid suppressing drug, such as antacids or H2RAs, might also be considered in RTR with ID. Potential clinical consequences associated with ID underscore this, including premature mortality [3] and severely disabling restless legs syndrome, which has a reported prevalence of 51.5% among RTR [47]. Since the majority of studies investigating the association between PPI use and ID are observational, randomized controlled clinical trials are needed to determine a causal effect of PPI use on iron status.

Supplementary Materials: The following are available online at http://www.mdpi.com/2077-0383/8/9/1382/s1. Supplemental Results: Description of excluded RTR receiving oral iron supplementation. Table S1: Logistic regression analyses investigating the association of PPI use with ID in 626 stable RTR (H2RA users excluded). Table S2: Logistic regression analyses investigating the association of PPI use with ID (TSAT < 20% and ferritin < 100 µg/L) in 646 RTR. Table S3: Logistic regression analyses investigating the effect of medication use on the association of PPI use with ID in 646 RTR. Table S4: Logistic regression analyses investigating the association of PPI use with ID (TSAT < 20% and ferritin < 300 µg/L) in 646 RTR. Table S5: Baseline characteristics of RTR with and without oral iron supplementation.

Author Contributions: Data curation, R.M.D., A.W.G.-N., E.v.d.B. and S.J.L.B.; formal analysis, R.M.D., A.W.G.-N. and S.J.L.B.; methodology, R.M.D., A.W.G.-N., M.F.E., J.S.J.V., M.H.d.B., S.P.B, D.J.T., E.H., H.B., G.N. and S.J.L.B.; writing—original draft preparation, R.M.D., A.W.G.-N.; writing—review and editing, R.M.D., A.W.G.-N., M.F.E., J.S.J.V., M.H.d.B., E.v.d.B., S.P.B., D.J.T., E.H., H.B., G.N. and S.J.L.B; supervision, H.B., G.N. and S.J.L.B.; funding acquisition, R.M.D., E.v.d.B., and S.J.L.B.

Funding: Generation of this study was funded by Top Institute Food and Nutrition (grant A-1003). R.M. Douwes is supported by NWO/TTW in a partnership program with DSM, Animal Nutrition and Health, The Netherlands; grant number: 14939.

Conflicts of Interest: Dr. De Borst is the principal investigator of a clinical trial supported by the Dutch Kidney Foundation (grant no 17OKG18) and Vifor Fresenius Medical Care Renal Pharma. He received consultancy fees (to employer) from Amgen, Astra Zeneca, Bayer, Kyowa Kirin, Sanofi Genzyme, and Vifor Fresenius Medical Care Renal Pharma. None of these entities had any role in the design, collection, analysis, and interpretation of data for the current study, nor in writing the report or the decision to submit the report for publication. The other authors declare that they have no other relevant financial interests.

References

1. Lorenz, M.; Kletzmayr, J.; Perschl, A.; Furrer, A.; Horl, W.H.; Sunder-Plassmann, G. Anemia and iron deficiencies among long-term renal transplant recipients. *J. Am. Soc. Nephrol.* **2002**, *13*, 794–797. [PubMed]

2. Yorgin, P.D.; Scandling, J.D.; Belson, A.; Sanchez, J.; Alexander, S.R.; Andreoni, K.A. Late post-transplant anemia in adult renal transplant recipients. An under-recognized problem? *Am. J. Transplant.* **2002**, *2*, 429–435. [CrossRef] [PubMed]

3. Eisenga, M.F.; Minovic, I.; Berger, S.P.; Kootstra-Ros, J.E.; van den Berg, E.; Riphagen, I.J.; Navis, G.; van der Meer, P.; Bakker, S.J.; Gaillard, C.A. Iron deficiency, anemia, and mortality in renal transplant recipients. *Transpl. Int.* **2016**, *29*, 1176–1183. [CrossRef] [PubMed]

4. Imoagene-Oyedeji, A.E.; Rosas, S.E.; Doyle, A.M.; Goral, S.; Bloom, R.D. Posttransplantation anemia at 12 months in kidney recipients treated with mycophenolate mofetil: Risk factors and implications for mortality. *J. Am. Soc. Nephrol.* **2006**, *17*, 3240–3247. [CrossRef] [PubMed]

5. Lim, A.K.H.; Kansal, A.; Kanellis, J. Factors associated with anaemia in kidney transplant recipients in the first year after transplantation: A cross-sectional study. *BMC Nephrol.* **2018**, *19*, 252. [CrossRef] [PubMed]

6. Jones, H.; Talwar, M.; Nogueira, J.M.; Ugarte, R.; Cangro, C.; Rasheed, H.; Klassen, D.K.; Weir, M.R.; Haririan, A. Anemia after kidney transplantation; its prevalence, risk factors, and independent association with graft and patient survival: A time-varying analysis. *Transplantation* **2012**, *93*, 923–928. [CrossRef] [PubMed]

7. Chhabra, D.; Grafals, M.; Skaro, A.I.; Parker, M.; Gallon, L. Impact of anemia after renal transplantation on patient and graft survival and on rate of acute rejection. *Clin. J. Am. Soc. Nephrol.* **2008**, *3*, 1168–1174. [CrossRef]

8. Tran-Duy, A.; Connell, N.J.; Vanmolkot, F.H.; Souverein, P.C.; de Wit, N.J.; Stehouwer, C.D.A.; Hoes, A.W.; de Vries, F.; de Boer, A. Use of proton pump inhibitors and risk of iron deficiency: A population-based case-control study. *J. Intern. Med.* **2019**, *285*, 205–214. [CrossRef]

9. Lam, J.R.; Schneider, J.L.; Quesenberry, C.P.; Corley, D.A. Proton Pump Inhibitor and Histamine-2 Receptor Antagonist Use and Iron Deficiency. *Gastroenterology* **2017**, *152*, 821–829. [CrossRef]

10. Sarzynski, E.; Puttarajappa, C.; Xie, Y.; Grover, M.; Laird-Fick, H. Association between proton pump inhibitor use and anemia: A retrospective cohort study. *Dig. Dis. Sci.* **2011**, *56*, 2349–2353. [CrossRef]

11. Hashimoto, R.; Matsuda, T.; Chonan, A. Iron-deficiency anemia caused by a proton pump inhibitor. *Intern. Med.* **2014**, *53*, 2297–2299. [CrossRef] [PubMed]

12. Charlton, R.W.; Bothwell, T.H. Iron absorption. *Annu. Rev. Med.* **1983**, *34*, 55–68. [CrossRef] [PubMed]

13. Lawen, A.; Lane, D.J. Mammalian iron homeostasis in health and disease: Uptake, storage, transport, and molecular mechanisms of action. *Antioxid. Redox Signal.* **2013**, *18*, 2473–2507. [CrossRef] [PubMed]

14. Ajmera, A.V.; Shastri, G.S.; Gajera, M.J.; Judge, T.A. Suboptimal response to ferrous sulfate in iron-deficient patients taking omeprazole. *Am. J. Ther.* **2012**, *19*, 185–189. [CrossRef] [PubMed]

15. Van den Berg, E.; Engberink, M.F.; Brink, E.J.; van Baak, M.A.; Joosten, M.M.; Gans, R.O.; Navis, G.; Bakker, S.J. Dietary acid load and metabolic acidosis in renal transplant recipients. *Clin. J. Am. Soc. Nephrol.* **2012**, *7*, 1811–1818. [CrossRef]

16. Van den Berg, E.; Geleijnse, J.M.; Brink, E.J.; van Baak, M.A.; van der Heide, J.J.H.; Gans, R.O.; Navis, G.; Bakker, S.J. Sodium intake and blood pressure in renal transplant recipients. *Nephrol. Dial. Transplant.* **2012**, *27*, 3352–3359. [CrossRef] [PubMed]

17. Eisenga, M.F.; van Londen, M.; Leaf, D.E.; Nolte, I.M.; Navis, G.; Bakker, S.J.L.; de Borst, M.H.; Gaillard, C.A.J.M. C-Terminal Fibroblast Growth Factor 23, Iron Deficiency, and Mortality in Renal Transplant Recipients. *J. Am. Soc. Nephrol.* **2017**, *28*, 3639–3646. [CrossRef]

18. Charytan, C.; Levin, N.; Al-Saloum, M.; Hafeez, T.; Gagnon, S.; Van Wyck, D.B. Efficacy and Safety of Iron Sucrose for Iron Deficiency in Patients With Dialysis-Associated Anemia: North American Clinical Trial. *Am. J. Kidney Dis.* **2001**, *37*, 300–307. [CrossRef]

19. Anker, S.D.; Comin Colet, J.; Filippatos, G.; Willenheimer, R.; Dickstein, K.; Drexler, H.; Lüscher, T.F.; Bart, B.; Banasiak, W.; Niegowska, J.; et al. Ferric Carboxymaltose in Patients with Heart Failure and Iron Deficiency. *N. Engl. J. Med.* **2009**, *361*, 2436–2448. [CrossRef]

20. Van den Berg, E.; Engberink, M.F.; Brink, E.J.; van Baak, M.A.; Gans, R.O.B.; Navis, G.; Bakker, S.J.L. Dietary protein, blood pressure and renal function in renal transplant recipients. *Br. J. Nutr.* **2013**, *109*, 1463–1470. [CrossRef]

21. Feunekes, I.J.; Van Staveren, W.A.; Graveland, F.; De Vos, J.; Burema, J. Reproducibility of a semiquantitative food frequency questionnaire to assess the intake of fats and cholesterol in The Netherlands. *Int. J. Food Sci. Nutr.* **1995**, *46*, 117–123. [CrossRef] [PubMed]

22. Dutch Food Composition Table NEVO-Tabel. *Nederlands Voedingsstoffenbestand*; RIVM/Netherlands Nutrition Centre: Bilthoven, The Netherlands, 2006.

23. Kirchheiner, J.; Glatt, S.; Fuhr, U.; Klotz, U.; Meineke, I.; Seufferlein, T.; Brockmoller, J. Relative potency of proton-pump inhibitors-comparison of effects on intragastric pH. *Eur. J. Clin. Pharmacol.* **2009**, *65*, 19–31. [CrossRef] [PubMed]

24. Locatelli, F.; Bárány, P.; Covic, A.; De Francisco, A.; Del Vecchio, L.; Goldsmith, D.; Hörl, W.; London, G.; Vanholder, R.; Van Biesen, W.; et al. Kidney Disease: Improving Global Outcomes guidelines on anaemia management in chronic kidney disease: A European Renal Best Practice position statement. *Nephrol. Dial. Transplant.* **2013**, *28*, 1346–1359. [CrossRef] [PubMed]

25. Ratcliffe, L.E.K.; Thomas, W.; Glen, J.; Padhi, S.; Pordes, B.A.J.; Wonderling, D.; Connell, R.; Stephens, S.; Mikhail, A.I.; Fogarty, D.G.; et al. Diagnosis and Management of Iron Deficiency in CKD: A Summary of the NICE Guideline Recommendations and Their Rationale. *Am. J. Kidney Dis.* **2016**, *67*, 548–558. [CrossRef] [PubMed]

26. Sharma, V.R.; Brannon, M.A.; Carloss, E.A. Effect of omeprazole on oral iron replacement in patients with iron deficiency anemia. *South. Med. J.* **2004**, *97*, 887–889. [CrossRef] [PubMed]

27. Abedini, S.; Holme, I.; Marz, W.; Weihrauch, G.; Fellstrom, B.; Jardine, A.; Cole, E.; Maes, B.; Neumayer, H.H.; Gronhagen-Riska, C.; et al. Inflammation in renal transplantation. *Clin. J. Am. Soc. Nephrol.* **2009**, *4*, 1246–1254. [CrossRef] [PubMed]

28. Schaefer, B.; Effenberger, M.; Zoller, H. Iron metabolism in transplantation. *Transpl. Int.* **2014**, *27*, 1109–1117. [CrossRef]

29. Zheng, S.; Coyne, D.W.; Joist, H.; Schuessler, R.; Godboldo-Brooks, A.; Ercole, P.; Brennan, D.C. Iron deficiency anemia and iron losses after renal transplantation. *Transpl. Int.* **2009**, *22*, 434–440. [CrossRef]

30. Hunfeld, N.G.; Touw, D.J.; Mathot, R.A.; Schaik, R.H.; Kuipers, E.J. A comparison of the acid-inhibitory effects of esomeprazole and rabeprazole in relation to pharmacokinetics and CYP2C19 polymorphism. *Aliment. Pharmacol. Ther.* **2012**, *35*, 810–818. [CrossRef]

31. Sim, S.C.; Risinger, C.; Dahl, M.-L.; Aklillu, E.; Christensen, M.; Bertilsson, L.; Ingelman-Sundberg, M. A common novel CYP2C19 gene variant causes ultrarapid drug metabolism relevant for the drug response to proton pump inhibitors and antidepressants. *Clin. Pharmacol. Ther.* **2006**, *79*, 103–113. [CrossRef]

32. Stewart, C.A.; Termanini, B.; Sutliff, V.E.; Serrano, J.; Yu, F.; Gibril, F.; Jensen, R.T. Iron absorption in patients with Zollinger-Ellison syndrome treated with long-term gastric acid antisecretory therapy. *Aliment. Pharmacol. Ther.* **1998**, *12*, 83–98. [CrossRef] [PubMed]

33. Koop, H.; Bachem, M.G. Serum iron, ferritin, and vitamin B12 during prolonged omeprazole therapy. *J. Clin. Gastroenterol.* **1992**, *14*, 288–292. [CrossRef] [PubMed]

34. Hutchinson, C.; Geissler, C.A.; Powell, J.J.; Bomford, A. Proton pump inhibitors suppress absorption of dietary non-haem iron in hereditary haemochromatosis. *Gut* **2007**, *56*, 1291–1295. [CrossRef] [PubMed]

35. Bezwoda, W.; Charlton, R.; Bothwell, T.; Torrance, J.; Mayet, F. The importance of gastric hydrochloric acid in the absorption of nonheme food iron. *J. Lab. Clin. Med.* **1978**, *92*, 108–116. [PubMed]

36. Henry, E.B.; Carswell, A.; Wirz, A.; Fyffe, V.; McColl, K.E. Proton pump inhibitors reduce the bioavailability of dietary vitamin C. *Aliment. Pharmacol. Ther.* **2005**, *22*, 539–545. [CrossRef] [PubMed]

37. Sridharan, K.; Sivaramakrishnan, G. Interaction of Citrus Juices with Cyclosporine: Systematic Review and Meta-Analysis. *Eur. J. Drug Metab. Pharmacokinet.* **2016**, *41*, 665–673. [CrossRef] [PubMed]

38. Sotomayor, C.G.; Eisenga, M.F.; Gomes Neto, A.W.; Ozyilmaz, A.; Gans, R.O.B.; de Jong, W.H.A.; Zelle, D.M.; Berger, S.P.; Gaillard, C.A.J.M.; Navis, G.J.; et al. Vitamin C Depletion and All-Cause Mortality in Renal Transplant Recipients. *Nutrients* **2017**, *9*, 568. [CrossRef] [PubMed]

39. Saha, P.; Yeoh, B.S.; Singh, R.; Chandrasekar, B.; Vemula, P.K.; Haribabu, B.; Vijay-Kumar, M.; Jala, V.R. Gut Microbiota Conversion of Dietary Ellagic Acid into Bioactive Phytoceutical Urolithin A Inhibits Heme Peroxidases. *PLoS ONE* **2016**, *11*, e0156811. [CrossRef] [PubMed]

40. González, A.; Gálvez, N.; Martín, J.; Reyes, F.; Pérez-Victoria, I.; Dominguez-Vera, J.M. Identification of the key excreted molecule by *Lactobacillus fermentum* related to host iron absorption. *Food Chem.* **2017**, *228*, 374–380. [CrossRef] [PubMed]

41. Hoppe, M.; Önning, G.; Berggren, A.; Hulthén, L. Probiotic strain *Lactobacillus plantarum* 299v increases iron absorption from 2 an iron-supplemented fruit drink: A double-isotope cross-over single-blind 3 study in women of reproductive age—Erratum. *Br. J. Nutr.* **2015**, *114*, 1948. [CrossRef] [PubMed]

42. Imhann, F.; Bonder, M.J.; Vila, A.V.; Fu, J.; Mujagic, Z.; Vork, L.; Tigchelaar, E.F.; Jankipersadsing, S.A.; Cenit, M.C.; Harmsen, H.J.; et al. Proton pump inhibitors affect the gut microbiome. *Gut* **2016**, *65*, 740–748. [CrossRef] [PubMed]

43. Pagès-Puigdemont, N.; Mangues, M.A.; Masip, M.; Gabriele, G.; Fernández-Maldonado, L.; Blancafort, S.; Tuneu, L. Patients' Perspective of Medication Adherence in Chronic Conditions: A Qualitative Study. *Adv. Ther.* **2016**, *33*, 1740–1754. [CrossRef] [PubMed]

44. Suliburska, J.; Skrypnik, K.; Szulińska, M.; Kupsz, J.; Markuszewski, L.; Bogdański, P. Diuretics, Ca-Antagonists, and Angiotensin-Converting Enzyme Inhibitors Affect Zinc Status in Hypertensive Patients on Monotherapy: A Randomized Trial. *Nutrients* **2018**, *10*, 1284. [CrossRef]

45. Van Raaij, S.E.G.; Rennings, A.J.; Biemond, B.J.; Schols, S.E.M.; Wiegerinck, E.T.G.; Roelofs, H.M.J.; Hoorn, E.J.; Walsh, S.B.; Nijenhuis, T.; Swinkels, D.W.; et al. Iron handling by the human kidney: Glomerular filtration and tubular reabsorption both contribute to urinary iron excretion. *Am. J. Physiol. Physiol.* **2019**, *316*, F606–F614. [CrossRef] [PubMed]

46. Bardet, V.; Junior, A.P.; Coste, J.; Lecoq-Lafon, C.; Chouzenoux, S.; Bernard, D.; Soubrane, O.; Lacombe, C.; Calmus, Y.; Conti, F. Impaired erythropoietin production in liver transplant recipients: The role of calcineurin inhibitors. *Liver Transpl.* **2006**, *12*, 1649–1654. [CrossRef]
47. Naini, A.E.; Amra, B.; Mahmoodnia, L.; Taheri, S. Sleep apnea syndrome and restless legs syndrome in kidney transplant recipients. *Adv. Biomed. Res.* **2015**, *4*, 206.

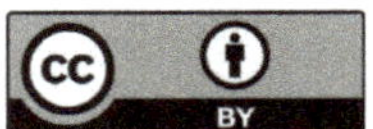

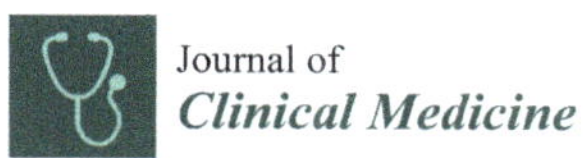

Journal of
Clinical Medicine

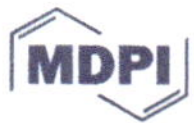

Article

Native Nephrectomy before and after Renal Transplantation in Patients with Autosomal Dominant Polycystic Kidney Disease (ADPKD)

Andreas Maxeiner [1,†], Anna Bichmann [2,†], Natalie Oberländer [1], Nasrin El-Bandar [1], Nesrin Sugünes [1], Bernhard Ralla [1], Nadine Biernath [1], Lutz Liefeldt [3], Klemens Budde [3], Markus Giessing [4], Thorsten Schlomm [1] and Frank Friedersdorff [1,*]

[1] Department of Urology, Charité–Universitätsmedizin Berlin, Corporate Member of Freie Universität Berlin, Humboldt-Universität zu Berlin, and Berlin Institute of Health, Charitéplatz 1, 10117 Berlin, Germany; Andreas.maxeiner@charite.de (A.M.); natalie.oberlaender@hotmail.de (N.O.); nasrin.el-bandar@charite.de (N.E.-B.); nesrin.suguenes@charite.de (N.S.); bernhard.ralla@charite.de (B.R.); nadine.biernath@charite.de (N.B.); thorsten.schlomm@charite.de (T.S.)

[2] Department of Anesthesiology and Operative Intensive Care Medicine, Campus Charité Mitte, Charité–Universitätsmedizin Berlin, Corporate Member of Freie Universität Berlin, Humboldt-Universität zu Berlin, and Berlin Institute of Health, Charitéplatz 1, 10117 Berlin, Germany; anna.bichmann@charite.de

[3] Department of Nephrology, Charité–Universitätsmedizin Berlin, Corporate Member of Freie Universität Berlin, Humboldt-Universität zu Berlin, and Berlin Institute of Health, Charitéplatz 1, 10117 Berlin, Germany; lutz.liefeldt@charite.de (L.L.); klemens.budde@charite.de (K.B.)

[4] Department of Urology, Heinrich-Heine-University, 40225 Düsseldorf, Germany; markus.giessing@med.uni-duesseldorf.de

[*] Correspondence: frank.friedersdorff@charite.de; Tel.: +4930450615219

[†] Contributed equally.

Received: 13 August 2019; Accepted: 27 September 2019; Published: 4 October 2019

Abstract: The aim of this study was 1) to evaluate and compare pre-, peri-, and post-operative data of Autosomal Dominant Polycystic Kidney Disease (ADPKD) patients undergoing native nephrectomy (NN) either before or after renal transplantation and 2) to identify advantages of optimal surgical timing, postoperative outcomes, and economical aspects in a tertiary transplant centre. This retrospective analysis included 121 patients divided into two groups—group 1: patients who underwent NN prior to receiving a kidney transplant ($n = 89$) and group 2: patients who underwent NN post-transplant ($n = 32$). Data analysis was performed according to demographic patient details, surgical indication, laboratory parameters, perioperative complications, underlying pathology, and associated mortality. There was no significant difference in patient demographics between the groups, however right-sided nephrectomy was performed predominantly within group 1. The main indication in both groups undergoing a nephrectomy was pain. Patients among group 2 had no postoperative kidney failure and a significantly shorter hospital stay. Higher rates of more severe complications were observed in group 1, even though this was not statistically significant. Even though the differences between both groups were substantial, the time of NN prior or post-transplant does not seem to affect short-term and long-term transplantation outcomes. Retroperitoneal NN remains a low risk treatment option in patients with symptomatic ADPKD and can be performed either pre- or post-kidney transplantation depending on patients' symptom severity.

Keywords: ADPKD; native nephrectomy; kidney transplantation; patient outcome; perioperative complications

1. Introduction

Autosomal dominant polycystic kidney disease (ADPKD) is the fourth most frequent cause of end-stage renal disease (ESRD) in Europe, accounting for around 10–15% of patients on dialysis and 9% to 10% of renal transplantation [1,2]. ADPKD patients develop progressive expansion of multiple bilateral cysts in the renal parenchyma, causing a deterioration of their glomerular filtration rate (GFR) [3]. Patients with ADPKD often develop recurrent urinary tract infections, nephrolithiasis, and back or abdominal pain. Approximately one-fifth of ADPKD patients will require unilateral or bilateral nephrectomy at some point in their life [4–6]. Due to a heterogeneous clinical presentation ranging from asymptomatic to very severe, treatment options are highly variable. In comparison to other forms of renal replacement therapy, kidney transplantation seems to be the option of choice in most ESRD patients, with improved survival and lower morbidity [7]. However, the optimal time for nephrectomy in ADPKD patients awaiting renal transplantation remains a matter of debate. Furthermore, the severity of clinical symptoms may also influence patients' wishes to undergo nephrectomy. Some previously published research does not recommend pre-transplant nephrectomy due to associated increased morbidity and mortality [8,9]. Others suggest a "sandwich technique", whereby the most severely affected native kidney is removed before, and the remaining polycystic kidney is removed after transplantation [10,11]. Concomitant nephrectomy and transplantation is another method that is described within the literature [6,12], which is predominantly used for ADPKD patients who are scheduled for living donor kidney transplants. The aim of this study was (1) to evaluate and compare pre-, peri-, and post-operative data of ADPKD patients undergoing native nephrectomy either before or after renal transplantation and (2) to identify advantages of optimal surgical timing, postoperative outcomes, and economical aspects in a tertiary transplant center.

2. Methods

2.1. Patient and Study Design

The retrospective analysis included 141 patients with ADPKD who underwent unilateral surgical nephrectomy between January 2005 and December 2018. Twenty patients were excluded due to incomplete data. Three patients underwent bilateral nephrectomy sequentially and were also excluded. Group 1 included nephrectomy patients who were on dialysis prior to kidney transplantation ($n = 89$) and group 2 represents patients who had post-transplant nephrectomy ($n = 32$). Data analysis was performed according to demographic patient details, surgical indication, laboratory parameters, perioperative complications, underlying pathology, and associated mortality. Patients in group 2 received a standard triple maintenance immunosuppression that consisted of tacrolimus or cyclosporin A in combination with mycophenolate mofetil and prednisolone.

2.2. Surgical Procedure

The operation procedure was performed by a unilateral flank incision of 20–25 cm with perioperative antibiotic treatment. A strictly extra-peritoneal surgical preparation was performed. If an intraoperative peritoneal laceration occurred, an immediate surgical reparation was done. The vessel hilum was sealed by using three Hem-o-lok clips. Surgical drains were placed at the time of transplant and were present postoperatively. Figure 1 shows a removed polycystic kidney preparation after retroperitoneal nephrectomy.

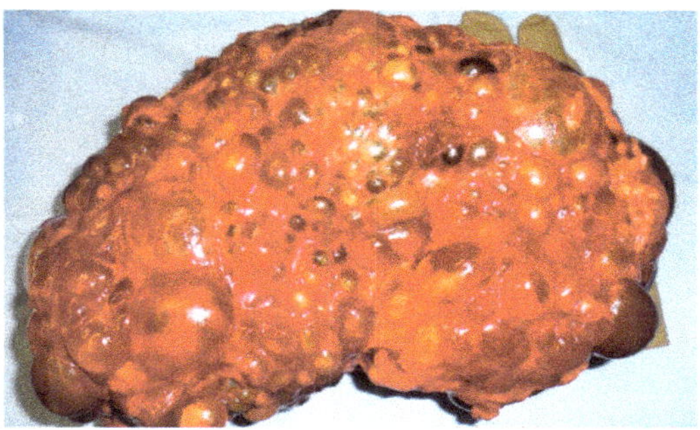

Figure 1. Polycystic kidney preparation after retroperitoneal nephrectomy.

2.3. Statistical Analysis

Statistical analyses were performed using SPSS (SPSS Inc., version 25, Armonk, NY, USA). Both univariate and multivariate analyses were applied to identify risk factors for complications following cystic kidney removal, both before and after kidney transplantation. Baseline characteristics were compared using the Chi-squared test and Fisher's exact test for categorical variables. Continuous variables were tested with the Student's t-test or Mann–Whitney U-test (if the assumption of Gaussian distribution was not fulfilled). Results were reported as means and standard deviations (SD) for continuous variables; categorical variables were reported as numbers and percentages. For all the statistical measures, a p-value <0.05 was considered significant. Odds ratio (OR) was calculated and statistical determinations were within the 95% confidence interval.

3. Results

3.1. Demographic Data

Out of the 121 included patients with ADPKD, 89 patients underwent nephrectomy prior to kidney transplantation (group 1) and 32 patients underwent nephrectomy post-transplant (group 2). Patient's demographic data is displayed in Table 1 below.

Table 1. Demographic data.

Parameter	Group 1 ($n = 89$)	Group 2 ($n = 32$)	p-Value
Age average in years	53.92	53.75	0.927
Male sex (%)	69.70	68.80	0.923
Right sided nephrectomy (%)	58.40	34.40	0.02 *
Left sided nephrectomy (%)	41.6	65.6	0.02 *
BMI (kg/m^{2}average)	25.93	25.31	0.445
Median duration of dialysis (months)	33.00	22.00	0.100
Median weight of the removed kidney	2600 g	1683 g	0.004

Group 1: pre-transplant, Group 2: post-transplant. *, statistically significant; BMI, body mass index.

There was no significant difference in the patient demographics between both groups, although right-sided nephrectomy was predominantly performed within group 1 ($p = 0.02$). The main comorbidities in both groups were cardiovascular diseases (group 1: 83.1% verus group 2: 81.3%; $p = 0.808$), which were represented most commonly by coronary artery disease, hypertension, and peripheral vascular disease.

3.2. Indications

Table 2 shows the individual indications for a nephrectomy.

Table 2. Indications for a nephrectomy.

Indications	Group 1 (*n* = 89)	Group 2 (*n* = 32)	*p*-Value
Renal pain (%)	50.6	59.4	0.392
Infection (%)	31.5	28.1	0.725
Urolithiasis (%)	11.2	6.3	0.514
Haematuria (%)	4.5	6.3	0.654
Gastrointestinal complaints (%)	2.2	0	1.000

Group 1: pre-transplant, group 2: post-transplant.

3.3. Patient Outcome Analysis

Comparing pre-operative serum creatinine levels in patients within group 2, a mild increase from an average pre-operative level of 1.47 mg/dL to 1.61 mg/dL postoperatively occurred. No patients had peri-operative kidney failure. In all 32 cases undergoing post-transplantation nephrectomy, the initially elevated creatinine levels postoperatively appeared stable (3 months: 1.62 mg/dL, 6 months: 1.64 mg/dL, 1 year: 1.69 mg/dL, and 3 years: 1.64 mg/dL). The difference between the pre- and post-operative haemoglobin levels was insignificant (group 1: 2.2 g/dL versus group 2: 2.5 g/d, $p = 0.468$). The difference in surgical time between both groups was insignificant (group 1: 175 min versus group 2: 170.5 min, $p = 0.541$), although a significant difference in the duration of hospital admission was observed (group 1: 7 days versus group 2: 6 days; $p = 0.001$). The pathological assessment of polycystic nephrectomy samples showed a 3% risk for renal cell carcinoma in both groups (group 1: 3.4% versus group 2: 3.1%; $p = 1.0$). No statistical difference was reported in the rates of acute inflammation in the pathological report (group 1: 15.6% versus group 2: 5.6%; $p = 0.127$). Furthermore, there was no significant difference between the chronic renal inflammation rates (group 1: 61.8% versus group 2: 71.9%; $p = 0.307$), which were defined as low-grade chronic systemic inflammation characterized by persistent, low to moderate levels of one or more circulating inflammation markers, such as white blood cells count, C-reactive protein, and procalcitonin. However, a significant difference was observed in the median weight of the removed kidney (group 1: 2600 g compared to 1683 g in group 2 ($p = 0.004$)). Concerning postoperative complication rates, group 1 had a higher prevalence of 43.8% compared to 37.5% within group 2, even though it was not statistically significant ($p = 0.936$). The complications within group 1 were classified as Clavien-Dindo 1 in 7.9% and as Clavien-Dindo 2 in 22.5%. Those categorized as Clavien-Dindo 3 (7.9%) included two patients suffering from a pneumothorax and one patient appeared with a pancreatic injury. Severe complications (Clavien-Dindo 4: 5.5%) included two patients of whom one required laparotomy on the second postoperative day due to a retroperitoneal abscess and one suffered a pulmonary embolism with subsequent cardiac arrest with a return of spontaneous circulation upon resuscitation. A total of three patients died within group 1 (3.4%), of which two suffered severe sepsis and one a hypoglycaemic shock. Complication rates within group 2 were mostly minor (Clavien-Dindo 1: 9.4%, Clavien-Dindo 2: 25%). Only one patient was classified as Clavien-Dindo 3. No patients in group 2 were categorized as Clavien-Dindo 4 or deceased. Among all outcome parameters, the multivariate analysis identified the following parameters as significant risk factors for a prolonged hospital stay: age ($p <0.001$) as well as undergoing native nephrectomy prior to transplantation (represented by group 1) ($p = 0.013$). Factors such as male sex, body mass index (BMI), organ weight, duration of operation, and time on dialyses were not significant risk factors for a prolonged hospital stay.

4. Discussion

ADPKD is the most common inherited disease with over 12 million patients with associated terminal renal failure, representing the fourth leading cause for dialysis worldwide. Patients suffering from ADPKD develop progressive expansion of multiple bilateral cysts in the renal parenchyma, causing a deterioration of GFR [3]. Patients with ADPKD often develop recurrent urinary tract infections, nephrolithiasis, and back or abdominal pain. Approximately one-fifth of ADPKD patients will require unilateral or bilateral nephrectomy at some point in their life [4–6]. It is still unclear if patients undergoing nephrectomy post-transplant have higher complication rates. This research was not able to display a significant difference between both groups, even though the prevalence of complications was higher within group 1 (43.8% versus 37.5%).

The indications for nephrectomy were often multiple for each patient and the major indications are listed in Table 2. Overall, the main nephrectomy indication was pain in over 50% of the patients. Further indications for nephrectomy need to be critically evaluated and can be based on intra-abdominal space issues, uncontrolled hypertension, and cystic bleeding [6,7,13]. Due to the often-present additional liver cysts in 80% of patients with ADPKD [14], a right-sided intra-abdominal space problem occurs, resulting in less affected contralateral kidneys. The statistically significant difference in organ weight, as stated previously (2600 g versus 1683 g, $p = 0.004$), seems to underline this hypothesis. In addition, kidney volume seems to be an early marker of severity of the disease and is shown to be a determinant of a reduction in kidney functions [3].

According to the literature, no difference in average age at the time of nephrectomy ($p = 0.927$) was observed [7,15] and, further, a higher rate of male patients was also reported in our cohort despite being an autosomal dominant disease [6,13,15]. Lifestyle and preventive factors also need to be addressed in ADPKD. Patients can prevent disease progression by controlling hypertension through a low salt diet [16,17]. These statements are of limited value for external validity as these publications involved low case numbers of patients with ADKPD who were reviewed at the time of nephrectomy. Nevertheless, the assumption can be made that disease progression can be delayed by a healthy lifestyle. Studies have shown that females have higher health awareness in their daily living [18], which could also explain the male dominant cohort. However, cyst expansion can cause ischemia within the kidney and, consequently, the activation of Renin-Angiotensin-Aldosterone-System (RAAS), leading to the development and/or maintenance of hypertension [19]. Hence, patients might benefit from native nephrectomy if hypertension is predominantly present. On the other hand, preserving patient's urine excretion might also preserve quality of life concerning daily fluid intake.

Research published focusing on patients who are positive for polycystic kidney disease 1 (PKD1) mutations prior to the age of 35 years show a worse and faster disease progression in the male sub-cohort and/or hypertension [20]. However, the average BMI within our cohort was around a normal range of 25 kg/m^2. A known disadvantage using BMI as a reference is the inconsideration of water and muscle mass, which is greatly variable in these patients. Hence, observing that the BMI does not increase in pre-transplant patients despite significant edemas has not yet been discussed in published research.

In all cases, only unilateral nephrectomy was carried out. This changed to bilateral nephrectomies prior to renal transplants in the 1970s and reduced infection-based complications [21]. Nevertheless, higher postoperative complications were observed, including worsening anemia and loss of diuresis [22]. Within the past few decades, bilateral nephrectomy case numbers decreased due to advanced medication and stricter surgical indication. Fuller et al. reviewed a small cohort of 32 patients who underwent simultaneous and sequential bilateral nephrectomy [6]. Out of the studied 25 patients, 6 had simultaneous bilateral native nephrectomy with higher rates of blood transfusions, increasing antibody production, and worsening post-transplant outcomes [6]. Hence, the authors concluded not to promote bilateral simultaneous intervention. Further, 3% of patients in both groups were found to have a histological diagnosis of coincidental cancer, which is in concurrence with literature published to date [6,7,13]. Histological analysis within the post-transplant group showed higher rates of inflammation, which is potentially due to the effects of immunosuppressive medication. These findings have not been published elsewhere. We suggest taking samples from potentially inflamed cysts intraoperatively. An extended antibiotic cover with lipophilic properties can then be discussed.

However, our study found no significant differences between patients undergoing native nephrectomy prior or post-transplant. Hence, the role of transplantation and subsequent immunosuppressive therapy seems to be irrelevant as group 2 had less severe and a smaller number of post-operative complications. The deceased patients within group 1 were patients without transplants. Chebib et al. had fewer complications in the cohort undergoing a nephrectomy post-transplant [15]. Similar observations were published by Kirkman et al. [7]. Thus, the presumed increased risk through immunosuppressive therapy concerning wound healing and increased infection rates post-operatively cannot be supported. The significantly shorter hospital stay of the post-transplant patients in our cohort also represents a fact that can be witnessed within the literature [6].

Despite our findings, we acknowledge limitations of the present study and potential sources of bias that need to be addressed. The retrospective analysis as well as the limited number of patients of group 2 might confound our results. Furthermore, the exclusion of 23 patients due to missing data may have also decreased the potential study cohort. In addition, analysis of short-term and long-term transplantation outcomes (graft loss, delayed graft function, acute rejection, bacterial and cytomegalovirus (CMV] infection, and post-transplant diabetes mellitus) between both groups was not included.

5. Conclusions

In conclusion, our study demonstrates that open retroperitoneal nephrectomies represent a low risk management option in patients with symptomatic ADPKD and post-transplant nephrectomy seems to not be associated with higher complication rates. Hence, timing and indication of native nephrectomy should be primarily based on symptom severity rather than on the date of transplantation.

Author Contributions: F.F., K.B., L.L., and B.R. designed the study; N.O. and N.S. analyzed the data; A.M., F.F., and A.B. wrote the manuscript; N.E.-B., N.B., M.G., F.F., and T.S. drafted and revised the paper; all authors approved the final version of the manuscript.

Conflicts of Interest: The authors declare no conflict of interest.

References

1. Spithoven, E.M.; Kramer, A.; Meijer, E.; Orskov, B.; Wanner, C.; Caskey, F.; Collart, F.; Finne, P.; Fogarty, D.G.; Groothoff, J.W.; et al. Analysis of data from the ERA-EDTA Registry indicates that conventional treatments for chronic kidney disease do not reduce the need for renal replacement therapy in autosomal dominant polycystic kidney disease. *Kidney Int.* **2014**, *86*, 1244–1252. [CrossRef] [PubMed]
2. Argyrou, C.; Moris, D.; Vernadakis, S. Tailoring the 'Perfect Fit' for Renal Transplant Recipients with End-stage Polycystic Kidney Disease: Indications and Timing of Native Nephrectomy. *In Vivo* **2017**, *31*, 307–312. [CrossRef] [PubMed]
3. Grantham, J.J.; Torres, V.E.; Chapman, A.B.; Guay-Woodford, L.M.; Bae, K.T.; King, B.F., Jr.; Wetzel, L.H.; Baumgarten, D.A.; Kenney, P.J.; Harris, P.C.; et al. CRISP Investigators: Volume progression in polycystic kidney disease. *N. Engl. J. Med.* **2006**, *354*, 2122–2130. [CrossRef] [PubMed]
4. Neeff, H.P.; Pisarski, P.; Tittelbach-Helmrich, D.; Karajanev, K.; Neumann, H.P.; Hopt, U.T.; Drognitz, O. One hundred consecutive kidney transplantations with simultaneous ipsilateral nephrectomy in patients with autosomal dominant polycystic kidney disease. *Nephrol. Dial. Transpl.* **2013**, *28*, 466–471. [CrossRef] [PubMed]
5. Bajwa, Z.H.; Gupta, S.; Warfield, C.A.; Steinman, T.I. Pain management in polycystic kidney disease. *Kidney Int.* **2001**, *60*, 1631–1644. [CrossRef] [PubMed]
6. Fuller, T.F.; Brennan, T.V.; Feng, S.; Kang, S.M.; Stock, P.G.; Freise, C.E. End stage polycystic kidney disease: Indications and timing of native nephrectomy relative to kidney transplantation. *J. Urol.* **2005**, *174*, 2284–2288. [CrossRef]
7. Kirkman, M.A.; van Dellen, D.; Mehra, S.; Campbell, B.A.; Tavakoli, A.; Pararajasingam, R.; Parrott, N.R.; Riad, H.N.; McWilliam, L.; Augustine, T. Native nephrectomy for autosomal dominant polycystic kidney disease: Before or after kidney transplantation? *BJU Int.* **2011**, *108*, 590–594. [CrossRef] [PubMed]
8. Akoh, J.A. Current management of autosomal dominant polycystic kidney disease. *World J. Nephrol.* **2015**, *4*, 468–479. [CrossRef]

9. Patel, P.; Horsfield, C.; Compton, F.; Taylor, J.; Koffman, G.; Olsburgh, J. Native nephrectomy in transplant patients with autosomal dominant polycystic kidney disease. *Ann. R. Coll. Surg. Engl.* **2011**, *93*, 391–395. [CrossRef]

10. Dinckan, A.; Kocak, H.; Tekin, A.; Turkyilmaz, S.; Hadimioglu, N.; Ertug, Z.; Gunseren, F.; Ari, E.; Dinc, B.; Gurkan, A.; et al. Concurrent unilateral or bilateral native nephrectomy in kidney transplant recipients. *Ann. Transpl.* **2013**, *18*, 697–704.

11. Cassuto-Viguier, E.; Quintens, H.; Chevallier, D.; Derrier, M.; Jambou, P.; Toubol, J.; Duplay, H. Transplantation and nephrectomy in autosomal dominant polycystic kidney disease. *Clin. Nephrol.* **1991**, *36*, 105–106. [PubMed]

12. Nunes, P.; Mota, A.; Alves, R.; Figueiredo, A.; Parada, B.; Macário, F.; Rolo, F. Simultaneous renal transplantation and native nephrectomy in patients with autosomal-dominant polycystic kidney disease. *Transpl. Proc.* **2007**, *39*, 2483–2485. [CrossRef] [PubMed]

13. Jankowska, M.; Kuzmiuk-Glembin, I.; Skonieczny, P.; Debska-Slizien, A. Native Nephrectomy in Renal Transplant Recipients with Autosomal Dominant Polycystic Kidney Disease. *Transpl. Proc.* **2018**, *50*, 1863–1867. [CrossRef] [PubMed]

14. Luciano, R.L.; Dahl, N.K. Extra-renal manifestations of autosomal dominant polycystic kidney disease (ADPKD): Considerations for routine screening and management. *Nephrol. Dial. Transpl.* **2014**, *29*, 247–254. [CrossRef] [PubMed]

15. Chebib, F.T.; Prieto, M.; Jung, Y.; Irazabal, M.V.; Kremers, W.K.; Dean, P.G.; Rea, D.J.; Cosio, F.G.; Torres, V.E.; El-Zoghby, Z.M. Native Nephrectomy in Renal Transplant Recipients with Autosomal Dominant Polycystic Kidney Disease. *Transpl. Direct.* **2015**, *1*, e43. [CrossRef] [PubMed]

16. Schrier, R.W.; Abebe, K.Z.; Perrone, R.D.; Torres, V.E.; Braun, W.E.; Steinman, T.I.; Winklhofer, F.T.; Brosnahan, G.; Czarnecki, P.G.; Hogan, M.C.; et al. Blood pressure in early autosomal dominant polycystic kidney disease. *N. Engl. J. Med.* **2014**, *371*, 2255–2266. [CrossRef]

17. Torres, V.E.; Abebe, K.Z.; Schrier, R.W.; Perrone, R.D.; Chapman, A.B.; Yu, A.S.; Braun, W.E.; Steinman, T.I.; Brosnahan, G.; Hogan, M.C.; et al. Dietary salt restriction is beneficial to the management of autosomal dominant polycystic kidney disease. *Kidney Int.* **2017**, *91*, 493–500. [CrossRef] [PubMed]

18. Regitz-Zagrosek, V. Sex and gender differences in health. Science & Society Series on Sex and Science. *EMBO Rep.* **2012**, *13*, 596–603.

19. Chapman, A.B. Approaches to testing new treatments in autosomal dominant polycystic kidney disease: Insights from the CRISP and HALT-PKD studies. *Clin. J. Am. Soc. Nephrol.* **2008**, *3*, 1197–1204. [CrossRef]

20. Cornec-Le Gall, E.; Audrézet, M.P.; Rousseau, A.; Hourmant, M.; Renaudineau, E.; Charasse, C.; Morin, M.P.; Moal, M.C.; Dantal, J.; Wehbe, B.; et al. The PROPKD Score: A New Algorithm to Predict Renal Survival in Autosomal Dominant Polycystic Kidney Disease. *J. Am. Soc. Nephrol.* **2016**, *27*, 942–951. [CrossRef]

21. Bennett, A.H.; Stewart, W.; Lazarus, J.M. Bilateral nephrectomy in patients with polycystic renal disease. *Surg. Gynecol. Obstet.* **1973**, *137*, 819–820. [PubMed]

22. Sanfilippo, F.P.; Vaughn, W.K.; Peters, T.G.; Bollinger, R.R.; Spees, E.K. Transplantation for polycystic kidney disease. *Transplantation* **1983**, *36*, 54–59. [CrossRef] [PubMed]

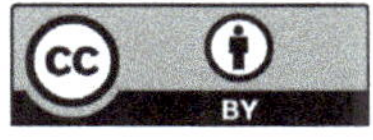

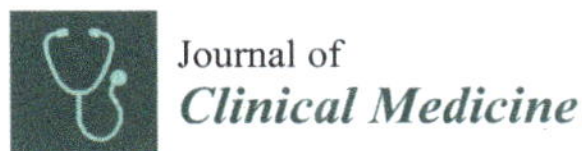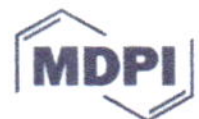

Article

Urinary Epidermal Growth Factor/Creatinine Ratio and Graft Failure in Renal Transplant Recipients: A Prospective Cohort Study

Manuela Yepes-Calderón [1], Camilo G. Sotomayor [1,*], Matthias Kretzler [2], Rijk O. B. Gans [3], Stefan P. Berger [1], Gerjan J. Navis [1], Wenjun Ju [2] and Stephan J. L. Bakker [1]

[1] Division of Nephrology, Department of Internal Medicine, University Medical Center Groningen, University of Groningen, 9700 RB Groningen, The Netherlands; manueyepes@gmail.com (M.Y.-C.); s.p.berger@umcg.nl (S.P.B.); g.j.navis@umcg.nl (G.J.N.); s.j.l.bakker@umcg.nl (S.J.L.B.)

[2] Department of Internal Medicine, Department of Computational Medicine and Bioinformatics, University of Michigan, Ann Arbor, MI 48109, USA; kretzler@umich.edu (M.K.); wenjunj@med.umich.edu (W.J.)

[3] Department of Internal Medicine, University Medical Center Groningen, University of Groningen, 9700 RB Groningen, The Netherlands; r.o.b.gans@umcg.nl

* Correspondence: c.g.sotomayor.campos@umcg.nl; Tel.: +31-061-921-0881

Received: 13 August 2019; Accepted: 12 October 2019; Published: 13 October 2019

Abstract: Graft failure (GF) remains a significant limitation to improve long-term outcomes in renal transplant recipients (RTR). Urinary epidermal growth factor (uEGF) is involved in kidney tissue integrity, with a reduction of its urinary excretion being associated with fibrotic processes and a wide range of renal pathologies. We aimed to investigate whether, in RTR, uEGF is prospectively associated with GF. In this prospective cohort study, RTR with a functioning allograft ≥1-year were recruited and followed-up for three years. uEGF was measured in 24-hours urine samples and normalized by urinary creatinine (Cr). Its association with risk of GF was assessed by Cox-regression analyses and its predictive ability by C-statistic. In 706 patients, uEGF/Cr at enrollment was 6.43 [IQR 4.07–10.77] ng/mg. During follow-up, 41(6%) RTR developed GF. uEGF/Cr was inversely associated with the risk of GF (HR 0.68 [95% CI 0.59–0.78]; $P < 0.001$), which remained significant after adjustment for immunosuppressive therapy, estimated Glomerular Filtration Rate, and proteinuria. C-statistic of uEGF/Cr for GF was 0.81 ($P < 0.001$). We concluded that uEGF/Cr is independently and inversely associated with the risk of GF and depicts strong prediction ability for this outcome. Further studies seem warranted to elucidate whether uEGF might be a promising marker for use in clinical practice.

Keywords: epidermal growth factor; creatinine; graft failure; renal transplantation.

1. Introduction

Although in recent decades short-term graft survival has seen great improvement, chronic graft failure remains a major clinical challenge for renal transplantation with no significant reduction achieved in the same time frame [1]. Graft failure is a culmination of several factors, including chronic rejection, toxicity of calcineurin inhibitors, infection, hypertension, oxidative stress, and proteinuria, together leading to progressive fibrosis and loss of renal function [2–5]. In clinical settings, most biomarkers used for follow-up, e.g., urinary albumin excretion and urinary protein excretion, are indicators of glomerular damage [6], improper of the development of fibrosis, which is an early event in the natural history of chronic rejection [3]. Finding non-invasive biomarkers that could reflect the pathophysiological changes in the renal tissue would be of remarkable utility as potential tools to monitor patients and timely identify those at high risk of graft failure [7], who could benefit from further interventions and stricter follow-up before structural damage is already present [8].

Epidermal growth factor (EGF) is a 53-amino acid peptide produced in the kidney at the ascending loop of Henle and the distal convoluted tubule [7,8]. It stimulates the proliferation and differentiation of epidermal and epithelial cells, and under normal conditions it has a critical role in renal development [7], maintenance of renal tubule integrity and tubular regenerative response to acute kidney injury [9–11]. However, the dysregulation and chronic activation of its receptor is known to promote pro-inflammatory response [12]; furthermore, it has been implicated in the development of interstitial fibrosis [13]. In clinical settings, the urinary excretion of EGF has shown to be decreased in a wide range of kidney pathologies—e.g., diabetic nephropathy and IgA nephropathy—suggesting that it could potentially work as a biomarker of a pathway which is common to several kidney tissue insults [14]. Although it would not be possible to summarize the complexity of the graft failure process with one biomarker, fibrosis is an important step towards graft failure development [2]; and suppression of urinary EGF (uEGF) is an early marker of this phenomenon [15]. It may be theorized that uEGF could also be altered in patients at high risk of graft failure; however, the potential association with outcome or predictive ability of uEGF for graft failure is yet to be evaluated.

In the current study, we aimed to investigate the hypothesis that uEGF is prospectively associated with the risk of graft failure in a large, well-phenotyped, cohort of stable renal transplant recipients (RTR). Furthermore, we aimed to evaluate the prediction ability of uEGF for graft failure.

2. Materials and Methods

2.1. Study Design and Patient Population

In this prospective cohort study, all adult RTR with a functioning graft for ≥1 year, without history of drug addiction, alcohol addiction or malignancy, who visited the outpatient clinic of the University Medical Center of Groningen (The Netherlands) between November 2008–May 2011 were invited to participate. In total 707 (86%) of the 817 eligible RTR signed a written informed consent. RTR with missing information about uEGF at enrollment (n = 57) were excluded, resulting in 649 RTR eligible for the statistical analyses (Figure 1). There were no significant differences in risk factors for graft failure between patients with complete data and patients with missing data (Table S1). The primary end point of the current study was death-censored graft failure, defined as restart of dialysis or need of re-transplantation. The patients were followed-up for a total of 3 years. We contacted general practitioners or referring nephrologists in cases where the status of a patient was unknown. No participants were lost to follow-up (Figure 1). The current study was approved by the institutional review board (METc 2008/186) and adhered to the Declarations of Helsinki and Istanbul.

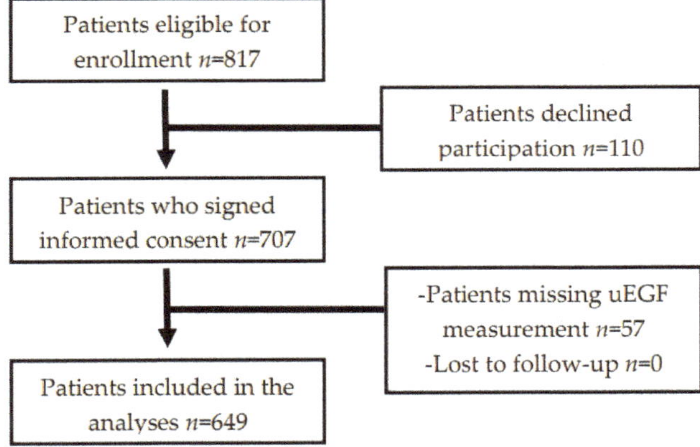

Figure 1. Participant flow diagram.

2.2. Data Collection

Data at enrollment were collected during a visit to the outpatient clinic, following a detailed protocol described elsewhere [16,17]. Systolic blood pressure (SBP) and diastolic blood pressure (DBP) were measured using a semiautomatic device (Dinamap 1846, Critikon, Tampa, Florida, USA) every minute for 15 minutes, following a strict protocol as described before [16].

Other relevant donor, recipient, and transplant information was extracted from the Groningen Renal Transplant Database [18]. Delayed graft function was defined as oliguria for 7 days or need for continuous ambulatory peritoneal dialisys or need for >2 sessions of hemodyalisis. Data collection is ensured by the continuous surveillance system of the outpatient clinic of our university hospital and close collaboration with affiliated hospitals.

2.3. Laboratory Measurements and Calculations

According to a strict protocol, all RTR were asked to collect a 24-hours urine sample during the day before to their visit to the outpatient clinic and on that day fasting blood samples were taken. Serum creatinine was determined using the Jaffé reaction (MEGA AU510, Merck Diagnostica, Germany); plasma glucose by the glucose oxidase method (YSI 2300 Stat Plus, Yellow Springs Instruments, Yellow Springs, OH, USA). uEGF concentration was measured by ELISA (R&D Systems, Minneapolis, MN, USA); the test has a range of detection of 3.9–250 pg/mL and the intra- and inter-plate coefficients of variation were less than 10% and 15%, respectively [15]. Urinary creatinine concentration was measured by colorimetric detection kit (Enzo, New York, NY, USA). Finally, the concentration of uEGF was normalized by the concentration of urinary creatinine, and a ratio was created and used for all analyses (uEGF/Cr).

Body surface area was calculated according to the Du Bois formula [19], estimated glomerular filtration rate (eGFR) by the serum creatinine based Chronic Kidney Disease EPIdemiology collaboration equation (CKD-EPI) [20] and the cumulative dose of prednisolone as the sum of the maintenance dose of prednisolone from transplantation until enrollment.

2.4. Statistical Analysis

Data analyses, computations, and graphs were performed with SPSS 22.0 software (IBM Corporation, Chicago, IL, USA) and GraphPad Prism version 7 software (GraphPad Software, San Diego, CA, USA). Descriptive statistics data are presented as mean ± standard deviation (SD) for normally distributed data, and as median (interquartile range [IQR]) for variables with a non-normal distribution. Categorical data are expressed as number (percentage). Differences in characteristics at enrollment between patients with and without data on uEGF, and among subgroups of RTR according to tertiles of uEGF/Cr were tested by one-way ANOVA for continuous variables with normal distribution, Mann–Whitney U test for continuous variables with skewed distribution and χ^2 test for categorical variables. We also performed linear regression analyses testing the association between time after transplantation and uEGF/Cr in crude and multivariable analyses with adjustment for use of cyclosporine inhibitors. For all statistical analyses, a statistical significance level of $P \leq 0.05$ (two-tailed) was used.

Graft failure development was visualized by Kaplan-Meier curves according to tertiles of uEGF/Cr, with statistical significance among curves tested by log-rank (Mantel–Cox) test. The prospective association of uEGF/Cr with risk of graft failure during follow-up was further examined, incorporating time to event, by means of uni- and multivariate Cox proportional-hazards regression analyses with time-dependent covariates to calculate hazard ratios (HR) and 95% confidence intervals (CI). First, we performed an unadjusted model. Afterwards we adjusted for age and sex, and the following variables: in model 2, transplant related data (transplant vintage, pre–emptive transplantation, age and sex of donor, type of donor and cold ischemia time); in model 3, renal transplant recipient characteristics (human leukocyte antigen [HLA] mismatch with donor and delayed graft function);

in model 4, we adjusted for the variables included in the model 2 and 3; in model 4, immunosuppressive therapy (usage of calcineurin inhibitors and proliferation inhibitors, and acute rejection treatment); in model 5, graft function (eGFR and urinary protein excretion); and the final model (model 6) was a combination of model 4 and 5. Schoenfeld residuals were calculated to assess whether proportionality assumptions were fulfilled. Furthermore, we tested the potential predictive ability of uEGF/Cr for graft failure by means of performing a receiver operating characteristics (ROC) curve. To investigate whether uEGF might be of additional value to urinary albumin excretion and protein excretion, we calculated the individual C-statistic of these variables, and then the C-statistic of them combined with uEGF/Cr. Moreover, we performed an F-test to check whether the difference between predictive models was significant. Positive and negative predictive value were calculated for the cut-off points of the uEGF/Cr tertiles.

As secondary analyses, we assessed potential effect-modifications by pre-specified variables of: age, sex, eGFR, plasma creatinine concentration, proteinuria, high-sensitivity C-reactive protein (hs-CRP), acute rejection, and transplantation without dialysis (pre-emptive) by fitting models containing both main effects and their cross-product terms. Finally, we performed sensitivity analyses in which we eliminated patients with extreme values of uEGF/Cr (outside −2 and 2 standard deviations).

3. Results

3.1. Characteristics at Enrollment

In total 649 RTR were included in the analyses with a mean ± SD age of 53 ± 13 years, 57% men. Patients were included at a median (IQR) of 5.28 (1.74–12.00) years after transplantation and uEGF/Cr ratio had a median of 6.43 (4.07–10.77) ng/mg. In crude linear regression analyses, there was no significant association between years after transplantation and uEGF/Cr (Std. $\beta = -0.015$; $P = 0.71$), however, the association became apparent after the adjustment for calcineurin inhibitors usage (Std. $\beta = -0.81$; $P = 0.046$). Characteristics at enrollment of the overall RTR population and according to tertiles of uEGF/Cr are shown in Table 1. In the highest uEGF/Cr tertile patients had older age ($P = 0.01$), smaller percentage of male population ($P < 0.001$), higher eGFR ($P < 0.001$), lower urinary protein excretion ($P < 0.001$), larger percentage of transplant from living donors ($P < 0.001$), younger donors age ($P < 0.001$), and higher percentage of donors were male ($P = 0.03$). Also, they used less cyclosporine ($P = 0.002$) and tacrolimus ($P < 0.001$) in their immunosuppressive regimens, but more mycophenolic acid ($P = 0.03$); and a smaller percentage of patients required acute rejection treatment ($P < 0.001$) (Table 1). Patients in the highest uEGF/Cr tertile also had higher glycated hemoglobin percentage (Table 1), independent of whether they were diabetic or non-diabetic subjects (Table S2).

Table 1. Characteristics at enrollment of the study population.

Characteristics	Overall RTR (n = 649)	Tertile 1 <4.78 ng/mg	Tertile 2 4.78–8.80 ng/mg	Tertile 3 >8.80 ng/mg	P
uEGF/Cr, ng/mg	6.43 (4.07–10.77)	3.18 (2.12–4.07)	6.43 (5.57–7.45)	12.91 (10.77–16.08)	—
Demographics					
Age, years	53 ± 13	51 ± 13	53 ± 13	55 ± 12	0.01
Sex (male), n (%)	373 (57)	149 (69)	124 (57)	100 (46)	<0.001
Caucasian ethnicity, n (%)	647 (99)	216 (100)	216 (100)	215 (99)	0.44
Renal allograft function					
eGFR, mL/min/1.73 m^2 [a]	52 ± 20	37 ± 14	53 ± 16	68 ± 17	<0.001
Urinary protein excretion, g/24 h [b]	0.20 (0.02–0.34)	0.25 (0.13–0.63)	0.19 (0.02–0.32)	0.08 (0.02–0.26)	<0.001
Urinary albumin excretion, mg/24 h [c]	38.27 (10.57–174.38)	94.00 (20.48–393.77)	37.52 (10.50–155.20)	19.35 (7.11–71.08)	<0.001
Renal transplantation characteristics					
Pre–emptive transplantation, n (%)	105 (16)	27 (13)	35 (16)	43 (20)	0.11
Living donor, n (%) [d]	230 (35)	30 (14)	95 (44)	75 (35)	0.002
Age of donor, years [e]	43 ± 15	47 ± 14	45 ± 15	37 ± 15	<0.001
Sex of donor (male), n (%) [f]	331 (51)	97 (45)	109 (50)	125 (58)	0.03
Cold ischemia time, hours [g]	15.2 (2.7–21.3)	15.6 (3.0–22.5)	14.0 (2.6–21.0)	15.4 (2.7–22.0)	0.03
Time since transplantation, years	5.28 (1.74–12.00)	5.07 (1.53–12.92)	5.26 (1.40–12.32)	5.45 (2.63–10.98)	0.96
Renal transplantation recipients' characteristics					
Delayed graft fuction, n (%)	47 (7)	24 (11)	13 (6)	10 (5)	0.02
HLA mismatch with donor, number [h]	2 (1–3)	2 (1–3)	2 (1–3)	2 (1–3)	0.10
Immunosuppressive therapy					
Cumulative prednisolone dose, g	17.4 (5.2–36.2)	17.0 (4.7–38.4)	16.8 (4.6–36.4)	18.1 (8.1–32.8)	0.78
Sirolimus or rapamune use, n (%) [i]	13 (2)	4 (2)	6 (3)	3 (1)	0.57
Type of calcineurin inhibitor					
Cyclosporine, n (%)	258 (40)	90 (42)	102 (47)	66 (31)	0.002
Tacrolimus, n (%)	120 (18)	66 (31)	32 (15)	22 (10)	<0.001
Type of proliferation inhibitor					
Mycophenolic acid, n (%)	424 (65)	126 (58)	147 (68)	151 (70)	0.03
Azathioprine, n (%)	112 (17)	41 (19)	32 (15)	39 (18)	0.47
Acute rejection treatment, n (%)	172 (27)	77 (36)	55 (25)	40 (19)	<0.001

Table 1. *Cont.*

Characteristics	Overall RTR (n = 649)	Tertile 1	Tertile 2	Tertile 3	P
		<4.78 ng/mg	4.78–8.80 ng/mg	>8.80 ng/mg	
Body composition					
Body surface area, m^2	1.94 ± 0.22	1.97 ± 0.23	1.94 ± 0.20	1.92 ± 0.21	0.06
Body mass index, kg/m^2	26.5 ± 4.7	26.4 ± 4.8	26.4 ± 4.4	26.8 ± 4.9	0.53
Cardiovascular history					
History of cardiovascular disease, n (%) [j]	281 (43)	88 (41)	96 (44)	97 (45)	0.65
Arterial pressure					
SBP, mmHg [a]	136 ± 17	138 ± 18	135 ± 17	135 ± 17	0.17
DBP, mmHg [a]	82 ± 11	84 ± 11	82 ± 11	82 ± 10	0.06
Use of antihypertensives, n (%)	573 (88)	202 (94)	194 (90)	177 (82)	0.001
Lifestyle					
Current smoker, n (%) [k]	78 (12)	31 (14)	25 (12)	22 (10)	0.48
Alcohol intake >30 g/day, n (%) [l]	29 (4)	9 (4)	11 (5)	9 (4)	0.60
SQUASH, intensity x hours	5050 (1950–8055)	5190 (1800–9105)	4750 (1700–7260)	5408 (2645–7301)	0.89
Diabetes and glucose homeostasis					
Diabetes mellitus, n (%)	160 (25)	50 (23)	58 (27)	52 (24)	0.53
Plasma glucose, mmol/L [a]	5.2 (4.8–6.0)	5.3 (4.8–5.9)	5.2 (4.8–6.1)	5.3 (4.7–6.1)	0.09
HbA1c, % [m]	5.8 (5.5–6.2)	5.7 (5.4–6.1)	5.8 (5.5–6.2)	5.9 (5.6–6.3)	0.004
Inflammation					
Leukocyte count, per 10^9/L [b]	8.2 ± 2.7	8.1 ± 2.8	8.2 ± 2.8	8.1 ± 2.4	0.97
hs-CRP, mg/L [n]	1.6 (0.7–4.6)	1.7 (0.8–4.9)	1.4 (0.7–3.7)	1.6 (0.7–5.1)	0.71

Differences were tested by ANOVA for continuous variables with normal distribution, Kruskal–Wallis test for continuous variables with non-normal distribution and by χ^2 test for categorical variables. Data available in [a] 647, [b] 648, [c] 637, [d] 649, [e] 633, [f] 636, [g] 623, [h] 638, [i] 608, [j] 567, [k] 607, [l] 581, [m] 627, [n] 613 patients. RTR, renal transplant recipients; uEGF, urinary epidermal growth factor; Cr, creatinine; eGFR, estimated glomerular filtration rate; SBP, systolic blood pressure; DBP, diastolic blood pressure; SQUASH, Short QUestionnaire to ASsess Health-enhancing physical activity; HDL, high–density lipoprotein cholesterol; LDL, low–density lipoprotein cholesterol; HbA1c, glycated hemoglobin; hs-CRP, high-sensitivity C-reactive protein.

3.2. Prospective Analyses on Graft Failure

During a follow-up of 3 years, 41 (6%) RTR developed graft failure. Thirty-three events (80%) were in the lowest tertile of uEGF/Cr, 4 (10%) in the intermediate tertile and 4 (10%) in the highest tertile. The curves were significantly different according to the log-rank (Mantel cox) test ($P < 0.001$). The corresponding Kaplan–Meier curves are shown in Figure 2.

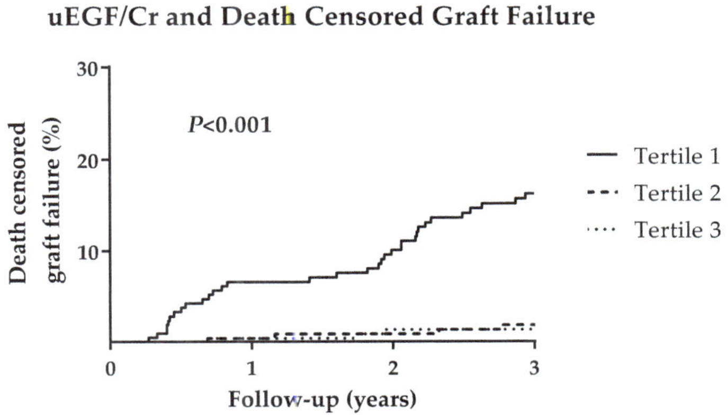

uEGF/Cr and Death Censored Graft Failure

Number at risk (Censored)				
Tertile 1	216	195 (11)	181 (3)	158 (2)
Tertile 2	217	215 (9)	209 (5)	196 (4)
Tertile 3	216	214 (11)	209 (10)	200 (7)

Figure 2. Kaplan–Meier curves by tertiles of uEGF/Cr on graft failure. Tertile 1: < 4.78 ng/mg; Tertile 2: 4.78–8.80 ng/mg; Tertile 3: > 8.80 ng/mg. *P* value was obtained from the log-rank (Mantel cox) test. uEGF/Cr, urinary epidermal growth factor/creatinine ratio.

Cox regression analyses showed that uEGF/Cr ratio is inversely associated with the risk of graft failure (HR 0.68 [95% CI 0.59-0.78] per ng/mg) and this association is highly significant ($P < 0.001$). Further adjustment for transplantation-related data, renal transplant recipient characteristics, immunosuppressive therapy, eGFR and urinary protein excretion did not materially change this finding. The association between uEGF/Cr and graft failure was still strongly significant in the final model which included adjustment for both immunosuppressive therapy and graft function, with a HR of 0.79 (95% CI 0.67-0.94; $P = 0.007$) (Table 2).

Table 2. Multivariable-adjusted associations between uEGF/Cr and graft failure in 649 RTRs.

Models	uEGF/Cr, ng/mg		
	HR	**95% CI**	**P**
Crude	0.68	0.59–0.78	<0.001
Model 1	0.67	0.58–0.78	<0.001
Model 2	0.70	0.58–0.77	<0.001
Model 3	0.67	0.58–0.78	<0.001
Model 4	0.66	0.57–0.77	<0.001
Model 5	0.78	0.66–0.93	0.005
Model 6	0.79	0.67–0.94	0.007

In total 41 (6%) patients developed graft failure. Model 1: adjusted for age, sex, and transplant related data. Model 2: adjusted for age, sex, and renal transplant recipient characteristics. Model 3: Model 1 + Model 2. Model 4: adjusted for age, sex, and immunosuppressive therapy. Model 5: adjusted for age, sex, and eGFR and urinary protein excretion. Model 6: model 4 + model 5. RTRs, renal transplant recipients; uEGF, urinary epidermal growth factor.

A ROC curve assessing the prediction ability of uEGF/Cr for graft failure is displayed in Figure 3. uEGF/Cr showed to be a good predictor of the development of graft failure up to the following three years (C-statistic = 0.81), with better predictive ability than urinary albumin excretion and urinary protein excretion (C-statistic = 0.78 and C-statistic = 0.76, respectively). The curve of uEGF/Cr was significantly different from the reference line ($P < 0.001$). Being on the first tertile of uEGF/Cr had a positive predictive value of 75% for the development graft failure, on the other hand, being in the third tertile had a negative predictive value of 81% (Table S3).

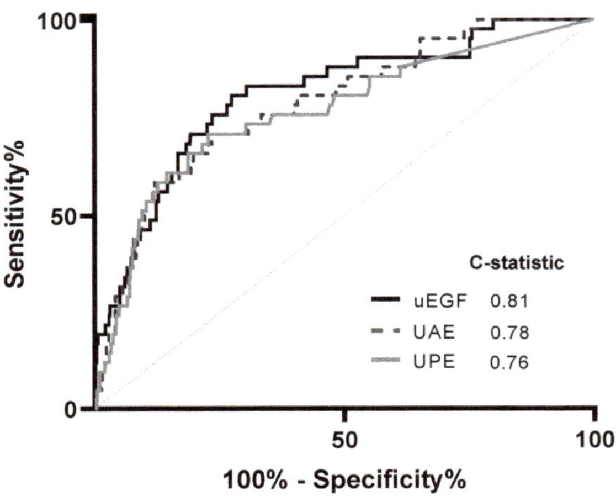

Figure 3. ROC curve of uEGF/Cr for graft failure. During a follow-up of 3 years, 41 (6%) patients developed graft failure. GF, graft failure; uEGF/Cr, urinary epidermal growth factor/creatinine ratio; UAE, urinary albumin excretion; UPE, urinary protein excretion.

Urinary protein excretion and urinary albumin excretion had a C-statistic of 0.76 and 0.78, respectively. The predictive value for both variables was significantly improved after the addition of uEGF/Cr (C-statistic = 0.82, F-test for difference among models = $P < 0.001$) (Table 3).

Table 3. Predictive value (C-statistic) for uEGF/Cr on top of established risk factors for graft failure

	C-Statistic	P *
Urinary protein excretion, g/24 h	0.76	Ref.
+ uEGF/Cr, ng/mg	0.82	<0.001
Urinary albumin excretion, mg/24 h	0.78	Ref.
+ uEGF/Cr, ng/mg	0.82	<0.001

* *P*-value of F-test for difference between the reference model and the model plus uEGF/Cr. uEGF/Cr, urinary epidermal growth factor/creatinine ratio.

3.3. Secondary and Sensitivity Analysis

In effect-modification analyses we found that none of the pre-specified variables we explored (age, sex, eGFR, plasma creatinine concentration, proteinuria, hs-CRP, acute rejection, and pre-emptive transplantation) was a significant effect-modifier of the association between uEGF/Cr and the risk of graft failure ($P > 0.10$), therefore we did not proceed with any subgroup analyses (Table S4).

Finally, in the sensitivity analyses in which we removed patients with extreme values of uEGF/Cr (patients outside of the −2 and +2 standard deviation), our findings remained materially unchanged. uEGF/Cr was strongly inversely associated with risk of graft failure (HR 0.68 (95% CI 0.59–0.78);

$P < 0.001$) and further adjustments analogous to models used in the primary analyses did not materially modified this association (Table S5).

4. Discussion

In a large cohort of stable RTR, we showed first, that patients with impaired renal function have significantly lower excretion of uEGF. Second, that uEGF/Cr is inversely associated with the risk of graft failure and that this association is independent of potential confounders, including immunosuppressive therapy, eGFR and urinary protein excretion. Finally, uEGF/Cr also appears to have good prediction ability for the development of graft failure, superior to urinary albumin excretion and urinary protein excretion. These findings are in agreement with previous evidence showing that uEGF is a biomarker altered in several kidney pathologies [15,21,22], and for the first time we provided evidence in the post-renal transplantation setting.

EGF is a 53-amino acid peptide which expression is restricted to the kidney [7,15,22], particularly to the thick ascending limb of Henle and the distal tubule [14], therefore it is found in higher concentrations in urine than in any other body fluid [23]. EGF and its receptor are involved in several processes within kidney tissue, mainly related to tubular cell proliferation [13] and pathways of cell survival [10,11], making EGF a critical component in promoting kidney recovery from acute injury [11]. Therefore, its dysregulation is involved in key pathogenic pathways that drive kidney disease progression independent of etiology, e.g., chronic inflammation [24], extracellular matrix modulation and tubular cell dedifferentiation [15].

EGF has gained interest as a biomarker of renal disease because its decreased urinary excretion has been observed in nearly all rodent kidney injury models [20] and in various human kidney diseases [25], including diabetic nephropathy, IgA nephropathy, and lupus nephritis [14]. Consistently, we found that our study population of RTR had a decreased uEGF/Cr ratio when compared to healthy subjects, and comparable ratios to those of patients with chronic kidney disease [15,26,27]. Its common clinical standardization by creatinine (uEGF/Cr) has shown several advantages as a biomarker of kidney tissue damage: (i) it is highly tissue specific, which makes it robust to extra renal events that may affect the accuracy of other nonspecific biomarkers; (ii) it is known that even in the normal creatinine range there is a significant influence of kidney function on uEGF/Cr [22]; and (iii) it shows only a weak correlation with markers of glomerular damage as urinary protein excretion, which shows that uEFG/Cr is a representation of a different independent pathophysiologic mechanism [12,14,27] and could complement these other parameters. Our study further supports the role of uEGF/Cr as a biomarker of damage to renal tissue, and more importantly, as a biomarker independently associated with risk of graft failure in stable renal transplant recipients. Furthermore, the strong prediction abilities of uEGF/Cr for risk of graft failure, even superior to those of urinary albumin excretion and urinary protein excretion, and of adding predictive value in combination with these variables, also supports the idea of uEGF/Cr being a marker of a different pathological aspect of graft failure which might be earlier than stablished glomerular damage.

Because risk of graft failure increases with time, one could speculate that uEGF decreases with time after transplantation. However, we did not observe such a relationship over increasing tertiles of uEGF. This finding may be explained by a confounding effect of use of cyclosporine resulting in lowering of uEGF, which is supported by the observation that an association between uEGF and time after transplantation became apparent after adjustment for use of cyclosporine in linear regression analyses. We also found in our population that the use of calcineurin inhibitors was higher among patients with lower uEGF/Cr. This is in agreement with previous studies showing an inverse association between uEGF and the use of calcineurin inhibitors [28,29] and a potential involvement of the EGF receptor in the alterations that lead to magnesium loss in renal transplant recipients receiving calcineurin inhibitors [29,30]. Nevertheless, the association between uEGF/Cr and graft failure was independent of the adjustment for the use of calcineurin inhibitors. This suggests that the association of uEGF/Cr is not mediated by a nephrotoxic effect of calcineurin inhibitors, but is mediated by other mechanisms, which may involve renal fibrosis. Furthermore, in contrast to previous results [31], no difference was observed in the prevalence of diabetes between the uEGF/Cr tertiles in our study population.

The present study has several strengths. We assessed not only the association but also the risk-prediction ability for graft failure of uEGF/Cr. Also, our extensively phenotyped cohort allowed us to control for several potential confounders, among which demographic and anthropometric variables, renal function and immunosuppressive therapy were accounted for. The following limitations should be considered in the interpretation of our results. This study was carried out in a single center with over-representation of Caucasian population, which calls prudence to extrapolation of our results to different populations regarding ethnicity. Also, we did not have repeated uEGF measurements, and the single measurement of the variable of interest could have given rise to the underestimation of the true effect [32,33]. Moreover, we used the Jaffé method to measure serum creatinine, which can generate false positive results in the presence of pesudochromogens such as ketones [34]. Next, only limited data were available regarding donors characteristics and therefore we could not adjust for donor variables such as donor serum creatinine or donor hepatitis C status. Finally, as with any observational study, residual confounding may occur despite the substantial number of potentially confounding factors for which we adjusted.

5. Conclusions

uEGF/Cr is inversely and independently associated with the risk of graft failure in stable RTR. This study provides for the first time relevant prospective data on a potential role of EGF in the pathophysiological changes that lead to graft failure. Furthermore, it appears that uEGF/Cr could be a biomarker of interest in the identification of patients at high risk of graft failure. Of note, to the best of our knowledge, current reference values for uEGF/Cr have not been established. Given our findings standardized assays for uEGF with reference values being generated are warranted. The potential utility of EGF directed therapies or the implementation of uEGF/Cr in clinical care of stable RTR requires further research and validation in a larger and more heterogeneous clinical studies.

Supplementary Materials: The following are available online at http://www.mdpi.com/2077-0383/8/10/1673/s1, Table S1: Comparison of characteristics between renal transplant recipients with and without data of urinary EGF concentration; Table S2: Glycated hemoglobin according to tertiles of uEGF/Cr ratio in diabetic and non-diabetic subjects; Table S3: Positive and negative predictive value by tertiles of uEGF/Cr; Table S4: Effect-modification of pre-specified characteristics on the associations of uEGF/Cr with graft failure; Table S5: Multivariable-adjusted associations between uEGF/Cr ratio and graft failure in RTR among the −2 and +2 standard deviations of uEGF/Cr.

Author Contributions: Data curation, M.K. and W.J.; Formal analysis, M.Y.-C. and C.G.S.; Funding acquisition, S.J.L.B.; Investigation, M.K., R.O.B.G., S.P.B., G.J.N., and W.J.; Methodology, M.K., W.J., and S.J.L.B.; Project administration, R.O.B.G., S.P.B., G.J.N., and S.J.L.B.; Supervision, S.J.L.B.; Writing—original draft, M.Y.-C. and C.G.S.; Writing—review and editing, R.O.B.G., S.P.B., G.J.N., W.J., and S.J.L.

Funding: This study was based on the TransplantLines Food and Nutrition Biobank and Cohort Study (TxL-FN), which was funded by the Top institute food and nutrition of The Netherlands, grant number A-1003.

Acknowledgments: The study is registered at clinicaltrials.gov under number NCT02811835. Dr. Sotomayor is supported by a doctorate studies grant from CONICYT (F 72190118). This paper is partially supported by NIDDK P30 DK081943 for University of Michigan O'Brien Kidney Translational Core Center. The authors thank Therese Roth for technical support.

Conflicts of Interest: The authors declare no conflict of interest.

References

1. Meier-Kriesche, H.-U.; Schold, J.D.; Srinivas, T.R.; Kaplan, B. Lack of Improvement in Renal Allograft Survival Despite a Marked Decrease in Acute Rejection Rates Over the Most Recent Era. *Am. J. Transplant.* **2004**, *4*, 378–383. [CrossRef] [PubMed]
2. Kloc, M.; Ghobrial, R.M. Chronic allograft rejection: A significant hurdle to transplant success. *Burn Trauma* **2014**, *2*, 3–10. [CrossRef] [PubMed]
3. Ponticelli, C. Progression of renal damage in chronic rejection. *Kidney Int.* **2000**, *75*, S62–S70. [CrossRef]

4. Schratzberger, G.; Gert, M. Chronic allograft failure: A disease we don't understand and can't cure? *Nephrol. Dial. Transplant.* **2002**, *17*, 1384–1390. [CrossRef] [PubMed]

5. McLaren, A.J.; Fuggle, S.V.; Welsh, K.I.; Gray, D.W.R.; Phil, D.; Morris, P.J. Chronic Allograft Failure in Human Renal Transplantation. A Multivariate Risk Factor Analysis. *Ann. Surg.* **2000**, *232*, 98–103. [CrossRef] [PubMed]

6. Nauta, F.L.; Bakker, S.J.L.; van Oeveren, W.; Navis, G.; van der Heide, J.J.H.; van Goor, H.; de Jong, P.E.; Gansevoort, R.T. Albuminuria, proteinuria, and novel urine biomarkers as predictors of long-term allograft outcomes in kidney transplant recipients. *Am. J. Kidney Dis.* **2011**, *57*, 733–743. [CrossRef] [PubMed]

7. Stein-Oakley, A.N.; Tzanidis, A.; Fuller, P.J.; Jablonski, P.; Thomson, N.M. Expression and distribution of epidermal growth factor in acute and chronic renal allograft rejection. *Kidney Int.* **1994**, *46*, 1207–1215. [CrossRef] [PubMed]

8. Worawichawong, S.; Radinahamed, P.; Muntham, D.; Sathirapongsasuti, N.; Nongnuch, A.; Assanatham, M.; Kitiyakara, C. Urine Epidermal Growth Factor, Monocyte Chemoattractant Protein-1 or Their Ratio as Biomarkers for Interstitial Fibrosis and Tubular Atrophy in Primary Glomerulonephritis. *Kidney Blood Press Res.* **2016**, *41*, 997–1007. [CrossRef]

9. Harskamp, L.R.; Gansevoort, R.T.; van Goor, H.; Meijer, E. The epidermal growth factor receptor pathway in chronic kidney diseases. *Nat. Rev. Nephrol.* **2016**, *12*, 496. [CrossRef]

10. Yarden, Y.; Sliwkowski, M.X. Untangling the ErbB signalling network. *Nat. Rev. Mol. Cell Biol.* **2001**, *2*, 127. [CrossRef]

11. Schlessinger, J. Ligand-Induced, Receptor-Mediated Dimerization and Activation of EGF Receptor. *Cell* **2002**, *110*, 669–672. [CrossRef]

12. Klein, J.; Bascands, J.-L.; Buffin-Meyer, B.; Schanstra, J.P. Epidermal growth factor and kidney disease: A long-lasting story. *Kidney Int.* **2016**, *89*, 985–987. [CrossRef] [PubMed]

13. Tang, J.; Liu, N.; Zhuang, S. Role of epidermal growth factor receptor in acute and chronic kidney injury. *Kidney Int.* **2013**, *83*, 804–810. [CrossRef] [PubMed]

14. Isaka, Y. Epidermal growth factor as a prognostic biomarker in chronic kidney diseases. *Ann. Transl. Med.* **2016**, *4* (Suppl. 1), S62. [CrossRef]

15. Ju, W.; Nair, V.; Smith, S.; Zhu, L.; Shedden, K.; Song, P.X.K.; Mariani, L.H.; Eichinger, F.H.; Berthier, C.C.; Randolph, A.; et al. Tissue transcriptome-driven identification of epidermal growth factor as a chronic kidney disease biomarker. *Sci. Transl. Med.* **2015**, *7*, 316ra193. [CrossRef] [PubMed]

16. van den Berg, E.; Geleijnse, J.M.; Brink, E.J.; van Baak, M.A.; Homan van der Heide, J.J.; Gans, R.O.B.; Navis, G.; Bakker, S.J.L. Sodium intake and blood pressure in renal transplant recipients. *Nephrol. Dial. Transplant.* **2012**, *27*, 3352–3359. [CrossRef]

17. van den Berg, E.; Engberink, M.; Brink, E.; van Baak, M.; Gans, R.; Navis, G.; Bakker, S. Dietary protein, blood pressure and renal function in renal transplant recipients. *Br. J. Nutr.* **2013**, *109*, 1463–1470. [CrossRef] [PubMed]

18. De Vries, A.P.J.; Bakker, S.J.L.; Van Son, W.J.; Van Der Heide, J.J.H.; Ploeg, R.J.; The, H.T.; De Jong, P.E.; Gans, R.O.B. Metabolic Syndrome Is Associated with Impaired Long-term Renal Allograft Function; Not All Component criteria Contribute Equally. *Am. J. Transplant.* **2004**, *4*, 1675–1683. [CrossRef]

19. Du Bois, D.; Du Bois, E.F. A formula to estimate the approximate surface area if height and weight be known. *Nutrition* **1989**, *5*, 303–311.

20. Levey, A.S.; Stevens, L.A.; Schmid, C.H.; Zhang, Y.L.; Castro, A.F.; Feldman, H.I.; Kusek, J.W.; Eggers, P.; Van Lente, F.; Greene, T.; et al. A new equation to estimate glomerular filtration rate. *Ann. Intern. Med.* **2009**, *150*, 604–612. [CrossRef]

21. Kok, H.M.; Falke, L.L.; Goldschmeding, R.; Nguyen, T.Q. Targeting CTGF, EGF and PDGF pathways to prevent progression of kidney disease. *Nat. Rev. Nephrol* **2014**, *10*, 700–711. [CrossRef] [PubMed]

22. Amado, J.A.; De-Francisco, A.L.M.; Botana, M.A.; Pesquera, C.; Vázquez-de-Prada, J.A.; Arias, M. Influence of kidney or heart transplantation on the urinary excretion of epidermal growth factor. *Transpl. Int.* **1994**, *7*, 127–130. [CrossRef] [PubMed]

23. Rayego-Mateos, S.; Rodrigues-Diez, R.; Morgado-Pascual, J.L.; Valentijn, F.; Valdivielso, J.M.; Goldschmeding, R.; Ruiz-Ortega, M. Role of Epidermal Growth Factor Receptor (EGFR) and Its Ligands in Kidney Inflammation and Damage. *Mediat. Inflamm.* **2018**, *2018*, e8739473. [CrossRef] [PubMed]

24. Azukaitis, K.; Ju, W.; Kirchner, M.; Nair, V.; Smith, M.; Fang, Z.; Thurn-Valsassina, D.; Bayazit, A.; Niemirska, A.; Canpolat, N.; et al. Low levels of urinary epidermal growth factor predict chronic kidney disease progression in children. *Kidney Int.* **2019**, *96*, 214–221. [CrossRef] [PubMed]

25. Meybosch, S.; De Monie, A.; Anné, C.; Bruyndonckx, L.; Jürgens, A.; De Winter, B.Y.; Trouet, D.; Ledeganck, K.J. Epidermal growth factor and its influencing variables in healthy children and adults. *PLoS ONE* **2019**, *14*, e0211212. [CrossRef] [PubMed]

26. Callegari, C.; Laborde, N.P.; Buenaflor, G.; Nascimento, C.G.; Brasel, J.A.; Fisher, D.A. The source of urinary epidermal growth factor in humans. *Eur. J. Appl. Physiol. Occup. Physiol.* **1988**, *58*, 26–31. [CrossRef]

27. Nath, K.A. Tubulointerstitial Changes as a Major Determinant in the Progression of Renal Damage. *Am. J. Kidney Dis.* **1992**, *20*, 1–17. [CrossRef]

28. Ledeganck, K.J.; Anné, C.; De Monie, A.; Meybosch, S.; Verpooten, G.; Vinckx, M.; Van Hoeck, K.; Van Eyck, A.; De Winter, B.; Trouet, D. Longitudinal Study of the Role of Epidermal Growth Factor on the Fractional Excretion of Magnesium in Children: Effect of Calcineurin Inhibitors. *Nutrients* **2018**, *10*, 677. [CrossRef]

29. Ledeganck, K.J.; De Winter, B.Y.; Van den Driessche, A.; Jurgens, A.; Bosmans, J.-L.; Couttenye, M.M.; Verpooten, G.A. Magnesium loss in cyclosporine-treated patients is related to renal epidermal growth factor downregulation. *Nephrol. Dial. Transplant.* **2014**, *29*, 1097–1102. [CrossRef]

30. Groenestege, W.M.; Thébault, S.; van der Wijst, J.; van den Berg, D.; Janssen, R.; Tejpar, S.; van den Heuvel, L.P.; van Cutsem, E.; Hoenderop, J.G.; Knoers, N.V.; et al. Impaired basolateral sorting of pro-EGF causes isolated recessive renal hypomagnesemia. *J. Clin. Investig.* **2007**, *117*, 2260–2267. [CrossRef]

31. Lev-Ran, A.; Hwang, D.L.; Miller, J.D.; Josefsberg, Z. Excretion of epidermal growth factor (EGF) in diabetes. *Clin. Chim. Acta* **1990**, *192*, 201–206. [CrossRef]

32. Koenig, W.; Sund, M.; Fröhlich, M.; Löwel, H.; Hutchinson, W.L.; Pepys, M.B. Refinement of the Association of Serum C-reactive Protein Concentration and Coronary Heart Disease Risk by Correction for Within-Subject Variation over TimeThe MONICA Augsburg Studies, 1984 and 1987. *Am. J. Epidemiol.* **2003**, *158*, 357–364. [CrossRef] [PubMed]

33. Danesh, J.; Wheeler, J.G.; Hirschfield, G.M.; Eda, S.; Eiriksdottir, G.; Rumley, A.; Lowe, G.D.O.; Pepys, M.B.; Gudnason, V. C-Reactive Protein and Other Circulating Markers of Inflammation in the Prediction of Coronary Heart Disease. *N. Engl. J. Med.* **2004**, *350*, 1387–1397. [CrossRef] [PubMed]

34. Lee, E.; Collier, C.P.; White, C.A. Interlaboratory Variability in Plasma Creatinine Measurement and the Relation with Estimated Glomerular Filtration Rate and Chronic Kidney Disease Diagnosis. *Clin. J. Am. Soc. Nephrol.* **2017**, *12*, 29–37. [CrossRef] [PubMed]

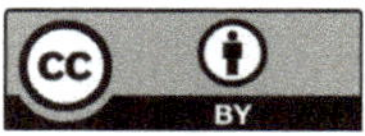

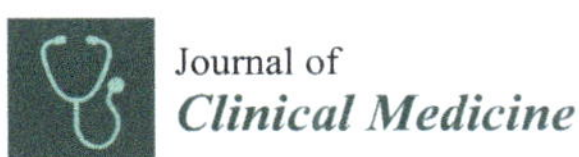
Journal of
Clinical Medicine

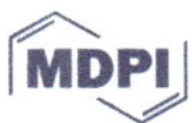

Review

BK Polyomavirus Virus Glomerular Tropism: Implications for Virus Reactivation from Latency and Amplification during Immunosuppression

Donald J. Alcendor

Center for AIDS Health Disparities Research, Meharry Medical College, 1005 Dr. D.B. Todd Jr. Blvd., Hubbard Hospital, 5th Floor, Rm. 5025, Nashville, TN 37208, USA; dalcendor@mmc.edu

Received: 12 August 2019; Accepted: 16 September 2019; Published: 17 September 2019

Abstract: BK polyomavirus (BKPyV), or BKV infection, is ubiquitous and usually non-pathogenic, with subclinical infections in 80–90% of adults worldwide. BKV infection is often associated with pathology in immunocompromised individuals. BKV infection often is associated with renal impairment, including ureteral stenosis, hemorrhagic cystitis, and nephropathy. BKV infection is less commonly associated with pneumonitis, retinitis, liver disease, and meningoencephalitis. BKV is known to replicate, establish latency, undergo reactivation, and induce clinical pathology in renal tubular epithelial cells. However, recent in vitro studies support the notion that BKV has expanded tropism-targeting glomerular parenchymal cells of the human kidney, which could impact glomerular function, enhance inflammation, and serve as viral reservoirs for reactivation from latency during immunosuppression. The implications of BKV expanded tropism in the glomerulus, and how specific host and viral factors that would contribute to glomerular inflammation, cytolysis, and renal fibrosis are related to BKV associated nephropathy (BKVAN), have not been explored. The pathogenesis of BKV in human glomerular parenchymal cells is poorly understood. In this review, I examine target cell populations for BKV infectivity in the human glomerulus. Specifically, I explore the implications of BKV expanded tropism in the glomerulus with regard viral entry, replication, and dissemination via cell types exposed to BKV trafficking in glomerulus. I also describe cellular targets shown to be permissive in vitro and in vivo for BKV infection and lytic replication, the potential role that glomerular parenchymal cells play in BKV latency and/or reactivation after immunosuppression, and the rare occurrence of BKV pathology in glomerular parenchymal cells in patients with BKVAN.

Keywords: polyomavirus; BKV; kidney; glomerulus; BKVAN; nephropathy; transplantation

---

1. Introduction

BK polyomavirus (BKPyV, hereafter referred to as BKV) is a member of the genus *Betapolyomavirus*, which belongs to the Polyomaviridae family of viruses that includes JC polyomavirus, or JCPyV, and Simian-virus 40 (SV40 virus) [1–6]. BKV was first isolated by Gardner in 1971, from the urine sample of a renal transplant patient diagnosed with ureteral stenosis with the initials "B.K." [7]. BKV is a small non-enveloped, icosahedral, circular, doubled-stranded DNA virus that is 40–45 nm in diameter, with a genome size of approximately 5 kb (kilobases) [8,9]. BKV was first reported in 1995 as being a cause of allograft failure in renal transplant patients [10]. It is now recognized as an emerging pathogen in renal transplant patients, with increased incidence that correlated with the use of more potent iatrogenic immunesuppressants such as tacrolimus (FK 506) and mycophenolate mofetil (Cellcept) [11–16].

While primary infection with BKV is usually asymptomatic and occurs early in life with a seroprevalence of 80–90% in adults worldwide, it is often associated with pathology in immunocompromised individuals [17,18]. BKV has a seroprevalence of 65% to 90% in children aged 5–9 years, and can be transmitted via respiratory, uro-oral, and feco-oral borne routes [19,20].

Because latent BKV is known to reactivate in patients who have immunocompromised incidence of conditions associated with BKV infection such as encephalitis, nephritis, hemorrhagic cystitis, retinitis, and pneumonia, it has also been reported in HIV-1 infected patients [21,22]. HIV-1 patients also experience a higher prevalence of BKV viruria than healthy individuals that show a positive correlation with the degree of immunosuppression [23].

BKV reactivation after immunosuppression in transplant recipients can result in clinical disease in the form of BKV associated nephropathy (BKVAN), leading to ureteral stenosis, tubular interstitial damage, as well as hemorrhagic cystitis in bone marrow transplant patients [24–26]. Primary BKV infection is accompanied by viral replication, followed by the establishment of latency in renal tissue [27]. BKV-associated pathology linked to immunosuppression includes diseases of the respiratory tract, urinary bladder, kidney, the central nervous system (CNS), eye, digestive tract, and endothelium [20]. BKV reactivation from latency is followed by viruria, which occurs in up to 20% of asymptomatic immunocompetent individuals, and in 20–60% of immunocompromised patients [28]. Approximately 80% of renal transplant recipients experience BK viruria and among those 5–10% develop BKVAN [28]. Virus infection leading to viremia, interstitial inflammation, graft rejection with the progression of interstitial fibrosis, and tubular atrophy, can lead to allograft failure and end stage renal disease (ESRD). ESRD represents an important health disparity among underserved populations [29–32]. Currently, there is no specific treatment for BKVAN. With no effective consistent antiviral therapy, pre-emptive reduction of maintenance immunosuppression and/or changes to the immunosuppressive regimen is recommended to control BKV replication, which may lead to an increased risk of allograft rejection [27]. The underlying mechanisms and kinetics of BKV infection in BKVAN remain largely unexplored. Primary infection of glomerular parenchymal cells could lead to progressive inflammation, injury, and cytolysis, which contribute to renal fibrosis and likely lead to ESRD.

2. BKV Infection and Post-Transplant Kidney Disease

In the adult population, there is a high prevalence of BKV infection and latency in renal tissue that usually remains asymptomatic in immunocompetent individuals, but predisposes renal transplant patients that require immunosuppression to BKV reactivation and replication. Approximately 50–80% of patients that develop BKVAN also experience graft failure [33]. The incidence of graft failure is dependent on the degree of glomerular inflammation caused by proinflammatory cytokines, the influx of immune effector cells, BKV lytic replication, and lysis of renal tubular epithelial cells that can lead renal fibrosis and subsequent graft failure [34–36]. In renal transplant patients, reactivation of BKV occurs in the graft and the infection is donor-derived [37], with higher rates of reactivation occurring with donors that are BKV seropositive [37]. BKV reactivation after renal transplantation is usually first observed by the appearance of virus-infected uroepithelial cells, known as decoy cells, that are found in the urine or BKV DNA in the urine, which is followed by a viremic phase that occurs approximately one month post-transplantation, according to Hirsch et al. [38]. BKV viremia precedes BKVAN. It is a better predictor of pathology associated with nephropathy than viruria, especially when accompanied by viral titers >10,000 copies/mL [39,40]. The timing of BKV reactivation and replication after transplant has been associated with several factors. These include the intensity of the immunosuppressive regimen involving the use of tacrolimus or mycophenolate mofetil, recipient-related factors (such as patient age, male sex, non-African American race), donor-related factors (such the degree of HLA mismatches, BKV seropositivity), and viral-related factors (such as the BKV genotype) [27,41]. In addition, other factors, such as renal injury associated with variation in cold ischemia time, delayed allograft function, and the placement of ureteral stents, have also been reported to influence BKV reactivation [42,43]. However, conclusive diagnosis of BKVAN requires the detection of viral inclusion bodies on renal biopsies, as well as confirmation of genome detection by in situ hybridization or viral antigen detection via immunohistochemical staining for the BKV large T antigen (LTAg) [44]. The BKV LTAg is known to cross-react with antibodies against the LTAg of simian virus 40 (SV40) that shares 70% genome sequence homology with BKV. While ultrastructural analysis by electron microscopy is highly sensitive for detecting BKV, and has been used to diagnose BKV infection, the presence of BKV alone may not be sufficient to confirm a BKVAN diagnosis. The reliability of these techniques varies due to non-specific binding of immunoglobulins and DNA oligomers in human tissue, hence, standardization is warranted.

BKVAN is divided to three histopathological grades: A, B, and C. Grade A BKVAN presents as inflammation in the tubular epithelial with the absence of tubular epithelial necrosis. Grade B BKVAN is defined as more progressive in pathology, involving both tubular epithelial cell necrosis as well as tubular epithelial cell lysis. Grade C BKVAN is defined as the presence of interstitial fibrosis that can ultimately lead to ESRD [45]. A strong correlation exists between graft survival based on histopathological grades of BKVAN, with Grade A having the best prognosis for graft survival at two years (90%) and Grade C having the worst (50%) [46].

Histological lesions in BKVAN are normally scored by the Banff 97 classification of renal allograft pathology to indicate severity [46–48]. Several biomarkers have been examined to predict the onset of BKVAN and the relationship to graft failure, which includes urine analysis by PCR amplification of BKV-VP1, or the presence of grandzyme B, proteinase inhibitor-9, plasminogen activator inhibitor-1, as well as the urine polyomavirus Haufen Test to determine the presence of urinary cast [49–56]. There is currently no specific universal screening biomarker that is widely used in clinical practice that consistently predicts the early onset of BKVAN and correlates strongly with graft survival. Furthermore, the characteristic changes reported for BKVAN-associated renal pathology may only exist in a fraction of infected patients in varying degrees.

Expanded BKV tropism for glomerular parenchymal cells or GVU cells that includes glomerular podocytes, mesangial cells, and glomerular endothelial cells, has been confirmed by vitro studies in my laboratory [34] (Figure 1). This finding will require further investigation.

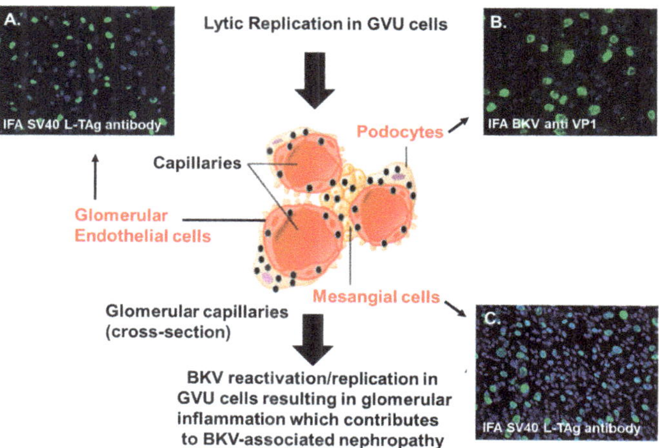

Figure 1. BK polyomavirus (BKV) infection of GVU cells. Immunofluorescent staining of GVU cells infected with BKV. (**A**) Primary human glomerular endothelial cells infected with BKV for 96 h and stained with a monoclonal antibodies against the SV40 Large T antigen (LTAg). (**B**) Human podocytes infected with BKV for 96 h and stained with monoclonal antibodies against the BKV major capsid protein VP1. (**C**) Primary human mesangial cells infected by BKV for 96 h and stained with a monoclonal antibody targeting the SV40 (LTAg). Nuclei were stained blue with 4′,6-diamidino-2-phenylindole (DAPI). All images were obtained using a Nikon TE2000S microscope mounted with a charge-coupled device (CCD) camera at ×200 magnification.

3. BKV Entry and Dissemination in the Glomerulus and the Cell Types Exposed to BKV Trafficking

In a hypothetical model proposed by Popik et al., BKV enters the glomerular parenchyma via the afferent arteriole during the viremic phase of infection, leading to viral dissemination and the initial exposure of glomerular mesangial cells to the virus (Figure 2). The virus then spreads from the mesangial cells to the glomerular podocytes and endothelial cells of glomerular capillaries. BKV may spread first to the parietal cells of the glomerular capsule and then to the proximal tubular cells before appearing in urine. The initial and continual dissemination track of BKV would also be influenced by the turbulence produced by blood flow and renal filtration. Most recently, a report by Popik et al. suggests that the tropism of BKV in the human kidney involves glomerular parenchymal cells, which have been shown to be permissive for BKV in vitro [34]. The potential role of these cells in viral latency, viral reactivation, viral load, viremic conversion, and BKVAN-associated renal pathology is unknown.

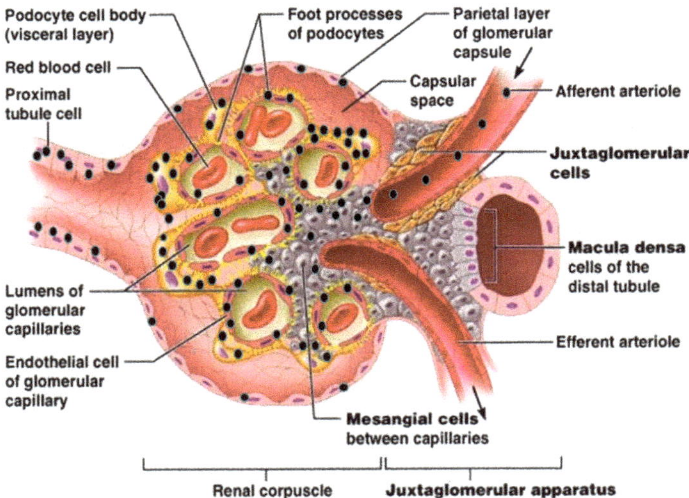

Figure 2. A hypothetical mode for BKV dissemination in the glomerular that includes GVU cells. BKV (black spheres) enters the glomerulus of the renal compartment via the afferent arteriole during the viremic phase of infection. This leads to the initial infection of GVU cells, namely the mesangial cells. Next, the virus spreads from mesangial cells to glomerular podocytes, and then locally to glomerular endothelial cells that are also highly permissive for infection in vitro and reported to be infected by BKV in vivo. The virus then encounters the parietal cells of the glomerular capsule that are reported to be permissive for BKV in vivo. Finally, the virus further disseminates and infects the proximal tubular epithelial cells that are highly permissive for BKV infection in vitro and in vivo. Widespread virus infection and replication in GVU targets cells, along with tubular epithelial cells and parietal glomerular capsular cells, would theoretically contributes to the viruria, viremia, inflammation, and nephropathy. Model of BKV entry and existence in the glomerulus (modified with permission from *Pearson Education Inc.* 2013 (unpublished data)).

4. Cellular Targets that are Permissive for BKV Infection and Lytic Replication

4.1. Tubular Epithelial Cells

A comprehensive examination of cellular targets for BKV infectivity in the proximal and distal glomerular compartments of the human kidney has not been reported. Rather, the focus of BKV infectivity and pathogenesis has been mainly on tubular epithelial cells, and most studies have proposed them as the primary viral reservoir and main driver of pathogenic pathways that lead to fibrosis in BKVAN [57,58]. These reports conclude that renal tubular epithelial cells are the major sites of viral persistence and reactivation in immunosuppressed kidney transplant patients [59]. Tubular epithelial cells are important in vitro and in vivo targets for BKV infection and replication. Findings from several studies support the notion that tubular epithelial cell infection, dysfunction, necrosis, and death are essential prerequisites for renal fibrosis associated with BKVAN. However, studies by de Kort H et al. suggest that rapid lytic replication of BKV occurs in tubular epithelial cells, because these cells are immunologically tolerant to BKV infection rendering them more susceptible to high levels of lytic replication when compared to other glomerular cells that are more immunologically responsive to BKV infection, as demonstrated by a robust induction of interferon beta (IFNβ) and CXCL10 in the latter, post-infection [60].

4.2. Bowman's Capsular Epithelial Cells (BCEC)

By examining renal biopsies from renal transplant patients with BKVAN, Celik and Randhawa detected cytopathic effects of BKV in Bowman's capsular epithelial cells (BCECs) at the parietal layer of Bowman's capsule [61]. The authors observed BKV cytopathology in BCECs in 36/124 biopsies (29%) from 83 patients examined with BKVAN in the allograft kidney, using H&E stained-light microscopy and immunohistochemistry [61]. The authors used in situ hybridization to confirm the presence of BKV DNA in BCECs [61]. Moreover, they also found that BKV cytopathology in BCECs correlated with high viral loads in the tubular epithelium [61]. Interestingly, tubular epithelial cells that are highly permissive for BKV lytic replication share the same embryologic origin as BCECs. Therefore, it is reasonable to speculate that BCECs are also permissive for BKV. However, the role for BCECs in BKV latency and reactivation is currently unknown. Comprehensive in vivo and in vitro studies of BCECs are warranted. The role of BCECs in viral latency and reactivation has not been explored. Results from studies that examine renal biopsies from transplant patients with BKVAN suggest that BKV infection of BCECs is rare. Nonetheless, it would be interesting to determine if BCECs play a similar role to that of tubular epithelial cells in BKVAN, due to their common origin.

4.3. Mesangial Cells

Until recently, there were no reports of BKV infection of mesangial cells. A study published in 2019 by Popik et al., shows that primary human renal mesangial cells are permissive for BKV infection in vitro. Specifically, the authors found that mesangial cells expressed BKV late genes 96 h post-infection, without exhibiting evidence of cytopathology [34]. However, immunofluorescent staining revealed high levels of virus replication in these cells, as demonstrated by nuclear staining of BKV-infected cells with an antibody against the SV40 LTAg, along with high levels of VP1 transcription [34]. The authors also observed significant induction of CXCL10 and IFNβ expression in BKV-infected cells that correlated with increased virus replication over a time course of infection. However, it is currently unclear if mesangial cells play a role in BKVAN progression in vivo. There are currently no reports of BKV-infected mesangial in biopsies from renal allograft patients with BKVAN. In a study by Celik et al., they report immune complex deposition in the mesangium and an increased mesangial cell matrix in renal biopsies from patients with BKVAN. However, the authors did not observe evidence of BKV infection in mesangial cells [61]. Since mesangial cells are immunologically responsive to BKV infection, as evidenced by induction of CXCL10 and IFNβ [34,35], they may be more effective at viral clearance than tubular epithelial cells. In addition, there could be host factors in the glomerular microenvironment induced in mesangial cells after infection that render them less permissive for BKV infection in vivo.

4.4. Glomerular Podocytes

Currently, there is only one report, by Brealey, describing a case study of BKVAN that shows evidence of viral particles in glomerular subepithelial humps. The author used transmission electron microscopy to analyze the glomeruli in a renal biopsy from a 59-year-old female kidney transplant patient who was experiencing symptoms of graft rejection [62]. There was clear clinical evidence from the examination of biopsy tissue to support a diagnosis of immune complex glomerulonephritis. Virus particles were observed in deposits in the cytoplasm of podocytes [62]. The authors confirmed the diagnosis of BKVAN by immunoperoxidase staining using BKV- specific antibodies. The author also observed evidence of cytoplasmic clearance of BKV by podocytes from the glomerular basement membrane [62]. However, this case study did not describe evidence of direct podocyte infection. Most recently, Popik et al., described BKV cytopathology and lytic replication in undifferentiated and differentiated podocytes in vitro, as demonstrated by high expression levels of VP1 total protein and mRNA post infection [34]. The authors also observed induction of CXCL10 and IFNβ transcriptional in BKV-infected podocytes that correlates with increased viral replication over the course of infection [34]. It is unclear if podocyte infection with BKV plays a direct role in BKVAN progression in vivo. Like mesangial cells, podocytes are immune responsive to BKV. Thus they may be able to clear BKV in vivo or avoid significant infection by the recruitment or of host factors that protect the cells against BKV infection, or by subverting those that enhance infection.

4.5. Glomerular Endothelial Cells

Until recently, there was only one case report of BKV-related polyomavirus vasculopathy in a renal transplant patient [63]. In this study, Petrogiannis-Haliotis et al. describes a 52-year-old male patient who had developed ESRD after undergoing a cadaveric renal transplantation [63]. The patient suffered from BKV vasculopathy resulting from virus infection of vascular endothelial cells [63]. BKV antigen expression was detected in endothelial cells by immunohistochemistry in renal biopsies and BKV DNA was identified in an extract of frozen kidney tissue by polymerase-chain-reaction (PCR) using BKV-specific primers [63]. Ultrastructural analysis by electron microscopy revealed BKV-infected endothelial cells in both the transplanted and native kidneys, but immunoperoxidase staining did not detect any virus in the renal tubules [63]. Recent, in vitro studies by Popik et al., using primary human glomerular endothelial cells (GECs), revealed that GECs are highly permissive for BKV infection and lytic replication, as demonstrated by BKV cytopathology as well as high expression levels of the BKV LTAg and VP1 [34]. They also observed the induction of a IFNβ transcription gene in BKV-infected GECs that correlates with increased viral replication over a time course of infection [34]. The authors also observed varying levels of CXCL10 induction over a time course of infection. In a recent study by An et al., the authors also observed an induction of CXCL10 and IFNβ expression in BKV-infected human GECs, along with the activation of IRF3 and STAT1 [64]. Findings from these studies support the notion that GECs can mount an immune protective response to BKV infection and may act as an immune barrier to BKV infection in vivo. These immune protective factors or receptors that may be suppressed or downregulated in vitro could render GECs more permissive for BKV infection and explain the rare occurrence GECs infection in vivo. Figure 2 shows a hypothetical model of cell types and routes of BKV dissemination in the proximal and distal compartments of the human glomerulus.

5. The Potential Role of Glomerular Parenchymal Cells (GVU cells) in BKV Latency/Reactivation and BKVAN

GVU cells have all been shown to be permissive for BKV infection in vitro. However, in vivo infection of GVU cells is rare in patients with BKVAN, possibly due to differential receptor expression, down regulation of the primary receptor, or induction of an antiviral host factors that promote viral clearance. Immunosuppression and concomitant suppression of T-cell immune surveillance trigger BKV reactivation from latency in renal transplant patients, subsequently leading to high levels of viral replication in the tubular epithelium. As a result, these patients develop BKV-associated nephropathy. The resulting denudation of the basement membrane, followed by robust viremia resulting in uncontrolled inflammation, can lead to nephropathy and fibrosis (Figure 3.) I propose that podocytes and mesangial cells may aid in the early phase recruitment of immune effector cells via the induction CXCL10 (Figure 3). In addition, the induction of IFNβ in these cells may be protective against BKV infection, due to the cytokine's antiviral and anti-proliferative effects [64,65]. Taken together, it is likely that GVU cells serve as potential latent BKV reservoirs that contribute to early events in BKV reactivation. Comprehensive studies that examine temporal events and early stages of BKV infection are needed to identify target cells in renal biopsies prior to development of BKVAN. Examination of renal biopsies to detect both BKV antigen and DNA would provide clues to the role that GVU cells play in BKVAN with respect to viral latency and reactivation.

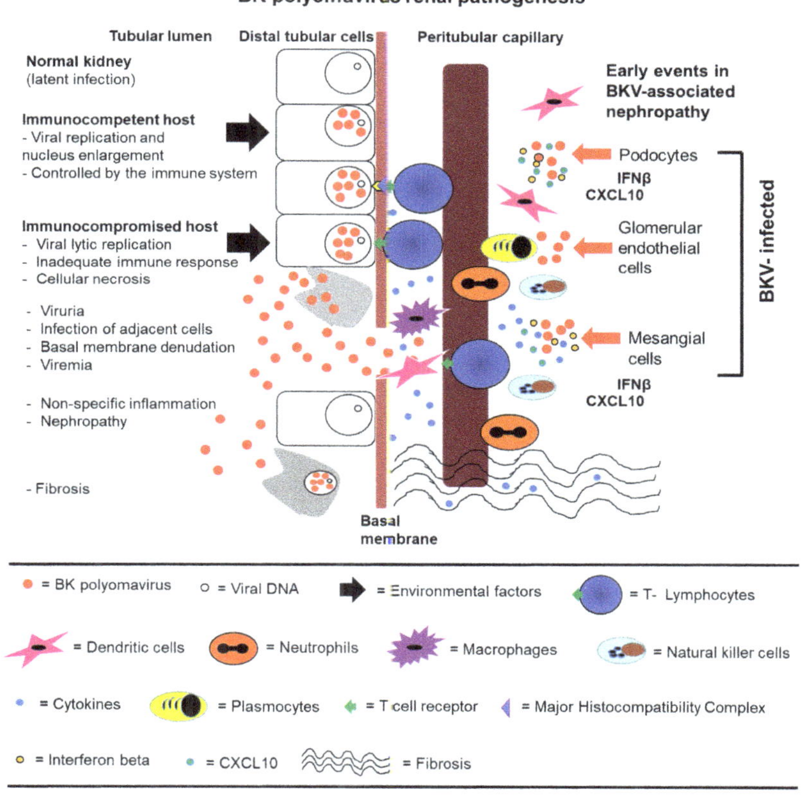

Figure 3. A hypothetical model for BKV pathogenesis that include infection of GVU cells. (**Left**) BKV (red spheres) infection of a normal kidney exists in the latent state in distal tubular epithelial cells. Initial BKV replication is then controlled by the immune system in an immunocompetent host. In the immunocompromised host, viral replication is not controlled, leading to extensive lytic replication and cellular necrosis. Viruria and viremia ensue, and the infection spreads to adjacent cells and the basement membrane is compromised. There is extensive inflammation and recruitment of immune effector cells. Nephropathy occurs followed by interstitial fibrosis. (**Right**) GVU cells are initially infected by BKV which leads to the induction of IFNβ and CXCL10. CXCL10 plays a role in the recruitment of immune effector cells that contribute to inflammation. The induction of IFNβ and IFNβ pathways may protect some GVU cells from BKV infection by establishing an immune barrier and promoting viral clearance. Model of BKV renal pathogenesis (modified with permission from Lamarche et al., BK polyomavirus and the transplanted kidney: Immunopathology and Therapeutic Approaches *Transplantation* 2016).

6. Rare Appearance of BKV in Glomerular Parenchymal Cells in Renal Biopsies of Patients with BKVAN

The role of BKV replication in glomerular parenchymal cells, as well as their contribution to viral latency, reactivation, and renal pathology associated with BKVAN, has been largely unexplored. Tubular epithelial cells may represent a selected cell type for BKV infection, because of their inability to mount an immune response against the virus. They also support high levels of viral replication. In other words, the tubular epithelium provides a functional microenvironment for BKV reactivation and provides an ideal site as a BKV reservoir for infection. GVU cells have all been shown to exhibit IFNβ induction in vitro, which may mount an antiviral response in uninfected cells during early stages of BKV reactivation. Elucidation of specific viral and host factor interactions required for BKV latency is warranted. Findings from these studies may explain why BKV infection is rarely detected in in GVU cells in vivo.

7. Discussion

BKV infection and reactivation following immunosuppression are important causes of renal allograft dysfunction and graft loss. These conditions eventually lead to BKVAN. Understanding the role of both proximal and distal glomerular cells in BKVAN progression will allow investigators to determine the pathogenic mechanisms involved in BKV trafficking and infection profiles, as well as additional viral reservoirs, and conditions required for the establishment of viral latency and reactivation. Future studies may help to advance the development of novel strategies to protect targeted cells in the glomerulus from BKV infection before and after immunosuppression. These studies may also contribute to novel strategies for early diagnosis and subsequent early interventions that aid in the recovery of renal function.

Funding: D.J.A. is supported by the Meharry Zika Startup Grant and the Research Centers in Minority Institutions (RCMI) grant (U54MD007586-01).

Acknowledgments: I thank Waldemar Popik and James E.K. Hildreth for reviewing the manuscript. I also thank the Meharry Office of Scientific Editing and Publications (NIH grant S21MD000104) for scientific editing support.

Conflicts of Interest: The author declares no conflict of interest.

References

1. Pinto, M.; Dobson, S. BK and JC virus: A review. *J. Infect.* **2014**, *68* (Suppl. 1), S2–S8. [CrossRef] [PubMed]
2. Neu, U.; Stehle, T.; Atwood, W.J. The Polyomaviridae: Contributions of virus structure to our understanding of virus receptors and infectious entry. *Virology* **2009**, *384*, 389–399. [CrossRef] [PubMed]
3. Shah, K.V. Polyomaviruses. In *Fields BN, Knipe*, 2nd ed.; Fields Virology; Knipe, D.M., Ed.; Lippincott-Raven: Philadelphia, PA, USA, 1996; pp. 2027–2043.
4. Assetta, B.; Atwood, W.J. The biology of JC polyomavirus. *Biol. Chem.* **2017**, *398*, 839–855. [CrossRef]
5. Padgett, B.L.; Walker, D.L.; ZuRhein, G.M.; Eckroade, R.J.; Dessel, B.H. Cultivation of papova-like virus from human brain with progressive multifocal leucoencephalopathy. *Lancet* **1971**, *297*, 1257–1260. [CrossRef]
6. Butel, J.S.; Lednicky, J.A. Cell and molecular biology of simian virus 40: Implications for human infections and disease. *J. Natl. Cancer. Inst.* **1999**, *91*, 119–134. [CrossRef] [PubMed]
7. Gardner, S.D.; Field, A.M.; Coleman, D.V.; Hulme, B. New human papovavirus (B.K.) isolated from urine after renal transplantation. *Lancet* **1971**, *279*, 1253–1257. [CrossRef]
8. Moens, U.; Calvignac-Spencer, S.; Lauber, C.; Ramqvist, T.; Feltkamp, M.C.W.; Daugherty, M.D.; Verschoor, E.J.; Ehlers, B. Ictv Report Consortium. ICTV Virus Taxonomy Profile: Polyomaviridae. *J. Gen. Virol.* **2017**, *98*, 1159–1160. [PubMed]
9. Cubitt, C.L. Molecular genetics of the BK virus. *Adv. Exp. Med. Biol.* **2006**, *577*, 85–95.
10. Purighalla, R.; Shapiro, R.; McCauley, J.; Randhawa, P. BK virus infection in a kidney allograft diagnosed by needle biopsy. *Am. Kidney Dis.* **1995**, *26*, 671–673. [CrossRef]
11. Hirsch, H.H. Polyomavirus BK nephropathy: A (re-)emerging complication in renal transplantation. *Am. J. Transplant.* **2002**, *2*, 25–30. [CrossRef]

12. Binet, I.; Nickeleit, V.; Hirsch, H.H.; Prince, O.; Dalquen, P.; Gudat, F.; Mihatsch, M.J.; Thiel, G. Polyomavirus disease under new immunosuppressive drugs: A cause of renal graft dysfunction and graft loss. *Transplantation* **1999**, *67*, 918–922. [CrossRef] [PubMed]

13. Mengel, M.; Marwedel, M.; Radermacher, J.; Eden, G.; Schwarz, A.; Haller, H.; Kreipe, H. Incidence of polyomavirus-nephropathy in renal allografts: Influence of modern immunosuppressive drugs. *Nephrol. Dial. Transplant.* **2003**, *18*, 1190–1196. [CrossRef] [PubMed]

14. Brennan, D.C.; Agha, I.; Bohl, D.L.; Schnitzler, M.A.; Hardinger, K.L.; Lockwood, M.; Torrence, S.; Schuessler, R.; Roby, T.; Gaudreault-Keener, M.; et al. Incidence of BK with tacrolimus versus cyclosporine and impact of preemptive immunosuppression reduction. *Am. J. Transplant.* **2005**, *5*, 582–594. [CrossRef] [PubMed]

15. Hirsch, H.H.; Vincenti, F.; Friman, S.; Tuncer, M.; Citterio, F.; Wiecek, A.; Scheuermann, E.H.; Klinger, M.; Russ, G.; Pescovitz, M.D.; et al. Polyomavirus BK replication in de novo kidney transplant patients receiving tacrolimus or cyclosporine: A prospective, randomized, multicenter study. *Am. J. Transplant.* **2013**, *13*, 136–145. [CrossRef] [PubMed]

16. Rahamimov, R.; Lustig, S.; Tovar, A.; Yussim, A.; Bar-Nathan, N.; Shaharabani, E.; Boner, J.; Shapira, Z.; Mor, E. BK polyoma virus nephropathy in kidney transplant recipient: The role of new immunosuppressive agents. *Transplant. Proc.* **2003**, *35*, 604–605. [CrossRef]

17. Knowles, W.A.; Pipkin, P.; Andrews, N.; Vyse, A.; Minor, P.; Brown, D.W.; Miller, E. Population-based study of antibody to the human polyomaviruses BKV and JCV and the simian polyomavirus SV40. *J. Med. Virol.* **2003**, *71*, 115–123. [CrossRef] [PubMed]

18. Egli, A.; Infanti, L.; Dumoulin, A.; Buser, A.; Samaridis, J.; Stebler, C.; Gosert, R.; Hirsch, H.H. Prevalence of polyomavirus BK and JC infection and replication in 400 healthy blood donors. *J. Infect. Dis.* **2009**, *199*, 837–846. [CrossRef] [PubMed]

19. Hirsch, H.H.; Snydman, D.R. BK virus: Opportunity makes a pathogen. *Clin. Infect. Dis.* **2005**, *41*, 354–360. [CrossRef] [PubMed]

20. Siguier, M.; Sellier, P.; Bergmann, J.F. BK-virus infections: A literature review. *Med. Mal. Infect.* **2012**, *42*, 181–187. [CrossRef] [PubMed]

21. Vago, L.; Cinque, P.; Sala, E.; Nebuloni, M.; Caldarelli, R.; Racca, S.; Ferrante, P.; Trabattoni, G.R.; Costanzi, G. JCV-DNA and BKV-DNA in the CNS tissue and CSF of AIDS patients and normal subjects. Study of 41 cases and review of the literature. *J. Acquir. Immune Defic. Syndr. Hum. Retrovirol.* **1996**, *12*, 139–146. [CrossRef]

22. Lesprit, P.; Chaline-Lehmann, D.; Authier, F.-J.; Ponnelle, T.; Gray, F.; Levy, Y. BK virus encephalitis in a patient with AIDS and lymphoma. *AIDS* **2001**, *15*, 1196–1199. [CrossRef] [PubMed]

23. Behzad-Behbahani, A.; Klapper, P.E.; Vallely, P.J.; Cleator, G.M.; Khoo, S.H. Detection of BK virus and JC virus DNA in urine samples from immunocompromised (HIV-infected) and immunocompetent (HIV-non-infected) patients using polymerase chain reaction and microplate hybridization. *J. Clin. Virol.* **2004**, *29*, 224–229. [CrossRef]

24. Smith, R.D.; Galla, J.H.; Skahan, K.; Anderson, P.; Linnemann, C.C., Jr.; Ault, G.S.; Ryschkewitsch, C.F.; Stoner, G.L. Tubulointerstitial nephritis due to a mutant polyomavirus BK virus strain, BKV(Cin), causing end-stage renal disease. *J. Clin. Microbiol.* **1998**, *36*, 1660–1665. [PubMed]

25. Barouch, D.H.; Faquin, W.C.; Chen, Y.; Koralnik, I.J.; Robbins, G.K.; Davis, B.T. BK virus-associated hemorrhagic cystitis in a human immunodeficiency virus-infected patient. *Clin. Infect. Dis.* **2002**, *35*, 326–329. [CrossRef] [PubMed]

26. Gluck, T.A.; Knowles, W.A.; Johnson, M.A.; Brook, M.G.; Pillay, D. BK virus-associated haemorrhagic cystitis in an HIV infected man. *AIDS* **1994**, *8*, 391–392. [CrossRef] [PubMed]

27. Dall, A.; Hariharan, S. BK virus nephritis after renal transplantation. *Clin. J. Am. Soc. Nephrol.* **2008**, *3* (Suppl. 2), S68–S75. [CrossRef] [PubMed]

28. Dalianis, T.; Hirsch, H.H. Human polyomaviruses in disease and cancer. *Virology* **2013**, *437*, 63–72. [CrossRef]

29. Burrows, N.R.; Li, Y.; Williams, D.E. Racial and ethnic differences in trends of end-stage renal disease: United States, 1995 to 2005. *Adv. Chronic Kidney Dis.* **2008**, *15*, 147–152. [CrossRef]

30. Palmer Alves, T.; Lewis, J. Racial differences in chronic kidney disease (CKD) and end-stage renal disease (ESRD) in the United States: A social and economic dilemma. *Clin. Nephrol.* **2010**, *74* (Suppl. 1), S72–S77.

31. Regunathan-Shenk, R.; Hussain, F.N.; Ganda, A. Chronic kidney disease and end-stage renal disease in disadvantaged communities of North America: An investigational challenge to limit disease progression and cardiovascular risk. *Clin. Nephrol.* **2016**, *86* (Suppl. 13), 37–40. [CrossRef]
32. Albertus, P.; Morgenstern, H.; Robinson, B.; Saran, R. Risk of ESRD in the United States. *Am. J. Kidney Dis.* **2016**, *68*, 862–872. [CrossRef]
33. Trofe, J.; Hirsch, H.H.; Ramos, E. Polyomavirus-associated nephropathy: Update of clinical management in kidney transplant patients. *Transpl. Infect. Dis.* **2006**, *8*, 76–85. [CrossRef] [PubMed]
34. Popik, W.; Khatua, A.K.; Fabre, N.F.; Hildreth, J.E.K.; Alcendor, D.J. BK Virus Replication in the Glomerular Vascular Unit: Implications for BK Virus Associated Nephropathy. *Viruses* **2019**, *11*, 583. [CrossRef] [PubMed]
35. Scadden, J.R.; Sharif, A.; Skordilis, K.; Borrows, R. Polyoma virus nephropathy in kidney transplantation. *World J. Transplant.* **2017**, *7*, 329–338. [CrossRef]
36. Kariminik, A.; Dabiri, S.; Yaghobi, R. Polyomavirus BK induces inflammation via up-regulation of CXCL10 at translation levels in renal transplant patients with nephropathy. *Inflammation* **2016**, *39*, 1514–1519. [CrossRef] [PubMed]
37. Andrews, C.A.; Shah, K.V.; Daniel, R.W.; Hirsch, M.S.; Rubin, R.H. A serological investigation of BK virus and JC virus infections in recipients of renal allografts. *J. Infect. Dis.* **1988**, *158*, 176–181. [CrossRef] [PubMed]
38. Hirsch, H.H.; Brennan, D.C.; Drachenberg, C.B.; Ginevri, F.; Gordon, J.; Limaye, A.P.; Mihatsch, M.J.; Nickeleit, V.; Ramos, E.; Randhawa, P.; et al. Polyomavirus associated nephropathy in renal transplantation: Interdisciplinary analyses and recommendations. *Transplantation* **2005**, *79*, 1277–1286. [CrossRef]
39. Hirsch, H.H.; Knowles, W.; Dickenmann, M.; Passweg, J.; Klimkait, T.; Mihatsch, M.J.; Steiger, J. Prospective study of polyomavirus type BK replication and nephropathy in renal-transplant recipients. *N. Engl. J. Med.* **2002**, *347*, 488–496. [CrossRef]
40. Randhawa, P.; Ho, A.; Shapiro, R.; Finkelstein, S.; Uhrmacher, J.; Weck, K. Correlates of quantitative measurement of BK polyomavirus (BKV) DNA with clinical course of BKV infection in renal transplant patients. *J. Clin. Microbiol.* **2004**, *42*, 1176–1180. [CrossRef]
41. Lee, H.M.; Jang, I.; Lee, D.; Kang, E.J.; Choi, B.S.; Park, C.W.; Choi, Y.J.; Yang, C.W.; Kim, Y.; Chung, B. Risk factors in the progression of BK virus-associated nephropathy in renal transplant recipients. *Korean J. Intern. Med.* **2015**, *30*, 865–872. [CrossRef]
42. Demey, B.; Tinez, C.; François, C.; Helle, F.; Choukroun, G.; Duverlie, G.; Castelain, S.; Brochot, E. Risk factors for BK virus viremia and nephropathy after kidney transplantation: A systematic review. *J. Clin. Virol.* **2018**, *109*, 6–12. [CrossRef]
43. Hashim, F.; Shehzad, R.; Gregg, J.A.; Dharnidharka, V.R. Ureteral Stent Placement Increases the Risk for Developing BK Viremia after Kidney Transplantation. *J. Transplant.* **2014**, *2014*, 459747. [CrossRef]
44. Randhawa, P.S.; Shapiro, R. Diagnosis and treatment of BK virus-associated transplant nephropathy. *Adv. Exp. Med. Biol.* **2006**, *577*, 213–227.
45. Adam, B.; Randhawa, P.; Chan, S.; Zeng, G.; Regele, H.; Kushner, Y.B.; Colvin, R.; Reeve, J.; Mengel, M. Banff Initiative for Quality Assurance in Transplantation (BIFQUIT): Reproducibility of polyomavirus immunohistochemistry in kidney allografts. *Am. J. Transplant.* **2014**, *9*, 2137–2147. [CrossRef]
46. Racusen, L.C.; Solez, K.; Colvin, R.B.; Bonsib, S.M.; Castro, M.C.; Cavallo, T.; Croker, B.P.; Demetris, A.J.; Drachenberg, C.B.; Fogo, A.B.; et al. The Banff 97 working classification of renal allograft pathology. *Kidney Int.* **1999**, *55*, 713–723. [CrossRef]
47. Bates, W.D.; Davies, D.R.; Welsh, K.; Gray, D.W.; Fuggle, S.V.; Morris, P.J. An evaluation of the Banff classification of early renal allograft biopsies and correlation with outcome. *Nephrol. Dial. Transplant.* **1999**, *14*, 2364–2369. [CrossRef]
48. Haas, M.; Kraus, E.S.; Samaniego-Picota, M.; Racusen, L.C.; Ni, W.; Eustace, J.A. Acute renal allograft rejection with intimal arteritis: Histologic predictors of response to therapy and graft survival. *Kidney Int.* **2002**, *61*, 1516–1526. [CrossRef]
49. Nickeleit, V.; Harsharan, K. Singh Polyomaviruses and disease: Is there more to know than viremia and viruria? *Curr. Opin. Organ Transplant.* **2015**, *20*, 348–358. [CrossRef]
50. Ding, R.; Medeiros, M.; Dadhania, D.; Muthukumar, T.; Kracker, D.; Kong, J.M.; Epstein, S.R.; Sharma, V.K.; Seshan, S.V.; Li, B.; et al. Noninvasive diagnosis of BK virus nephritis by measurement of messenger RNA for BK virus VP1 in urine. *Transplantation* **2002**, *74*, 987–994. [CrossRef]

51. Hirsch, H.H.; Babel, N.; Comoli, P.; Friman, V.; Ginevri, F.; Jardine, A.; Lautenschlager, I.; Legendre, C.; Midtvedt, K.; Muñoz, P.; et al. ESCMID Study Group of Infection in Compromised Hosts. European perspective on human polyomavirus infection, replication and disease in solid organ transplantation. *Clin. Microbiol. Infect.* **2014**, *20* (Suppl. 7), 74–88. [CrossRef]

52. Ambalathingal, G.R.; Francis, R.S.; Smyth, M.J.; Smith, C.; Khanna, R. BK Polyomavirus: Clinical Aspects, Immune Regulation, and Emerging Therapies. *Clin. Microbiol. Rev.* **2017**, *30*, 503–528. [CrossRef]

53. Heng, B.; Li, Y.; Shi, L.; Du, X.; Lai, C.; Cheng, L.; Su, Z. A Meta-analysis of the Significance of Granzyme B and Perforin in Noninvasive Diagnosis of Acute Rejection After Kidney Transplantation. *Transplantation* **2015**, *99*, 1477–1486. [CrossRef]

54. Rowshani, A.T.; Florquin, S.; Bemelman, F.; Kummer, J.A.; Hack, C.E.; Ten Berge, I.J. Hyperexpression of the granzyme B inhibitor PI-9 in human renal allografts: A potential mechanism for stable renal function in patients with subclinical rejection. *Kidney Int.* **2004**, *66*, 1417–1422. [CrossRef]

55. Katayama, S.; Nunomiya, S.; Koyama, K.; Wada, M.; Koinuma, T.; Goto, Y.; Tonai, K.; Shima, J. Markers of acute kidney injury in patients with sepsis: The role of soluble thrombomodulin. *Crit. Care* **2017**, *21*, 229. [CrossRef]

56. Singh, H.K.; Andreoni, K.A.; Madden, V.; True, K.; Detwiler, R.; Weck, K.; Nickeleit, V. Presence of urinary Haufen accurately predicts polyomavirus nephropathy. *J. Am. Soc. Nephrol.* **2009**, *20*, 416–427. [CrossRef]

57. Moriyama, T.; Sorokin, A. Intracellular trafficking pathway of BK virus in human renal proximal tubular epithelial cells. *Virology* **2008**, *371*, 336–349. [CrossRef]

58. Moriyama, T.; Marquez, J.; Wakatsuki, T.; Sorokin, A. Caveolar endocytosis is critical for BK virus infection of human renal proximal tubular epithelial cells. *J. Virol.* **2007**, *81*, 8552–8562. [CrossRef]

59. Mbianda, C.; El-Meanawy, A.; Sorokin, A. Mechanisms of BK virus infection of renal cells and therapeutic implications. *J. Clin. Virol.* **2015**, *71*, 59–62. [CrossRef]

60. De Kort, H.; Heutinck, K.M.; Ruben, J.M.; Silva, A.E.V.; Wolthers, K.C.; Hamann, J.; Ten Berge, I.J.M. Primary Human Renal-Derived Tubular Epithelial Cells Fail to Recognize and Suppress BK Virus Infection. *Transplantation* **2017**, *101*, 1820–1829. [CrossRef]

61. Celik, B.; Randhawa, P.S. Glomerular changes in BK virus nephropathy. *Hum Pathol.* **2004**, *35*, 367–370. [CrossRef]

62. Brealey, J.K. Ultrastructural observations in a case of BK virus nephropathy with viruses in glomerular subepithelial humps. *Ultrastruct. Pathol.* **2007**, *31*, 1–7. [CrossRef]

63. Petrogiannis-Haliotis, T.; Sakoulas, G.; Kirby, J.; Koralnik, I.J.; Dvorak, A.M.; Monahan-Earley, R.; De Girolami, P.C.; De Girolami, U.; Upton, M.; Major, E.O.; et al. BK-related polyomavirus vasculopathy in a renal-transplant recipient. *N. Engl. J. Med.* **2001**, *345*, 1250–1255. [CrossRef]

64. An, P.; Sáenz Robles, M.T.; Duray, A.M.; Cantalupo, P.G.; Pipas, J.M. Human polyomavirus BKV infection of endothelial cells results in interferon pathway induction and persistence. *PLoS Pathog.* **2019**, *15*, e1007505. [CrossRef]

65. Assetta, B.; De Cecco, M.; O'Hara, B.; Atwood, W.J. JC Polyomavirus Infection of Primary Human Renal Epithelial Cells Is Controlled by a Type I IFN-Induced Response. *MBio* **2016**, *7*, e00903–e00916. [CrossRef]

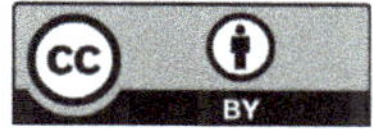

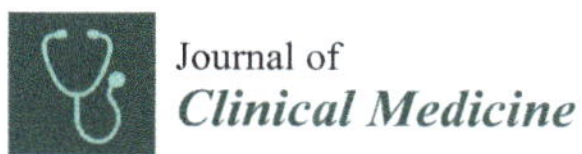

Journal of
Clinical Medicine

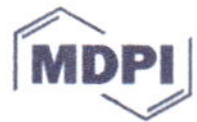

Article

Fast Tac Metabolizers at Risk—It is Time for a C/D Ratio Calculation

Katharina Schütte-Nütgen [1,†], Gerold Thölking [1,†], Julia Steinke [1], Hermann Pavenstädt [1], René Schmidt [2], Barbara Suwelack [1] and Stefan Reuter [1,*]

[1] Department of Medicine D, Division of General Internal Medicine, Nephrology and Rheumatology, University Hospital of Münster, 48149 Münster Germany; katharina.schuette-nuetgen@gmx.de (K.S.-N.); gerold.thoelking@ukmuenster.de (G.T.); j_steinke@ymail.com (J.S.); hermann.pavenstaedt@ukmuenster.de (H.P.); barbara.suwelack@ukmuenster.de (B.S.)

[2] Institute of Biostatistics and Clinical Research, University Hospital of Münster, 48149 Münster, Germany; rene.schmidt@ukmuenster.de

* Correspondence: Stefan.Reuter@ukmuenster.de; Tel.: +49-251-83-50607; Fax: +49-251-83-56973

† These authors contributed equally to this work.

Received: 31 March 2019; Accepted: 26 April 2019; Published: 28 April 2019

Abstract: Tacrolimus (Tac) is a part of the standard immunosuppressive regimen after renal transplantation (RTx). However, its metabolism rate is highly variable. A fast Tac metabolism rate, defined by the Tac blood trough concentration (C) divided by the daily dose (D), is associated with inferior renal function after RTx. Therefore, we hypothesize that the Tac metabolism rate impacts patient and graft survival after RTx. We analyzed all patients who received a RTx between January 2007 and December 2012 and were initially treated with an immunosuppressive regimen containing Tac (Prograf®), mycophenolate mofetil, prednisolone and induction therapy. Patients with a Tac C/D ratio <1.05 ng/mL × 1/mg at three months after RTx were characterized as fast metabolizers and those with a C/D ratio ≥1.05 ng/mL × 1/mg as slow metabolizers. Five-year patient and overall graft survival were noticeably reduced in fast metabolizers. Further, fast metabolizers showed a faster decline of eGFR (estimated glomerular filtration rate) within five years after RTx and a higher rejection rate compared to slow metabolizers. Calculation of the Tac C/D ratio three months after RTx may assist physicians in their daily clinical routine to identify Tac-treated patients at risk for the development of inferior graft function, acute rejections, or even higher mortality.

Keywords: kidney transplantation; tacrolimus; C/D-ratio; pharmacokinetics

---

1. Introduction

Tacrolimus (Tac) is recommended by The Kidney Disease: Improving Global Outcomes (KDIGO) guideline as the immunosuppressant of choice after renal transplantation (RTx) [1]. Although it is very effective in terms of preventing organ rejection, its highly inter-individual variable metabolism rate can be a challenging factor for physicians as many factors can impact on Tac metabolism [2]. Different approaches have largely failed to predict the dosing and Tac clearance or could not show the advantages pertaining to safety or outcomes [3–5]. Even though genetic polymorphisms have been shown to significantly influence Tac metabolism, genetic testing strategies did not improve clinical outcomes [6,7], and require effort in terms of cost and the interpretation of results and therefore have not found their way into clinical practice yet. Thus, therapeutic drug monitoring is essential for directing the therapy.

We recently proposed a classification of patients receiving Tac into two major metabolism groups. Our stratification is based on the calculation of the C/D ratio (expressed as the trough level concentration normalized by the dose). A C/D ratio <1.05 ng/mL × 1/mg identifies fast metabolizers, whereas a C/D ratio $\geq$1.05 ng/mL $\times$ 1/mg indicates a slow metabolism [8]. Alternative definitions of the metabolic state category, such as dose requirements [9], clearance rate, or calculation of the D/C ratio, exist [10,11]. Interestingly, fast Tac metabolizers have been found as being more prone to developing BK viremia [12], calcineurin-inhibitor toxicity [8,9], and acute rejections [10,13,14] after RTx. In congruence, kidney function (three to 24 months after RTx and 36 months after liver transplantation, respectively) was lower in fast than in slow metabolizers [8,9,15,16]. Based on these findings, suggesting an influence of fast Tac metabolism on adverse events and inferior renal function after renal transplantation, the aim of this study was to analyze whether Tac metabolism type might even impact on definite outcomes such as patient and graft survival and to identify whether fast Tac metabolism constitutes an independent risk factor that physicians should consider besides already known determinants of kidney transplant patients' long-term outcome. Hypothesizing that Tac metabolism-dependent effects on mortality might become discernable in the long-term, the present study was performed in a patient cohort with a complete five-year follow-up.

2. Methods

2.1. Patients

Prior to analysis, all patient data was anonymized and de-identified. The local ethics committee (Ethik Kommission der Ärztekammer Westfalen-Lippe und der Medizinischen Fakultät der Westfälischen Wilhelms-Universität, No. 2014-381-f-N) approved the study. The methods used in this study were carried out in accordance with the current transplantation guidelines and the Declarations of Istanbul and Helsinki. Written informed consent with regard to recording their clinical data was given by all participants at the time of transplantation.

We retrospectively analyzed all patients who underwent RTx between January 2007 and December 2012 at the University Hospital Münster and were initially treated with an immunosuppressive regimen containing Tac (Prograf®), mycophenolate mofetil, prednisolone, and induction therapy. Oral CMV-prophylaxis with valganciclovir was administered for 100 days for D+/R+, D−/R+ and D+/R− recipients, and none if both the donor and the recipient were negative for CMV. Recipients aged < 18 years, with combined transplants, and for whom the three month C/D ratio could not be adequately calculated (due to Tac-free immunosuppressive regimen, missing data, or simultaneous higher dosage of prednisolone ($\geq$20 mg/day, which is known to induce CYP3A activity)) were excluded. The Tac target trough level was 6–10 ng/mL. Recipient and donor data was collected from the patient files. The following parameters were examined: Patient and donor demographics, recipient body mass index (BMI), recipient history of hypertension or diabetes mellitus, cause of end-stage renal disease (ESRD), number of prior kidney transplants, time on dialysis, donor type of transplantation, degree of human leukocyte antigen (HLA)-mismatching, current panel-reactive antibodies (PRA), cold and warm ischemia time and incidence of new-onset diabetes after transplantation (NODAT) and cytomegalovirus (CMV) DNAaemia (a number of >600 copies/mL was considered as relevant corresponding to the threshold value given by the manufacturer (TaqMan-PCR, QIAamp DNA Blood Kit, Qiagen, Hilden, Germany)). CMV screening was performed monthly during the first six months after RTx, every second month during months 6–12, and on indication.

2.2. Tacrolimus Metabolism Rate

Tac metabolism rates were calculated at three months after RTx by dividing the Tac blood trough concentration (C) by the corresponding daily Tac dose (D), as published before [8,16].

$$\text{C/D ratio (ng/mL} \times \text{1/mg)} = \text{blood Tac trough concentration (ng/mL)/daily Tac dose (mg)} \qquad (1)$$

As inpatient values are more prone to errors due to coexisting factors like diarrhea, anaemia and CYP3A4 interfering drugs as azoles, e.g., only outpatient tacrolimus concentrations were considered.

Measurements with exceptional high Tac trough concentrations (>15 ng/mL) were not considered to exclude false-high values due to Tac ingestion prior blood sampling.

For 50 randomly selected patients we additionally calculated the Tac C/D ratio at one and six months as an average C/D ratio and compared it to the three-month C/D ratio to account for further potential factors that can influence the C/D ratio and might affect single-time point measurements. As the 3-month C/D ratio strongly correlated with the average C/D ratio at month one and six, we applied the 3-month C/D ratio for the following patient categorization:

As defined previously, patients with a Tac C/D ratio <1.05 ng/mL × 1/mg were categorized as fast metabolizers. Patients with a C/D ratio of 1.05–1.54 ng/mL × 1/mg or a C/D ratio ≥1.55 ng/mL × 1/mg were defined as intermediate metabolizers and slow metabolizers, respectively [8]. For simplification, intermediate and slow metabolizers were summarized as slower metabolizers in this study.

2.3. Outcome Measures

The main outcome measures were patient and overall graft survival. Patient survival was defined as time from RTx to death (from any cause) or last contact for alive patients. Overall graft survival was defined as the time from RTx to death (from any cause), graft failure, or last contact, whichever occurred first. Graft failure was defined as the reinitiation of dialysis treatment.

Further outcome parameters were serum creatinine and estimated glomerular filtration rate (eGFR) at years one to five after transplantation as well as the frequency of biopsy-proven acute rejection episodes (defined by Banff classification) and the rejection-free survival. Patients were subjected to kidney biopsy in case of a relevant rise in creatinine (≥0.3 mg/dL). Biopsies were evaluated by two pathologists.

Whole blood was analyzed for creatinine (enzymatic assay; Creatinine-Pap, Roche Diagnostics, Mannheim, Germany) and Tac (automated tacrolimus (TACR) assay; Dimension Clinical Chemistry System; Siemens Healthcare Diagnostic GmbH; Eschborn; Germany). Only 12 h Tac trough levels were used for analysis. Renal function was determined by calculating the eGFR using the CKD-EPI equation.

2.4. Statistical Analysis

Statistical analysis was performed using IBM SPSS® Statistics 25 for Windows (IBM Corporation, Somers, NY, USA). Normally distributed continuous variables are shown as mean ± standard deviation (SD) and non-normally distributed continuous variables as median and 1st and 3rd quartiles (interquartile range, IQR). Absolute and relative frequencies have been given for categorical variables. Pairs of independent groups were compared using the Student's t-test for normally distributed data, Mann–Whitney U test for non-normal data, and Fisher's exact test for categorical variables. To compare paired data, we used the Wilcoxon test for continuous variables and the McNemar test for categorical variables.

Survival analyses were based on a maximum follow-up of five years after RTx. Patient survival, overall allograft survival as well as rejection-free survival were analyzed using the Kaplan-Meier method [17], and the groups were compared using the log-rank test. Cox proportional hazards regression models [18] were built using a stepwise variable selection procedure to assess the association between C/D ratio metabolism status and survival while simultaneously adjusting for potential confounding factors (inclusion: p-value of the score test ≤ 0.05, exclusion: p-value of the likelihood ratio test > 0.1). Results have been presented as hazard ratios (HR) with 95% confidence interval (95% CI) and p-value of likelihood ratio test. The p-value of score test is given for non-selected variables in multivariable analyses.

Mixed models with AR (1) covariance structure were fitted to analyze the impact of biological and clinical markers on the time course of eGFR between year one and five after the transplantation based on the eGFR values observed at annual intervals during this period. Univariable analyses included each marker separately along with its interaction with time since baseline measurement (at year one after transplantation) in order to assess (i) the baseline eGFR and/or (ii) whether potential time trends of eGFR differ between the subgroups defined by the marker. Multivariable models were built using a stepwise variable selection procedure in order to assess the impact of C/D ratio metabolism status on baseline eGFR and time trends of eGFR while adjusting for potential confounding factors. Models included (i) C/D ratio metabolism status and its interaction with time since baseline measurement in a first block and (ii) potential confounding factors along with their interactions with time since baseline measurement in a second block with forwards variable selection (inclusion/exclusion criterion: *p*-value of Wald test ≤0.05/>0.1).

No adjustment for multiple testing was made, and all analyses were regarded as explorative. *p*-values ≤ 0.05 were considered statistically noticeable.

3. Results

3.1. Patient Cohort

The enrollment flow chart for the study population is shown in Figure 1. Between January 2007 and December 2012, 633 kidney transplants were performed at our center. After the exclusion of 50 patients aged <18 years and 25 patients with combined transplantation, data on immunosuppressive therapy was extracted from the remaining 558 adult kidney-only transplant recipients. From these, 401 patients with an initial Tac-based immunosuppressive therapy and complete data on the 3-month C/D ratio were included. From all patients, 253 recipients (63.1%) were categorized as slow metabolizers and 148 recipients (36.9%) as fast metabolizers. The average C/D ratio of month one and six for 50 randomly selected patients did not differ from the three-month C/D ratio (*p* = 0.765, Table S1) and categorization of slow and fast Tac metabolizers was similar when applying the three-month C/D ratio or the average C/D ratio of months one and six (*p* = 1.000, Table S2), suggesting that three-month C/D ratio strongly correlated with the average C/D ratio during months one and six.

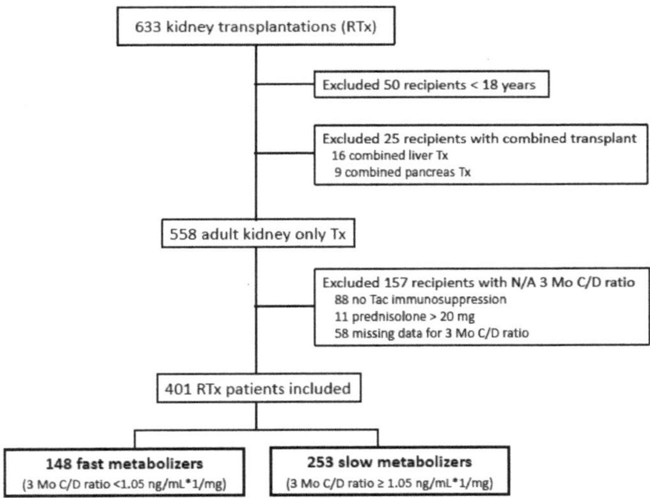

Figure 1. Enrollment flow chart for the study population. RTx = Renal transplantation; N/A: not available.

Baseline patient characteristics for donors and recipients and transplantation-associated parameters are shown in Table 1. Tac mean trough levels and daily doses were noticeably different between the groups. The two groups were similar with respect to all other baseline characteristics that were analyzed.

Table 1. Baseline patient characteristics.

	Slow Metabolizers ($n = 253$)	Fast Metabolizers ($n = 148$)	p-Value
Tac mean trough level at 3 months (ng/mL)	8.6 ± 2.8	7.1 ± 2.7	<0.001 [a]
Tac daily dose at 3 months (mg/day)	4.9 ± 2.3	10.3 ± 4.3	<0.001 [a]
Age (years, mean ± SD)	53.0 ± 13.4	50.2 ± 13.8	0.051 [a]
Male sex, n (%)	156 (61.7)	80 (54.1)	0.142 [c]
BMI (kg/m^2, mean ± SD)	25.2 ± 4.0	25.2 ± 4.1	0.944 [a]
Pre-existing recipient hypertension, n (%)	239 (94.5)	139 (94.6)	1.000 [c]
Pre-existing recipient diabetes, n (%)	33 (13.0)	16 (10.9)	0.636 [c]
Diagnosis of ESRD, n (%)			
Hypertension	20 (7.9)	11 (7.4)	
Diabetes	11 (4.3)	1 (0.7)	
Polycystic kidney disease	36 (14.2)	26 (17.6)	
Obstructive Nephropathy	20 (7.9)	14 (9.5)	0.411 [c]
Glomerulonephritis	103 (40.7)	53 (35.8)	
FSGS	6 (2.4)	5 (3.4)	
Interstitial nephritis	4 (1.6)	2 (1.4)	
Vasculitis	5 (2.0)	2 (1.4)	
Other	45 (17.8)	34 (23.0)	
Time on dialysis (months, median (IQR))	60.5 (25.5, 90.3)	52.5 (24.9, 87.1)	0.323 [b]
≥ 1 prior kidney transplant, n (%)	39 (15.4)	19 (12.8)	0.557 [c]
Living donor transplantation	58 (22.9)	44 (29.7)	0.4 [c]
Number HLA mismatch, n (%)			
0–3	169 (67.1)	98 (66.7)	1.000 [c]
4–6	83 (32.9)	49 (33.3)	
Current PRA, n (%)			
0–20%	248 (98.0)	145 (98.0)	1.000 [c]
> 20%	5 (2.0)	3 (2.0)	
Induction, n (%)			
Basiliximab	233 (92.1)	130 (87.8)	0.163 [c]
Thymoglobulin	20 (7.9)	18 (12.2)	
Cold ischaemia time (hours, mean ± SD)	8.7 ± 4.9	8.2 ± 5.4	0.419 [a]
Warm ischaemia time (min, mean ± SD)	31.8 ± 6.9	32.2 ± 8.0	0.684 [a]
Donor age (years, mean ± SD)	53.4 ± 16.6	54.7 (13.7)	0.394 [a]
Donor male sex, n (%)	121 (47.8)	63 (42.6)	0.350 [c]

Demographic characteristics of the study population by the Tac metabolization status. Results are presented as mean ± standard deviation (SD) or median and first and third quartile (IQR), respectively, or as absolute and relative frequencies. BMI = body mass index; ESRD = end-stage renal disease; FSGS = focal segmental glomerulosclerosis; HLA = human leukocyte antigen; PRA = panel reactive antibodies. [a] Student's *t*-test, [b] Mann-Whitney U test, [c] Fisher's exact test.

3.2. Patient and Overall Allograft Survival

Kaplan-Meier curves for patient and overall allograft survival by Tac metabolism status are shown in Figure 2. Five-year patient survival was noticeably reduced in fast metabolizers as compared to slow metabolizers (89.9% vs. 95.3%, log-rank $p = 0.036$, Figure 2). The Cox regression analysis revealed a noticeable association between a fast Tac metabolism and patient survival in both univariable (HR 2.209 (95% CI 1.034–4.719), $p = 0.041$) as well as multivariable analysis (HR 5.749 (95% CI 1.556–21.242), $p = 0.004$) (Table 2). Overall allograft survival was affected by the Tac metabolism status as well: Fast metabolizers showed a noticeably reduced 5-year allograft survival rate as compared to slow metabolizers (83.8% vs. 90.5%, log-rank $p = 0.044$, Figure 2). HR was 1.772 (95% CI 1.006–3.121, $p = 0.047$)) for fast metabolizers in univariable Cox regression and 2.715 (95% CI 1.231–5.989, $p = 0.012$) after adjustment for potential confounders (Table 3).

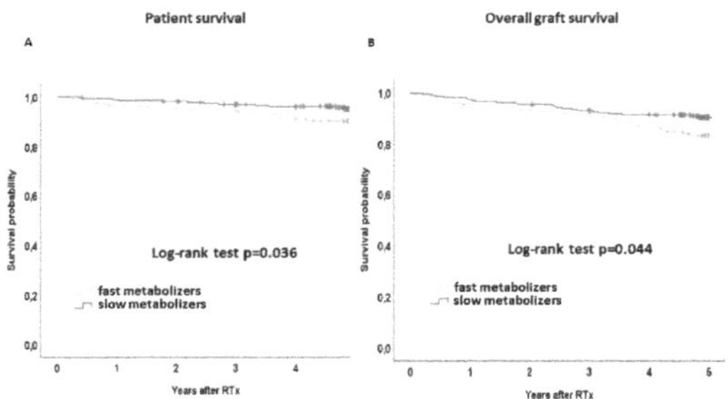

Figure 2. (**A**) Kaplan-Meier curves for patient survival and (**B**) overall graft survival. Survival rates of slow (red lines) and fast metabolizers (blue lines) were analyzed by the Kaplan–Meier method and compared using the log-rank test. Fast metabolizers showed a noticeably reduced patient and overall graft survival.

Table 2. Univariable and multivariable analyses of patient survival using Cox regression.

Parameters	Univariable		Multivariable	
	HR (95% CI)	*p*-Value	HR (95% CI)	*p*-Value
Fast metabolizers vs. slow metabolizers (ref.)	2.209 (1.034–4.719)	0.041	5.749 (1.556–21.242)	0.004
Age (years)	1.057 (1.023–1.093)	0.001	-	0.081
Recipient sex Male vs. female (ref.)	1.631 (0.714–3.727)	0.246	-	0.262
Recipient BMI (kg/m^2)	0.942 (0.852–1.042)	0.248	-	0.213
Pre-existing recipient hypertension yes vs. no (ref.)	1.512 (0.205–11.142)	0.685	-	0.635
Pre-existing recipient diabetes yes vs. no (ref.)	2.206 (0.890–5.468)	0.087	-	0.691
Cause of ESRD	-	0.852	-	0.738
Time on dialysis (months)	1.002 (0.993–1.011)	0.714	-	0.553
Prior kidney transplantation ≥1 vs. 0 (ref.)	1.379 (0.522–3.641)	0.517	-	0.707
Donor type Postmortal vs. living donor (ref.)	2.832 (0.853–9.405)	0.089	-	0.936
Number HLA mismatch 4–6 vs. 0–3	2.335 (1.097–4.968)	0.028	-	0.053
Current PRA >20% vs. 0–20%	1.951 (0.265–14.387)	0.512	-	0.709
Cold ischemia time (hours)	1.042 (0.972–1.118)	0.245	-	0.668
Donor age (years)	1.043 (1.014–1.074)	0.004	-	0.540
Donor sex Male vs. female (ref.)	0.928 (0.434–1.982)	0.847	-	0.266
NODAT yes vs. no (ref.)	2.983 (1.396–6.373)	0.005	5.150 (1.550–17.110)	0.005
CMV DNAaemia yes vs. no (ref.)	0.832 (0.352–1.968)	0.676	-	0.629
Acute rejection within 1 year yes vs. no (ref.)	1.610 (0.680–3.807)	0.279	-	0.947
eGFR at month 3 (mL/min/1.73m^2)	0.979 (0.960–0.998)	0.028	-	0.999
eGFR at month 12 (mL/min/1.73m^2)	0.968 (0.937–1.000)	0.047	-	0.166

Results are presented as hazard ratios (HR) with their 95% confidence interval (CI) and *p*-value of likelihood ratio test. For non-selected variables in multivariable analyses, *p*-value of score test is given. HR = hazard ratio; CI = confidence interval.

Table 3. Univariable and multivariable analyses of overall graft survival using Cox regression.

Parameters	Univariable		*p*-Value	
	HR (95% CI)	*p*-Value	HR (95% CI)	*p*-Value
Fast metabolizers vs. slow metabolizers (ref.)	1.772 (1.006–3.121)	0.047	2.715 (1.231–5.989)	0.012
Age (years)	1.056 (1.030–1.082)	<0.001	-	0.673
Recipient sex Male vs. female (ref.)	0.957 (0.539–1.698)	0.880	-	0.354
Recipient BMI (kg/m^2)	1.018 (0.949–1.092)	0.619	-	0.715
Pre-existing recipient hypertension yes vs. no (ref.)	2.797 (0.386–20.272)	0.309	-	0.401
Pre-existing recipient diabetes yes vs. no (ref.)	2.044 (1.018–4.102)	0.044	-	0.827
Cause of ESRD	-	0.717	-	0.942
Time on dialysis (months)	0.999 (0.992–1.007)	0.833	-	0.376
Prior kidney transplantation ≥1 vs. 0 (ref.)	0.702 (0.278–1.772)	0.454	-	0.331
Donor type Postmortem vs. living donor (ref.)	3.121 (1.236–7.879)	0.016	-	0.774
Number HLA mismatch 4–6 vs. 0–3	1.814 (1.028–3.201)	0.040	-	0.504
Current PRA >20% vs. 0–20%	1.073 (0.148–7.780)	0.944	-	0.709
Cold ischemia time (hours)	1.060 (1.006–1.116)	0.028	-	0.427
Donor age (years)	1.052 (1.029–1.075)	<0.001	-	0.485
Donor sex Male vs. female (ref.)	0.567 (0.311–1.034)	0.064	-	0.140
NODAT yes vs. no (ref.)	3.163 (1.787–5.596)	<0.001	3.203 (1.451–7.072)	0.003
CMV DNAaemia yes vs. no (ref.)	1.331 (0.737–2.404)	0.344	-	0.443
Acute rejection within one year yes vs. no (ref.)	1.909 (1.024–3.558)	0.042	-	0.943
eGFR at month 3 (mL/min/1.73m^2)	0.958 (0.941–0.976)	<0.001	-	0.851
eGFR at month 12 (mL/min/1.73m^2)	0.941 (0.916–0.967)	<0.001	0.943 (0.915–0.971)	<0.001

Results are presented as hazard ratios (HR) with their 95% confidence interval (CI) and *p*-value of likelihood ratio test. For non-selected variables in multivariable analyses, *p*-value of score test is given. HR = hazard ratio; CI = confidence interval.

Causes of death are given in Table 4. While fast metabolizers mostly died from cardiovascular diseases (40%), the most common cause of death in slow metabolizers were infectious diseases (41.7%). In summary, a fast Tac metabolism noticeably affects patient as well as overall allograft survival after kidney transplantation.

Table 4. Causes of death for slow and fast metabolizers.

	Slow Metabolizers (*n* = 12)	Fast Metabolizers (*n* = 15)
Cardiovascular	4 (33.3)	6 (40)
Infection	5 (41.7)	4 (26.7)
Tumor disease	2 (16.7)	-
Unknown	1 (8.3%)	5 (33.3)

3.3. Renal Function

Renal function was assessed yearly within the first five years after transplantation. Figure 3 shows the development of the eGFR between year one and five after renal transplantation in slow and fast metabolizers. A linear mixed model was applied to estimate the time-dependent course of eGFR. Fast metabolizers showed a noticeably faster decline of the eGFR within five years after transplantation as compared to slow metabolizers in both univariable ($p = 0.040$) and multivariable analysis ($p = 0.032$) (Table 5a,b).

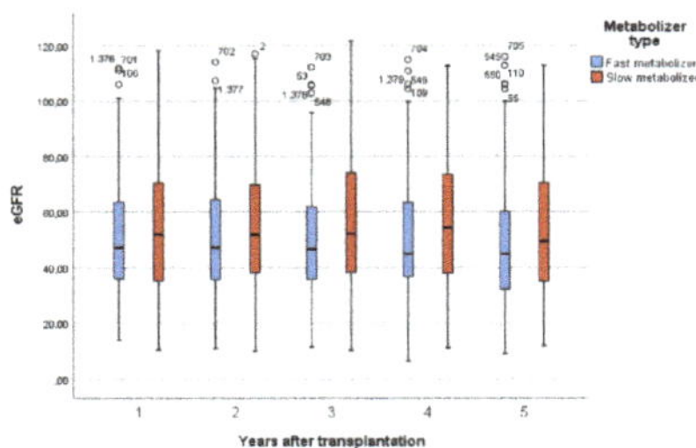

Figure 3. Time course of the eGFR within five years after renal transplantation. Fast metabolizers show a faster decline in the eGFR as compared to slow metabolizers over the first five years.

Table 5. (a) Univariable Analysis: eGFR at month 12 and linear time-trends of eGFR (between months 12 and 60) by subgroup/marker. (b) Multivariable Analysis: eGFR at month 12 and linear time-trends of eGFR (between month 12 and 60) by subgroup/marker.

(a)				
	Variable	**B**	**95% CI**	**p**
Metabolizer type				
	Fast vs. slow (at month 12)	−3.54	−8.57 to 1.49	0.167
	Fast vs slow (time-trends)	−1.07	−2.10 to −0.05	0.040
R_Sex				
	Male vs. female (at month 12)	−16.21	−1.26 to −11.61	<0.001
	Male vs. female (time-trends)	0.49	−0.49 to 1.47	0.325
PreHypertension				
	No vs. yes (at month 12)	0.78	−9.63 to 11.19	0.883
	No vs. yes (time-trends)	1.26	−0.79 to 0.20	0.240
PreDiabetes				
	No vs. yes (at month 12)	4.52	−3.04 to 12.08	0.241
	No vs. yes (time-trends)	0.91	−0.68 to 2.51	0.262
Cause of ESRD				
	Cause of ESRD (at month 12)	-	-	0.010 *
	Diabetes vs. Hypertension (at month 12)	3.72	−15.38 to 22.82	0.703
	Polycystic kidney disease vs. Hypertension (at month 12)	8.30	−1.90 to 18.50	0.111
	Obstructive Nephropahty vs. Hypertension (at month 12)	16.20	4.91 to 27.48	0.005
	Glomerulonephritis vs. Hypertension (at month 12)	5.82	−3.12 to 14.76	0.202
	FSGS vs. Hypertension (at month 12)	7.14	−10.58 to 24.85	0.429
	Interstitial nephritis vs. Hypertension (at month 12)	11.40	−8.85 to 31.65	0.269
	Vasculitis vs. Hypertension (at month 12)	2.51	−16.28 to 21.32	0.792
	Other vs. Hypertension (at month 12)	16.81	7.14 to 26.48	0.001
	Cause of ESRD (time-trends)	-	-	0.998 *
PriorTx				
	No vs. yes (at month 12)	−8.67	−15.48 to −1.86	0.013
	No vs. yes (time-trends)	0.25	−1.13 to 1.63	0.719
DonorType				
	Postmortal vs. Living (at month 12)	−11.15	−16.40 to −5.90	<0.001
	Postmortal vs. Living (time-trends)	0.47	−0.60 to 1.55	0.387

Table 5. *Cont.*

(a)

	Variable	B	95% CI	*p*
HLA Mismatch				
	0–3 vs. 4–6 (at month 12)	5.45	0.37 to 10.53	0.035
	0–3 vs. 4–6 (time-trends)	−0.21	−1.25 to 0.83	0.696
CurrentPRA				
	0–20 vs. >20 (at month 12)	−14.81	−32.19 to 2.57	0.095
	0–20 vs. >20 (time-trends)	−0.80	−4.15 to 2.54	0.638
D_Sex				
	Male vs. female (at month 12)	4.31	−0.47 to 9.09	0.077
	Male vs. female (time-trends)	−0.36	−1.32 to 0.62	0.470
NODAT				
	No vs. yes (at month 12)	6.50	1.31 to 11.69	0.014
	No vs. yes (time-trends)	0.52	−0.56 to 1.60	0.342
CMV DNAaemia				
	No vs. yes (at month 12)	4.46	−0.74 to 9.66	0.093
	No vs. yes (time-trends)	−0.26	−1.32 to 0.80	0.629
Acute rejection 1 year post RTx				
	No vs. yes (at month 12)	16.23	10.34 to 22.13	<0.001
	No vs. yes (time-trends)	0.09	−1.18 to 1.35	0.893
R-Age (years)				
	R-Age (at month 12)	−0.47	−0.63 to −0.32	<0.001
	R-Age (time-trends)	−0.004	−0.013 to 0.005	0.415
R-BMI				
	R-BMI (at month 12)	−1.12	−1.67 to −0.57	<0.001
	R-BMI (time-trends)	−0.008	−0.027 to 0.011	0.405
Time on Dialysis (month)				
	Time on Dialysis (at month 12)	−0.05	−0.11 to 0.01	0.112
	Time on Dialysis (time-trends)	−0.012	−0.008 to 0.006	0.743
CIT (hours)				
	CIT (at month 12)	−0.43	−0.86 to 0.004	0.052
	CIT (time-trends)	−0.014	−0.064 to 0.034	0.565
D_Age (years)				
	D-Age (at month 12)	−0.65	−0.78 to −0.52	<0.001
	D-Age (time-trends)	−0.006	−0.015 to 0.002	0.152

(b)

	Variable	Estimate	95% CI	*p*
At month 12				
	Metabolizer type: fast vs. slow	−2.48	−6.47 to 1.51	0.222
	D_Age (years)	−0.60	−0.71 to −0.48	<0.001
	R_Sex: male vs. female	−12.27	−15.75 to −8.79	<0.001
	Donor type: postmortem vs. living	−10.03	−13.94 to −6.12	<0.001
	R_BMI (kg/m^2)	−0.58	−1.03 to −0.14	0.010
	PreHypertension: no vs. yes			N/S: 0.051
	PreDiabetes: no vs. yes			N/S: 0.914
	Cause of ESRD			0.010 *
	• Diabetes vs. Hypertension	10.79	−2.08 to 23.65	0.100
	• Polycystic kidney disease vs. Hypertension	4.72	−2.57 to 12.02	0.204
	• Obstructive Nephropathy vs. Hypertension	11.34	3.11 to 19.56	0.007
	• Glomerulonephritis vs. Hypertension	2.83	−3.53 to 9.19	0.382
	• FSGS vs. Hypertension	5.16	−6.98 to 17.31	0.404
	• Interstitial nephritis vs. Hypertension	2.23	−14.60 to 19.06	0.794
	• Vasculitis vs. Hypertension	−0.31	−13.54 to 12.93	0.964
	• Other vs. Hypertension	11.26	4.30 to 18.22	0.002

Table 5. *Cont.*

(b)			
Variable	**Estimate**	**95% CI**	***p***
PriorTx: no vs yes			N/S: 0.225
HLAMismatch: 0–3 vs. 4–6			N/S: 0.713
CurrentPRA: 0–20 vs. >20			N/S: 0.272
D_Sex: male vs. female			N/S: 0.107
NODAT: no vs. yes			N/S: 0.995
CMV DNAaemia: no vs. yes			N/S: 0.417
Acute rejection 1 year post RTx: no vs. yes	14.00	9.64 to 18.36	<0.001
R_Age (years)			N/S: 0.495
Time Dialysis (months)			N/S: 0.112
CIT (hours)			N/S: 0.771
Time trends			
Metabolizer type: fast vs. slow	−1.07	−2.05 to −0.09	0.032
D_Age (years)			N/S: 0.121
R_Sex: male vs. female			N/S: 0.240
Donor Type: postmortem vs. living			N/S: 0.666
R_BMI (kg/m^2)			N/S: 0.810
PreHypertension: no vs. yes			N/S: 0.366
PreDiabetes: no vs. yes			N/S: 0.354
Cause of ESRD			N/S: 0.997 *
PriorTx: no vs. yes			N/S: 0.635
HLAMismatch: 0–3 vs. 4–6			N/S: 0.299
CurrentPRA: 0–20 vs. >20			N/S: 0.708
D_Sex: male vs. female			N/S: 0.293
NODAT: no vs. yes			N/S: 0.368
CMV DNAaemia: no vs. yes			N/S: 0.519
Acute rejection1 year post RTx: no vs. yes			N/S: 0.913
R_Age (years)			N/S: 0.332
Time Dialysis (months)			N/S: 0.840
CIT (hours)			N/S: 0.400

* *p*-value of F-test (global test).

3.4. Rejections

The Kaplan-Meier curve for rejection-free survival is shown in Figure 4A. The 5-year rejection-free survival was noticeably lower in fast metabolizers as compared to slow metabolizers (69.6% vs. 78.8%, log-rank $p = 0.032$, Figure 4A). The Cox regression analysis revealed a noticeable association between a fast Tac metabolism and rejection-free survival in univariable (HR 1.536 (95% CI 1.034–2.282), $p = 0.035$) as well as multivariable analysis (HR 1.622 (95% CI 1.085–2.424), $p = 0.020$) (Table 6). Table 7 shows the frequency of patients with ≥ 1 acute biopsy-proven rejection during the 5-year follow-up. While 45/148 (30.4%) fast metabolizers experienced at least one acute rejection, only 54/253 (21.3%) slow metabolizers were affected. Of note, the subtype analysis of the first rejection episode within the first five years after transplantation revealed an increased frequency of humoral and mixed rejections in fast metabolizers ($n = 10$, 6.8% vs. $n = 9$, 3.6% and $n = 10$, 6.8% vs. $n = 6$, 2.4%, respectively) (Table 7, Figure 4B), whereas slow metabolizers were mainly affected by borderline rejections.

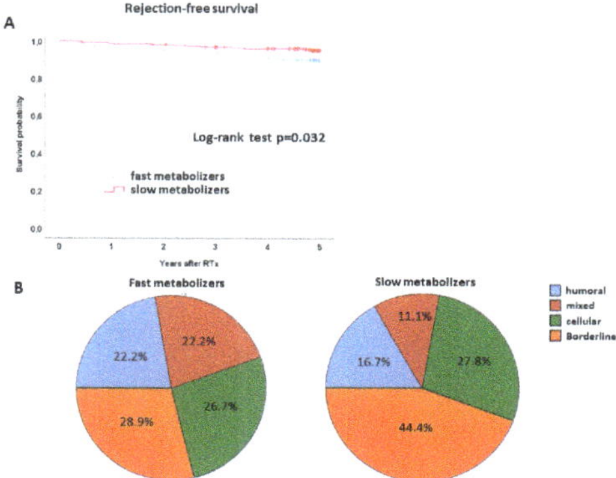

Figure 4. (**A**) Kaplan-Meier curves for rejection-free survival of slow (red lines) and fast metabolizers (blue lines), analyzed by the Kaplan–Meier method and compared using the log-rank test. Fast metabolizers showed a noticeably reduced rejection-free survival. (**B**) Subtype analysis of the first rejection episode within the first five years after transplantation. Fast metabolizers experienced increased frequencies of humoral and mixed acute rejection, whereas slow metabolizers were mainly affected by borderline rejections.

Table 6. Cox regression model for rejection-free survival. Univariable and multivariable analyses of rejection-free survival using Cox regression. Results are presented as hazard ratios (HR) with their 95% confidence interval (CI) and *p*-value of likelihood ratio test. For non-selected variables in multivariable analyses, *p*-value of score test is given.

Parameters	Univariable		Multivariable	
	HR (95% CI)	*p*-Value	HR (95% CI)	*p*-Value
Fast metabolizers vs. slow metabolizers (ref.)	1.536 (1.034–2.282)	0.035	1.622 (1.085–2.424)	0.020
Age (years)	0.996 (0.981–1.010)	0.547	-	0.615
Recipient sex Male vs. female (ref.)	1.432 (0.943–2.176)	0.092	-	0.122
Recipient BMI (kg/m^2)	1.057 (1.007–1.110)	0.026	1.073 (1.021–1.128)	0.006
Pre-existing recipient hypertension yes vs. no (ref.)	1.379 (0.507–3.751)	0.529	-	0.695
Pre-existing recipient diabetes yes vs. no (ref.)	1.032 (0.564–1.887)	0.919	-	0.716
Cause of ESRD	-	0.999	-	0.998
Time on dialysis (months)	1.000 (0.996–1.005)	0.862	-	0.746
Prior kidney transplantation ≥1 vs. 0 (ref.)	1.632 (0.999–2.665)	0.051	1.850 (1.109–3.087)	0.027
Donor type Postmortem vs. living donor (ref.)	0.765 (0.498–1.174)	0.220	-	0.249
Number HLA mismatch 4–6 vs. 0–3	1.043 (0.683–1.593)	0.845	-	0.905
Current PRA >20% vs. 0–20%	1.033 (0.255–4.189)	0.964	-	0.830
Cold ischaemia time (hours)	0.986 (0.948–1.026)	0.489	-	0.620
Donor age (years)	1.002 (0.989–1.014)	0.788	-	0.846
Donor sex Male vs. female (ref.)	0.936 (0.629–1.391)	0.742	-	0.632

HR = hazard ratio; CI = confidence interval.

Table 7. Frequencies of acute rejections and subtype analysis of the first rejection after RTx within five years after transplantation. Fast metabolizers showed increased frequencies of acute biopsy-proven rejections as compared to slow metabolizers. The *p*-value from Fisher's exact test is given.

	Slow Metabolizers ($n = 253$)	Fast Metabolizers ($n = 148$)	*p*-Value
Type of acute rejection			0.084
No rejection	199 (78.7)	103 (69.6)	
Humoral	9 (3.6)	10 (6.8)	
Mixed	6 (2.4)	10 (6.8)	
Cellular	15 (5.9)	12 (8.1)	
Borderline	24 (9.5)	13 (8.8)	

4. Discussion

Herein, we first described a significant influence of the Tac metabolism type on mortality after renal transplantation in a study population with a long-term observation period. A higher five-year mortality in fast metabolizers was accompanied by a higher rejection rate and inferior kidney function. Our study highlights the importance of a risk stratification strategy of RTx patients including information on individuals' Tac metabolism rate which turned out to be an independent risk factor for a lower patient survival after renal transplantation. The C/D ratio is a simple tool that can be easily applied for this purpose.

Based on our previous findings revealing an impact of fast Tac metabolism (C/D ratio < 1.05 ng/mL × 1/mg) on inferior renal function in a two-and three-year follow-up after RTx or LTx [8,16] we herein could demonstrate that this effect persists in the long term and that fast Tac metabolism also impacts on the time-dependent course of renal function in both univariable and multivariable analysis. Moreover, we identified fast Tac metabolism as an independent risk factor for a decreased graft survival.

In congruence, Kuypers et al. observed that patients with high early Tac dose requirements (namely, fast metabolism) had a significantly reduced kidney function at three-months post-RTx [9]. This was attributed to an increased rate of calcineurin inhibitor (CNI)-related toxicity, which is in line with the observations of our previous study [8]. High-dose requirement in Kuyper's study was associated with CYP3A5*1 genotype carriage in only 1/3 of cases, suggesting further factors impacting a patient's Tac metabolism rate [2]. Notably, the area under the curve and the Tac trough level were not different between patients with and without CNI toxicity. The connection between different dose requirements and comparable trough levels in groups–although not calculated–hints at different C/D ratio categories of patients in both groups. Further, Genvigir et al. showed in a Brazilian cohort of CYP3A genotyped RTx patients that expression of CYP3A4/5 alleles leading to fast Tac metabolism (they also calculated the C/D ratio but did not calculate a cut-off) was associated with a lower eGFR at 3-months after RTx [15]. Again, no association was found between Tac exposure and the genetic score. By applying a multiple linear regression analysis, they showed that genetic variants and age impacted the C/D ratio. This is consistent with the literature – metabolism rate usually decreases with age – and with our findings that show tendencies of slow metabolizers being older age [8] (Table 1). Given the limitations of genetic testing-based strategies, we refrained from genotyping our patients but rather searched for a simple and cost-effective tool, as the C/D ratio, that can assist physicians in the daily routine to individualize their patients' immunosuppressive therapy and stratify individuals with high risk for Tac-related side effects independent from complex genotyping-based methods.

In both aforementioned studies, rejection rates were calculated but not related to the C/D ratio or the dose requirements. However, as Kuypers et al. observed significantly higher rates of graft failure (32.3% vs. 13.7%) and lower rates of patients discontinuing steroids (5.8% vs. 23.7%) in patients requiring higher Tac doses, one can assume a higher rejection rate in these patients. We herein firstly describe a significant effect of the C/D ratio on acute rejections in a long-term follow up. In our study, rejection-free survival was increased in slow metabolizers, with higher frequencies of humoral and mixed rejections in fast than in slow metabolizers. In multivariable regression analysis, the BMI and the number of prior transplantations were associated with rejection as well. Recently, Barraclough et al. stated that the outcome of RTx patients depends on the immunosuppression within the first week after transplantation, although a relation between the AUC or Tac trough level and rejection was not detected [19]. Of note, as mentioned before, Tac AUC and trough levels are usually similar in slow and fast metabolizers and the C/D ratio was not calculated in their study. In a meta-analysis including data from the FDCC, Symphony, and OptiCept studies, Boumar et al. reported that the Tac trough concentration was not different between patients with and without acute rejection within the first 6 months after RTx [20]. Again, information regarding the Tac doses or the C/D ratio was not provided. In this regard, Egeland et al. observed that a high Tac clearance (or a fast metabolism) was associated with an increased risk of developing an acute rejection within the first few days after RTx [10]. Patients with a high Tac clearance might not reach the trough levels in time and suffer under-immunosuppression (at least at some time of the day).

Mortality in fast metabolizers over the five-year observation period was consistently higher than in slow metabolizers, despite a tendency towards an older age in slow metabolizers. Overall, graft failure was low in both groups but aligned with the data from the literature [21,22]. In a recently published large registry analysis from England, the main reasons of death within the first year after RTX were stated as infection (21.6%), cardiovascular events (18.3%), and malignancy (7.4%) [21]. The main reasons of death in our cohort were cardiovascular diseases in fast metabolizers and infections in slow metabolizers, respectively, but did not differ between groups. Unfortunately, the reason of death remained unclear in 33.3% of cases in fast and 8.3% cases in slow metabolizers. As previously observed, fast metabolizers are more prone to developing BK virus infection than slow metabolizers. Thus, one can speculate that over-immunosuppression is an issue in these patients [12]. However, other infections, e.g., urinary tract infections, have not been shown to be related to the C/D ratio [23], and deaths due to infection were not different between groups in our cohort. This aligns with the fact that Tac mainly suppresses T-cell activity while the host's defense to bacterial infections, which are more fatal in RTx patients than viral infections, is mainly based on innate immune cells [24]. Interestingly, 20% of death certificates in the English registry study stated "renal" as the cause of death within the first year after RTx [21]. Lastly, we were unable to identify a difference in reasons of death between groups. One reason for this could be the low mortality rate. However, factors that have been previously associated with increased risk of death, such as age at transplantation, diabetes, time on dialysis, or postmortal donation were not different between groups but rather distributed in favor of the fast metabolizer group (Table 1). Patient demographics associated with kidney function after RTx, such as living donation, number of transplants, cold ischemia time, hypertension, diabetes, donor age, and gender, did not differ between groups. This implies that the differences in renal function are likely to be related to Tac metabolism and rejection. Consequently, an inferior renal function is associated with higher mortality as cardiovascular events, infections as well as malignancies are related to kidney function [25].

We recognize that a study of this nature has limitations because of its retrospective design and potential errors inherent to maintaining a single-center database. Moreover, due to the relatively small patient size, inaccuracies in the data collection might affect the results; though data acquisition was performed thoroughly to avoid inconsistency or entry errors. The analyses are based on the assumption that coding errors and missing data are stochastic. Although we attempted to include as many relevant confounding parameters as possible there might still be residual factors that were not accounted for like the non-adherence of patients for example, which is difficult to measure. Prospective studies are needed to confirm our findings. We conclude from our data that the calculation of the C/D ratio, as a simple, cost-effective tool, can assist physicians in their daily clinical routine to identify Tac-treated patients at risk of developing an inferior graft function, acute rejections, or even higher mortality. This information should be used to individualize and optimize immunosuppressive therapy.

Supplementary Materials: The following are available online at http://www.mdpi.com/2077-0383/8/5/587/s1, Table S1: The average C/D ratio of month one and six for 50 randomly selected patients did not differ from the 3-month C/D ratio, suggesting that 3-month C/D ratio strongly correlated with the average C/D ratio during month one and six. P-value of Mann-Whitney U test is given, Table S2: Categorization of slow and fast Tac metabolizers was similar when applying the 3-month C/D ratio or the average C/D ratio of month one and six ($p = 1.000$, Fisher's exact test).

Author Contributions: Conceptualization, G.T., K.S.-N., and S.R.; methodology, G.T., K.S.-N., R.S.; formal analysis, K.S.-N., G.T., J.S. and R.S.; data curation, K.S.-N. and J.S.; writing—original draft preparation, K.S.-N., G.T., R.S., H.P., S.R.; writing—review and editing, H.P., B.S.; supervision, H.P., B.S., S.R.; project administration, H.P., B.S. and S.R.; funding acquisition, K.S.-N.

Funding: This work was fully funded by the Open Access Publication Fund of University of Münster and by the Interdisciplinary Centre for Clinical Research (IZKF), University of Münster (Katharina Schütte-Nütgen).

Conflicts of Interest: SR received travel support from Astellas, Chiesi, and Pfizer and lecture fees from Chiesi.

References

1. KDIGO clinical practice guideline for the care of kidney transplant recipients. *Am. J. Transplant.* **2009**, *9*. [CrossRef]

2. Schutte-Nutgen, K.; Tholking, G.; Suwelack, B.; Reuter, S. Tacrolimus - Pharmacokinetic Considerations for Clinicians. *Curr. Drug. Metab.* **2018**, *19*, 342–350. [CrossRef]

3. Chen, S.-Y.; Li, J.-L.; Meng, F.-H.; Wang, X.-D.; Liu, T.; Li, J.; Liu, L.-S.; Fu, Q.; Huang, M.; Wang, C.-X. Individualization of tacrolimus dosage basing on cytochrome P450 3A5 polymorphism—a prospective, randomized, controlled study. *Clin. Transplant.* **2013**, *27*, E272–E281. [CrossRef]

4. Boughton, O.; Borgulya, G.; Cecconi, M.; Fredericks, S.; Moreton-Clack, M.; MacPhee, I.A.M. A published pharmacogenetic algorithm was poorly predictive of tacrolimus clearance in an independent cohort of renal transplant recipients. *Br. J. Clin. Pharmacol.* **2013**, *76*, 425–431. [CrossRef] [PubMed]

5. Picard, N.; Bergan, S.; Marquet, P.; van Gelder, T.; Wallemacq, P.; Hesselink, D.A.; Haufroid, V. Pharmacogenetic Biomarkers Predictive of the Pharmacokinetics and Pharmacodynamics of Immunosuppressive Drugs. *Ther. Drug Monit.* **2016**, *38* (Suppl. 1), S57–S69. [CrossRef]

6. Mourad, M.; Wallemacq, P.; De Meyer, M.; Brandt, D.; van Kerkhove, V.; Malaise, J.; Chaïb Eddour, D.; Lison, D.; Haufroid, V. The influence of genetic polymorphisms of cytochrome P450 3A5 and ABCB1 on starting dose- and weight-standardized tacrolimus trough concentrations after kidney transplantation in relation to renal function. *Clin. Chem. Lab. Med.* **2006**, *44*, 1192–1198. [CrossRef]

7. Pallet, N.; Etienne, I.; Buchler, M.; Bailly, E.; Hurault de Ligny, B.; Choukroun, G.; Colosio, C.; Thierry, A.; Vigneau, C.; Moulin, B.; et al. Long-Term Clinical Impact of Adaptation of Initial Tacrolimus Dosing to CYP3A5 Genotype. *Am. J. Transplant.* **2016**, *16*, 2670–2675. [CrossRef] [PubMed]

8. Thölking, G.; Fortmann, C.; Koch, R.; Gerth, H.U.; Pabst, D.; Pavenstädt, H.; Kabar, I.; Hüsing, A.; Wolters, H.; Reuter, S.; et al. The tacrolimus metabolism rate influences renal function after kidney transplantation. *PLoS ONE* **2014**, *9*, e111128, eCollection 2014. [CrossRef]

9. Kuypers, D.R.J.; Naesens, M.; de Jonge, H.; Lerut, E.; Verbeke, K.; Vanrenterghem, Y. Tacrolimus dose requirements and CYP3A5 genotype and the development of calcineurin inhibitor-associated nephrotoxicity in renal allograft recipients. *Ther. Drug Monit.* **2010**, *32*, 394–404. [CrossRef] [PubMed]

10. Egeland, E.J.; Robertsen, I.; Hermann, M.; Midtvedt, K.; Størset, E.; Gustavsen, M.T.; Reisæter, A.V.; Klaasen, R.; Bergan, S.; Holdaas, H.; et al. High Tacrolimus Clearance Is a Risk Factor for Acute Rejection in the Early Phase After Renal Transplantation. *Transplantation* **2017**, *101*, e273–e279. [CrossRef]

11. Ohtani, H.; Barter, Z.; Minematsu, T.; Makuuchi, M.; Sawada, Y.; Rostami-Hodjegan, A. Bottom-up modeling and simulation of tacrolimus clearance: prospective investigation of blood cell distribution, sex and CYP3A5 expression as covariates and assessment of study power. *Biopharm. Drug Dispos.* **2011**, *32*, 498–506. [CrossRef] [PubMed]

12. Thölking, G.; Schmidt, C.; Koch, R.; Schuette-Nuetgen, K.; Pabst, D.; Wolters, H.; Kabar, I.; Hüsing, A.; Pavenstädt, H.; Reuter, S.; et al. Influence of tacrolimus metabolism rate on BKV infection after kidney transplantation. *Sci. Rep.* **2016**, *6*, 32273. [CrossRef]

13. Taber, D.J.; Gebregziabher, M.G.; Srinivas, T.R.; Chavin, K.D.; Baliga, P.K.; Egede, L.E. African-American race modifies the influence of tacrolimus concentrations on acute rejection and toxicity in kidney transplant recipients. *Pharmacotherapy* **2015**, *35*, 569–577. [CrossRef] [PubMed]

14. Cheng, Y.; Li, H.; Meng, Y.; Liu, H.; Yang, L.; Xu, T.; Yu, J.; Zhao, N.; Liu, Y. Effect of CYP3A5 polymorphism on the pharmacokinetics of tacrolimus and acute rejection in renal transplant recipients: Experience at a single centre. *Int. J. Clin. Pract. Suppl.* **2015**, *183*, 16–22. [CrossRef] [PubMed]

15. Genvigir, F.D.V.; Salgado, P.C.; Felipe, C.R.; Luo, E.Y.F.; Alves, C.; Cerda, A.; Tedesco-Silva, H.; Medina-Pestana, J.O.; Oliveira, N.; Rodrigues, A.C.; et al. Influence of the CYP3A4/5 genetic score and ABCB1 polymorphisms on tacrolimus exposure and renal function in Brazilian kidney transplant patients. *Pharmacogenet. Genomics* **2016**, *26*, 462–472. [CrossRef]

16. Thölking, G.; Siats, L.; Fortmann, C.; Koch, R.; Hüsing, A.; Cicinnati, V.R.; Gerth, H.U.; Wolters, H.H.; Anthoni, C.; Pavenstädt, H.; et al. Tacrolimus Concentration/Dose Ratio is Associated with Renal Function After Liver Transplantation. *Ann. Transplant.* **2016**, *21*, 167–179. [CrossRef] [PubMed]

17. Kaplan, E.L.; Meier, P. Nonparametric estimation from incomplete observations. *J. Am. Stat. Assoc.* **1958**, *53*, 457–481. [CrossRef]

18. Cox, D.R. Regression Models and Life-Tables. *J. Roy. Statisti. Soc. Ser. B Metho.* **1972**, *34*, 187–220. [CrossRef]

19. Barraclough, K.A.; Staatz, C.E.; Johnson, D.W.; Lee, K.J.; McWhinney, B.C.; Ungerer, J.P.; Hawley, C.M.; Campbell, S.B.; Leary, D.R.; Isbel, N.M. Kidney transplant outcomes are related to tacrolimus, mycophenolic acid and prednisolone exposure in the first week. *Transpl. Int.* **2012**, *25*, 1182–1193. [CrossRef]

20. Bouamar, R.; Shuker, N.; Hesselink, D.A.; Weimar, W.; Ekberg, H.; Kaplan, B.; Bernasconi, C.; van Gelder, T. Tacrolimus predose concentrations do not predict the risk of acute rejection after renal transplantation: A pooled analysis from three randomized-controlled clinical trials(†). *Am. J. Transplant.* **2013**, *13*, 1253–1261. [CrossRef]

21. Farrugia, D.; Cheshire, J.; Begaj, I.; Khosla, S.; Ray, D.; Sharif, A. Death within the first year after kidney transplantation–an observational cohort study. *Transpl. Int.* **2014**, *27*, 262–270. [CrossRef]

22. Hart, A.; Smith, J.M.; Skeans, M.A.; Gustafson, S.K.; Wilk, A.R.; Robinson, A.; Wainright, J.L.; Haynes, C.R.; Snyder, J.J.; Kasiske, B.L.; et al. OPTN/SRTR 2016 Annual Data Report: Kidney. *Am. J. Transplant.* **2018**, *18 Suppl 1*, 18–113. [CrossRef]

23. Thölking, G.; Schuette-Nuetgen, K.; Vogl, T.; Dobrindt, U.; Kahl, B.C.; Brand, M.; Pavenstädt, H.; Suwelack, B.; Koch, R.; Reuter, S. Male kidney allograft recipients at risk for urinary tract infection? *PLoS ONE* **2017**, *12*, e0188262.

24. Kinnunen, S.; Karhapää, P.; Juutilainen, A.; Finne, P.; Helanterä, I. Secular Trends in Infection-Related Mortality after Kidney Transplantation. *Clin. J. Am. Soc. Nephrol.* **2018**, *13*, 755–762. [CrossRef] [PubMed]

25. Abeling, T.; Scheffner, I.; Karch, A.; Broecker, V.; Koch, A.; Haller, H.; Schwarz, A.; Gwinner, W. Risk factors for death in kidney transplant patients: Analysis from a large protocol biopsy registry. *Nephrol. Dial. Transplant.* **2018**, *13*, 755–762. [CrossRef] [PubMed]

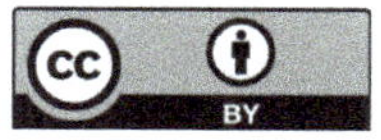

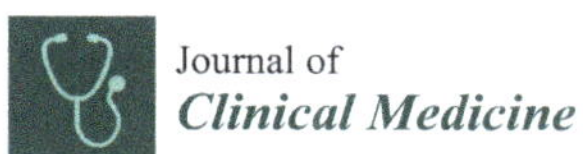

Journal of
Clinical Medicine

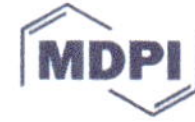

Review

Machine Perfusion for Abdominal Organ Preservation: A Systematic Review of Kidney and Liver Human Grafts

Maria Irene Bellini [1,*,†], **Mikhail Nozdrin** [2], **Janice Yiu** [3] and **Vassilios Papalois** [4,5]

1. Renal Transplant Centre, Belfast City Hospital, Belfast BT97AB, UK
2. School of Medicine, Imperial College London, London SW72AZ, UK
3. School of Medicine, University College London, London WC1E 6BT, UK
4. Renal and Transplant Directorate, Imperial College Healthcare NHS Trust, London W120HS, UK
5. Department of Surgery and Cancer, Imperial College London, London SW72AZ, UK
*   Correspondence: m.irene.bellini@gmail.com
†   Meeting Presentation: European Society of Organ Transplantation Congress, 15–18 September 2019, Copenhagen, Denmark.

Received: 19 July 2019; Accepted: 12 August 2019; Published: 15 August 2019

Abstract: Introduction: To match the current organ demand with organ availability from the donor pool, there has been a shift towards acceptance of extended criteria donors (ECD), often associated with longer ischemic times. Novel dynamic preservation techniques as hypothermic or normothermic machine perfusion (MP) are increasingly adopted, particularly for organs from ECDs. In this study, we compared the viability and incidence of reperfusion injury in kidneys and livers preserved with MP versus Static Cold Storage (SCS). Methods: Systematic review and meta-analysis with a search performed between February and March 2019. MEDLINE, EMBASE and Transplant Library were searched via OvidSP. The Cochrane Library and The Cochrane Central Register of Controlled Trials (CENTRAL) were also searched. English language filter was applied. Results: the systematic search generated 10,585 studies, finally leading to a total of 30 papers for meta-analysis of kidneys and livers. Hypothermic MP (HMP) statistically significantly lowered the incidence of primary nonfunction (PMN, $p = 0.003$) and delayed graft function (DGF, $p < 0.00001$) in kidneys compared to SCS, but not its duration. No difference was also noted for serum creatinine or eGFR post-transplantation, but overall kidneys preserved with HMP had a significantly longer one-year graft survival (OR: 1.61 95% CI: 1.02 to 2.53, $p = 0.04$). Differently from kidneys where the graft survival was affected, there was no significant difference in primary non function (PNF) for livers stored using SCS for those preserved by HMP and NMP. Machine perfusion demonstrated superior outcomes in early allograft dysfunction and post transplantation AST levels compared to SCS, but however, only HMP was able to significantly decrease serum bilirubin and biliary stricture incidence compared to SCS. Conclusions: MP improves DGF and one-year graft survival in kidney transplantation; it appears to mitigate early allograft dysfunction in livers, but more studies are needed to prove its potential superiority in relation to PNF in livers.

Keywords: machine perfusion; organ preservation; temperature; hypothermic; normothermic; transplant

1. Introduction

The increasing demand for allografts and growing waiting lists have led to the utilisation of organs from extended criteria donors (ECDs) or organs with prolonged ischemic times [1]. These organs are associated with higher rates of discard due to an anticipated increased risk of primary non function (PNF) or delayed graft function (DGF); therefore, novel dynamic preservation technologies are increasingly being adopted with the aim to allow organ utilisation in these circumstances.

Dynamic preservation is not a novel concept yet: ex situ organ perfusion was introduced in 1934 by Charles Lindbergh and Alexis Carrel, who developed the first machine perfusion (MP) to preserve animal organs, but the first application in a human kidney was performed by Belzer in 1967. Although the initial result was successful, the concept of dynamic preservation was not pursued forward at that time, with a progressive utilisation of static cold storage (SCS) mainly for logistic and economic reasons.

In the last thirty years instead, with the change in demographics of the donor population and the idea of tailoring the preservation method to the single graft, the debate as to what is the optimal organ treatment prior to transplantation, along with the possibility to ideally let the parenchymal cells continue their metabolic activity before implantation, has led to a re-investigation of the technique of dynamic preservation [2]. In this scenario, where the temperature setting seems to be a main determinant for the subsequent cell activity, and with no evidence for the gold standard temperature to store retrieved grafts before implantation, there are two main modalities as alternatives to SCS: hypothermic (0–4 °C) or normothermic (34–37 °C) machine perfusion.

The aim of this study is to provide evidence with a systematic review and metanalysis of the outcomes in terms of organ viability and incidence of reperfusion injury in hypothermic/normothermic MP in comparison to SCS in kidney and liver human grafts.

2. Methods

The following search algorithm was adopted (Table 1):

Table 1. Search Algorithm.

Step	Input
1	Machine perfusion and (Hypothermic or Normothermic)
2	(Organ* or kidney or liver) and (Preserv*)
3	1 and 2
4	Temperature and cell metabolism
5	3 or 4
6	Transplant*
7	exp Transplantation/
8	6 or 7
9	Renal* or kidney or liver or hepat*
10	(university of wisconsin or UW or HTK or histidine* or collins or hyperosmolar citrate or HOC or celsior or IGL-1 or institut-George* or custodial or belzer or MPS or KPS or marshall* or hypertonic citrate or soltran or ross)
11	8 and 9 and 10
12	5 or 11

2.1. Inclusion Criteria

All published studies including: abstracts from conferences, primary research on new preservation strategies, clinical trials (randomised controlled trials, non-randomised trials), retrospective studies (single centre study, cohort study), and case-controlled studies on organ transplantation of kidney and liver comparing normothermic machine perfusion (NMP) and/or hypothermic machine perfusion (HMP) to CS. To be included, the study had to analyse and discuss the effects of preservation temperatures on ≥1 following post-transplant outcomes. For kidneys: PNF, incidence and duration of DGF, serum creatinine post-surgery, one year graft survival, acute rejection, and estimated glomerular filtration rate (eGFR). For livers: PNF, serum bilirubin post-surgery, biliary stricture incidence, 1–7 day post-surgery peak AST and early allograft dysfunction (EAD).

2.2. Primary Objectives

- Compare DGF in transplanted kidneys (defined as the need for dialysis within 7 days post-transplantation) and EAD (defined using Olthoff [3] criteria) in transplanted livers preserved by MP to SCS.
- Compare PNF in kidneys and livers preserved by machine perfusion and simple cold storage.
- Compare post-transplantation estimated glomerular filtration rate (eGFR) and serum creatinine levels in kidneys preserved via HMP and SCS.
- Compare post-transplantation bilirubin and AST levels in serum in livers preserved via MP and SCS.

2.3. Secondary Objectives

- Where sufficient data existed, to compare one-year graft survival of organs perfused by MP and SCS.
- Compare acute organ rejection of organs preserved via MP and SCS.
- Indirectly compare the effectiveness of preserving liver grafts with HMP and NMP through evaluating studies that compared HMP to SCS and NMP to SCS.

2.4. Data Extraction and Review

Studies identified by the search strategy were screened for meeting the inclusion criteria using the titles and abstracts. Short-listed studies were further checked by reading the whole paper to exclude any ineligible studies, on the basis of the primary and secondary objectives.

2.5. Risk of Bias Assessment

The two reviewers (MN and JY) assessed the risk of bias independently. Randomised controlled trials (RCTs) and retrospective studies in humans were assessed by the Jadad scale. Where there was a disagreement about a Jadad score, advice from a third party (MIB) was sought.

2.6. Data Analysis

Meta-analysis was performed in Revman 5.3 [4]. The effect estimate was calculated together with 95% CI, studies were weighted by sample size, and heterogeneity was assessed with an I^2 test. When $I^2 > 50\%$, a random effects model was used to account for heterogeneity, otherwise a fixed effects model was used. The summary effect was determined using the p-value calculated from the Z test. Odds ratio (OR) was used to compare dichotomous data in organs perfused by HMP/NMP to SCS.

Standardised mean difference (SMD) was used to compare continuous data. For the papers that did not report mean and standard deviation, the method suggested by the Wan et al. 2014 paper [5] was used to approximate mean and standard deviation values using the median and either the interquartile range or range reported in those papers. Studies where this method was used are marked by * in the forest plots.

3. Results

The systematic search generated 10,585 studies of which 672 abstracts and papers were shortlisted by reading the abstract title, and they were further reduced to 102 after reading the abstract. Finally, after reading the full article, a total of 30 papers were selected for meta-analysis (Figure 1).

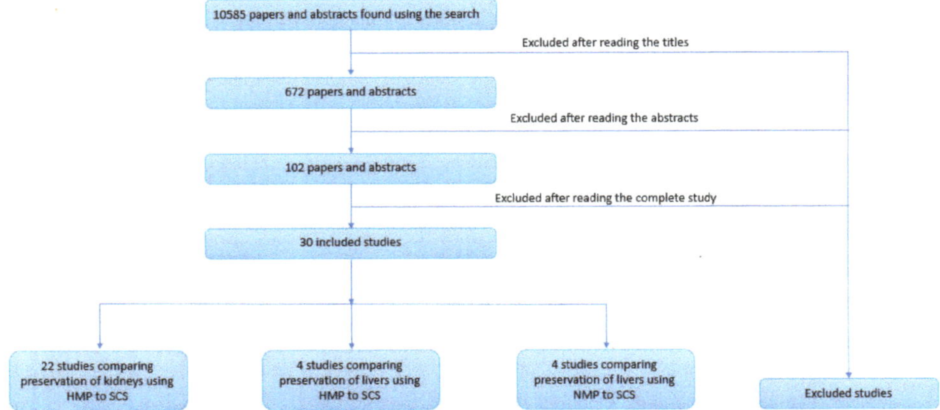

Figure 1. Flow diagram of the systematic literature search.

3.1. Selected Study Characteristics

Twenty-two studies [6–27] identified by the systematic search were included into the analysis (Table 2); fifteen were published papers and seven were abstracts. Ten were RCTs [6,11,12,15,16,18,19, 21,24,25], seven studies were retrospective [7–10,17,22,23], and five were prospective [13,14,20,26,27]. Predominantly, the studies used a LifePort® kidney transporter for hypothermic machine preservation; there was a large variation in cold storage solution type, with some studies not mentioning the specific cold storage preservation solution, but instead referring to local guidelines.

The main difference between LifePort® and RM3® is that the latter provides oxygen by sweeping air over the membrane within the circuit.

Table 2. Studies comparing HMP and SCS in kidneys. Abbreviations: HTK: Histidine-tryptophan-ketoglutarate, UW: University Wisconsin, KPS-1: Kidney Perfusion Solution 1 (Organ recovery systems), SPS-1: Static Preservation Solution 1 (Organ recovery systems), ECD: expanded criteria donors, DBD: donation after brain death, and DCD: donation after cardiac death.

Study	Study Type	Machine	Cold Storage Preservation Solution	Donor Type	HMP Grafts (N)	Cold Storage Grafts (N)
Amaduzzi 2011(abstract) [6]	RCT	?	?	DCD	48	59
Bellini 2019 [7]	Retrospective	RM3® Waters Medical System	?	DBD, DCD	33	33
Dion 2015 [8]	Retrospective	LifePort Kidney transporter®	?	DBD, DCD, ECD	15	15
Forde 2012 (abstract) [9]	Retrospective	LifePort Kidney transporter®	UW	DBD, ECD	88	88
Forde 2016 [10]	Retrospective	LifePort Kidney transporter®	UW	ECD	93	93

Table 2. *Cont.*

Study	Study Type	Machine	Cold Storage Preservation Solution	Donor Type	HMP Grafts (N)	Cold Storage Grafts (N)
Gallinat 2012 [12]	RCT	LifePort Kidney transporter®	HTK or UW	DBD and DCD	85	85
Gallinat 2015 (abstract) [11]	RCT	?	?	ECD	50	44
Gallinat 2017 [13]	Prospective	LifePort Kidney transporter®	HTK or UW	DBD	43	43
Guy 2015 [14]	Prospective	LifePort Kidney transporter®	?	DCD, ECD	74	101
Jochmans 2010 [15]	RCT	LifePort Kidney transporter®	HTK or UW	DBD and DCD	82	82
Kox 2018 [16]	RCT	LifePort Kidney transporter®	HTK or CS-UW	DBD, DCD, ECD	376	376
Kuo 2011 (abstract) [17]	Retrospective	?	?	DCD, DBD	2155	2155
Merion 1990 [18]	RCT	MOX-100	Euro-Collins	DBD	51	51
Moers 2009 [19]	RCT	LifePort Kidney transporter®	HTK or UW or Euro-Collins	DBD and DCD	336	336
Moustafellos 2007 [20]	Prospective	LifePort Kidney transporter®	UW	DCD	18	18
Paul 2008 (abstract) [21]	RCT	?	?	ECD	118	118
Plata-Munoz 2010 (abstract) [22]	Retrospective	?	?	DCD	83	34
Sedigh 2013 [23]	Retrospective	LifePort Kidney transporter®	HTK, UW, Euro-Collins, Custodiol-N	ECD	52	87
Tedesco-Silva 2017 [24]	RCT	LifePort Kidney transporter®	SPS-1, Celsior preservation solution	DBD	80	80
Wang 2017 [25]	RCT	LifePort Kidney transporter®	?	DCD	24	24
Yao 2016 [26]	Prospective	LifePort Kidney transporter®	UW	DCD	39	34
Yuan 2014 (abstract) [27]	Prospective	LifePort Kidney transporter®	?	DCD	32	32

Four studies identified in the systematic search were focused on comparing the effects of HMP and SCS in liver preservation [28–31] (Table 3). There was a lot of heterogeneity in the type of machine used for HMP of liver grafts; however, almost all studies had used the University Wisconsin solution for SCS.

Table 3. Studies comparing HMP and SCS in liver.

Study	Study Type	Machine	Cold Storage Preservation Solution	Donor Type	HMP Grafts (N)	Cold Storage Grafts (N)
Dutkowski 2015 [28]	Observational	ECOPS device (Organ Assist)®	University Wisconsin	DCD, DBD	25	50
Guarrera 2010 [29]	Observational	Modified Medtronic PBS®	University Wisconsin	DCD, ECD	20	20
Guarrera 2015 [30]	Observational	Modified Medtronic PBS®	University Wisconsin	ECD	31	30
Van Rijn 2017 [31]	Observational	Liver Assist (Organ Assist)®	According to local guidelines	DCD, DBD	10	20

Four normothermic perfusion of the liver vs SCS studies [32–35] were included in the meta-analysis (Table 4). The predominant machine perfusion device was OrganOx metra®. There were a variety of cold storage preservation solutions, and the most prevalent donor type was DBD (Table 4).

Table 4. Studies comparing NMP and SCS in liver.

Study	Study Type	Machine	Cold Storage Preservation Solution	Donor Type	NMP Grafts (N)	Cold Storage Grafts (N)
Ghinolfi 2019 [35]	RCT	Liver Assist (Organ Assist)®	Celsior solution	DBD	10	10
Jassem 2018 [34]	Observational	OrganOx metra®	University Wisconsin	DBD	12	27
Nasralla 2018 [32]	RCT	OrganOx metra®	According to local guidelines	DBD, DCD	121	101
Ravikumar 2016 [33]	Observational	OrganOx metra®	University Wisconsin	DBD, DCD	20	39

3.2. Risk of Bias Assessment

Overall studies had a poor Jadad score, and this is explained by many retrospective studies where organs preserved with MP were matched with organs preserved via SCS, so therefore no randomisation or blinding was possible. There was a significant proportion of RCT's in the meta-analyses of HMP vs SCS in kidneys (Table 5) and NMP vs SCS in livers (Table 6); however, all of the studies comparing HMP to SCS in liver were retrospective studies and therefore had poor Jadad scales (Table 7).

Table 5. Risk of bias assessment of studies comparing HMP and SCS preservation in kidney.

Study	Randomisation	Randomisation Description	Inappropriate Randomisation	Double Blind	Double Blinding Description	Inappropriate Double Blinding	Description of Losses	Total Jadad Score
Gallinat 2017	0	0	0	0	0	0	1	1
Forde 2016	0	0	0	0	0	0	1	1
Dion 2015	1	0	−1	0	0	0	1	1
Guy 2015	0	0	0	0	0	0	1	1
Gallinat 2012	1	0	0	0	0	0	1	2
Jochmans 2010	1	1	0	0	0	0	1	3
Merion 1990	1	1	0	0	0	0	1	3
Moers 2009	1	1	0	0	0	0	1	3
Moustafellos 2007	0	0	0	0	0	0	1	1
Sedigh 2013	0	0	0	0	0	0	1	1
Tedesco-Silva 2017	1	1	0	0	0	0	1	3
Bellini 2019	0	0	0	0	0	0	1	1
Wang 2017	1	0	−1	0	0	0	1	1
Yao 2016	0	0	0	0	0	0	1	1
Kox 2018	1	0	0	0	0	0	1	2
Gallinat 2015	1	0	0	0	0	0	1	2
Forde 2012	0	0	0	0	0	0	1	1
Amaduzzi 2011	1	0	0	0	0	0	1	2
Kuo 2011	0	0	0	0	0	0	1	1
Paul 2008	1	0	0	1	1	0	1	4
Plata-Munoz 2010	0	0	0	0	0	0	1	1
Yuan 2014	0	0	0	0	0	0	1	1

Table 6. Risk of bias assessment of studies comparing HMP and SCS in liver.

Study	Randomisation	Randomisation Described	Inappropriate Randomisation	Double Blind	Double Blinding Description	Inappropriate Double Blinding	Description of Losses	Total Jadad Score
Dutkowski 2015	0	0	0	0	0	0	1	1
Guarrera 2010	0	0	0	0	0	0	1	1
Van Rijn 2017	0	0	0	0	0	0	1	1
Guarrera 2015	0	0	0	0	0	0	1	1

Table 7. Risk of bias assessment of studies comparing NMP and SCS in liver.

Study	Randomisation	Randomisation Described	Inappropriate Randomisation	Double Blind	Double Blinding Description	Inappropriate Double Blinding	Description of Losses	Total Jadad Score
Nasralla 2018	1	1	0	1	1	0	1	5
Ravikumar 2016	0	0	0	0	0	0	1	1
Jassem 2018	0	0	0	0	0	0	1	1
Ghinolfi 2019	1	1	0	0	0	0	1	3

3.3. Kidney Transplant Outcomes

PNF, DGF (incidence and duration), acute rejection, serum Creatinine, one-year graft survival, and e-GFR were meta-analysed.

3.4. Primary Non-Function

Five studies [12,13,15,21,24] which reported PNF (816 patients), demonstrated that HMP significantly decreased primary nonfunction compared to SCS (OR: 0.35 95% CI 1.02 to 2.53, p = 0.003) (Figure 2).

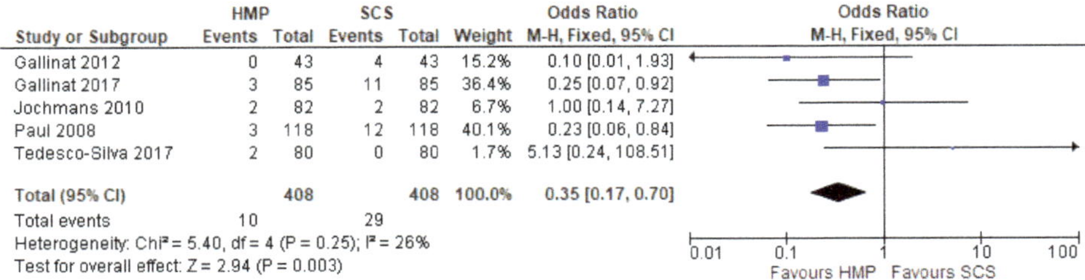

Figure 2. Primary nonfunction in kidneys preserved via HMP and SCS.

3.5. Delayed Graft Function

Twenty-two studies [6–27] comparing HMP and SCS described the incidence of DGF (Figure 3), and its duration (Figure 4), with a total of 7963 patients. The overall OR was 0.57 (0.45, 0.72, 95% CI), with p < 0.00001, favouring a statistically significantly lower prevalence of DGF in kidneys preserved by HMP.

Study or Subgroup	HMP Events	HMP Total	SCS Events	SCS Total	Weight	Odds Ratio M-H, Random, 95% CI
Amaduzzi 2011	18	48	18	59	4.6%	1.37 [0.61, 3.06]
Bellini 2019	8	33	16	33	3.3%	0.34 [0.12, 0.97]
Dion 2015	3	15	5	15	1.7%	0.50 [0.10, 2.63]
Forde 2012	15	88	21	88	5.0%	0.66 [0.31, 1.38]
Forde 2016	16	93	24	93	5.2%	0.60 [0.29, 1.22]
Gallinat 2012	25	85	29	85	5.7%	0.80 [0.42, 1.54]
Gallinat 2015	6	50	9	44	3.0%	0.53 [0.17, 1.63]
Gallinat 2017	5	43	9	43	2.8%	0.50 [0.15, 1.63]
Guy 2015	20	74	47	101	5.7%	0.43 [0.22, 0.81]
Jochmans 2010	44	82	57	82	5.7%	0.51 [0.27, 0.96]
Kox 2018	92	376	118	376	8.4%	0.71 [0.51, 0.98]
Kuo 2011	543	2155	610	2155	9.6%	0.85 [0.75, 0.98]
Merion 1990	21	51	16	51	4.6%	1.53 [0.68, 3.45]
Moers 2009	70	336	89	336	8.1%	0.73 [0.51, 1.04]
Moustafellos 2007	5	18	16	18	1.5%	0.05 [0.01, 0.29]
Paul 2008	26	118	37	118	6.2%	0.62 [0.35, 1.11]
Plata-Munoz 2010	15	83	27	34	3.6%	0.06 [0.02, 0.16]
Sedigh 2013	6	52	18	87	3.6%	0.50 [0.18, 1.35]
Tedesco-Silva 2017	36	80	49	80	5.8%	0.52 [0.28, 0.97]
Wang 2017	4	24	9	24	2.3%	0.33 [0.09, 1.29]
Yao 2016	1	39	6	34	1.1%	0.12 [0.01, 1.08]
Yuan 2014	5	32	6	32	2.5%	0.80 [0.22, 2.95]
Total (95% CI)		3975		3988	100.0%	0.57 [0.45, 0.72]
Total events	984		1236			

Heterogeneity: Tau² = 0.15; Chi² = 57.62, df = 21 (P < 0.0001); I² = 64%
Test for overall effect: Z = 4.68 (P < 0.00001)

Figure 3. DGF in kidneys preserved by hypothermic machine perfusion and cold storage.

Four of the studies [15,19,24,26] reporting DGF were included in a meta-analysis comparing the duration of DGF (352 patients) (Figure 4). There was no difference in duration of DGF in kidneys preserved with HMP and SCS (SMD: −0.04 CI 95% −0.25 to 0.17, p = 0.72) (Figure 4).

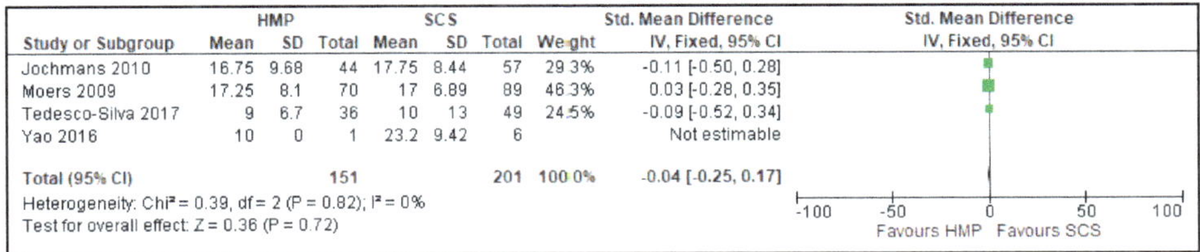

Figure 4. DGF duration in kidneys preserved by HMP and SCS. DGF duration was measured in days. In papers marked with "*", mean and standard deviation were calculated using the method described by Wan 2014 [5].

3.6. Acute Rejection

There was no significant difference in the prevalence of acute rejection in kidneys preserved by HMP or SCS (OR: 0.91 95% CI 0.66 to 1.27, $p > 0.05$). Five studies [12,15,19,23,25] were used for the meta-analysis of a total of 1193 patients (Figure 5).

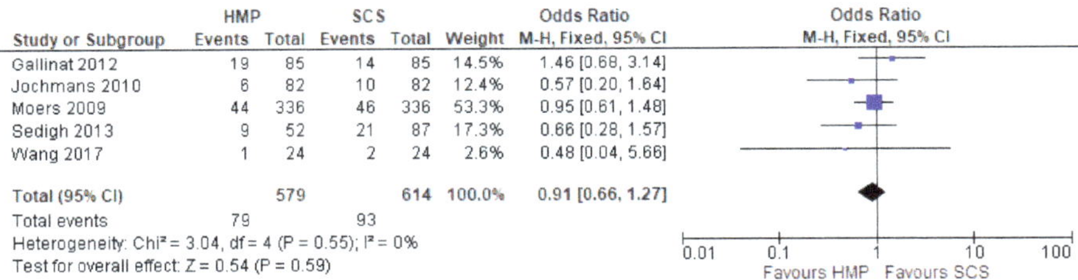

Figure 5. Acute rejection in Kidneys preserved via HMP and SC.

3.7. Comparison of Serum Creatinine One Month after Kidney Transplantation

Three studies [15,24,26] reported one-month post-transplantation serum creatinine (397 patients). There was no significant difference in serum creatinine values (SMD: −0.16 95% CI −0.62 to 0.31) (Figure 6).

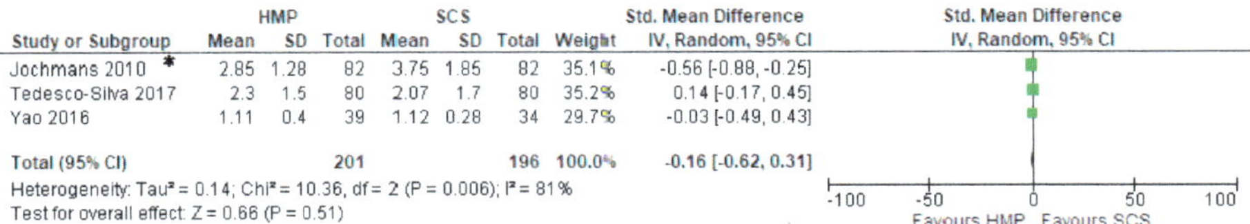

Figure 6. Comparison of one month post transplantation serum creatinine in kidneys preserved via HMP and SCS. In papers marked with "*", mean and standard deviation were calculated using the method described by Wan 2014 [5].

3.8. One-Year Graft Survival

Seven studies [7,10,11,13,15,19,23] that had data on graft survival (1397 patients) were meta-analysed. Overall, kidneys preserved with HMP had a significantly longer one-year graft survival (OR: 1.61 95% CI: 1.02 to 2.53, $p = 0.04$) (Figure 7).

Study or Subgroup	HMP Events	HMP Total	SCS Events	SCS Total	Weight	Odds Ratio M-H, Fixed, 95% CI
Bellini 2019	32	33	30	33	3.0%	3.20 [0.32, 32.48]
Forde 2016	91	93	90	93	6.5%	1.52 [0.25, 9.29]
Gallinat 2015	49	50	38	44	2.7%	7.74 [0.89, 67.02]
Gallinat 2017	42	43	38	43	3.0%	5.53 [0.62, 49.45]
Jochmans 2010	77	82	78	82	15.9%	0.79 [0.20, 3.05]
Moers 2009	316	336	302	326	61.1%	1.26 [0.68, 2.32]
Sedigh 2013	50	52	81	87	7.8%	1.85 [0.36, 9.53]
Total (95% CI)		**689**		**708**	**100.0%**	**1.61 [1.02, 2.53]**
Total events	657		657			

Heterogeneity: Chi² = 5.31, df = 6 (P = 0.51); I² = 0%
Test for overall effect: Z = 2.04 (P = 0.04)

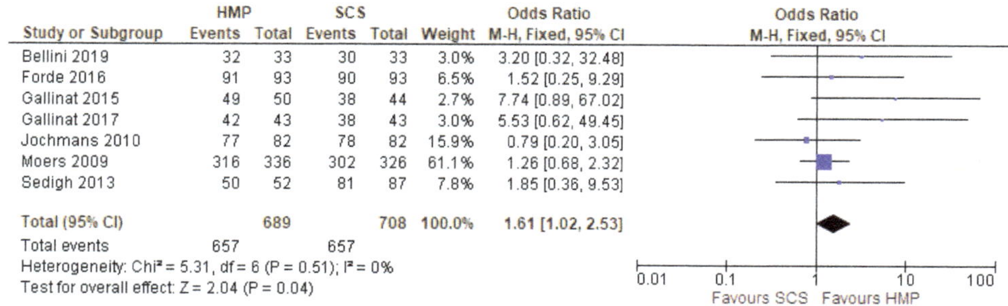

Figure 7. One year graft survival in kidneys preserved via HMP and SCS.

3.9. Post-Transplant Estimated Glomerular Filtration Rate in HMP and SCS Kidneys

One of our previous studies [7] as well as the one from Tedesco et al. [24] were the only two that reported eGFR at more than one time point after the surgery. Combined meta-analyses of 200 patients demonstrate that HMP increased eGFR only on day 7 post surgery (SMD: 0.39 95% CI 0.11 to 0.67, $p = 0.007$) (Figure 8). There was no significant difference in eGFR of kidneys preserved with HMP and SCS both on day 14 (SMD: 0.99 95% CI −0.26 to 2.24, $p > 0.05$) (Figure 9) and day 365 (SMD: 0.6 95% CI −0.19 to 1.38, $p > 0.05$) (Figure 10).

Study or Subgroup	HMP Mean	HMP SD	HMP Total	SCS Mean	SCS SD	SCS Total	Weight	Std. Mean Difference IV, Fixed, 95% CI
Bellini 2019	27.4	4.8	20	24.7	4.1	20	19.5%	0.59 [-0.04, 1.23]
Tedesco-Silva 2017	25	21.6	80	17.8	20.7	80	80.5%	0.34 [0.03, 0.65]
Total (95% CI)			**100**			**100**	**100.0%**	**0.39 [0.11, 0.67]**

Heterogeneity: Chi² = 0.50, df = 1 (P = 0.48); I² = 0%
Test for overall effect: Z = 2.72 (P = 0.007)

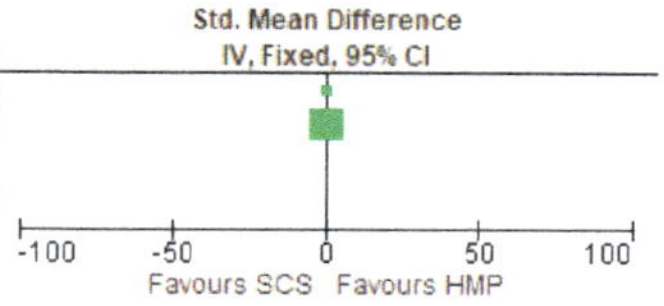

Figure 8. Estimated glomerular filtration rate (eGFR) in kidneys preserved via HMP and SCS; eGFR day 7.

Study or Subgroup	HMP Mean	HMP SD	HMP Total	SCS Mean	SCS SD	SCS Total	Weight	Std. Mean Difference IV, Random, 95% CI
Bellini 2019	34.6	4.1	20	28	3.6	20	46.5%	1.68 [0.95, 2.41]
Tedesco-Silva 2017	38.4	28.6	80	28.3	21.4	80	53.5%	0.40 [0.08, 0.71]
Total (95% CI)			**100**			**100**	**100.0%**	**0.99 [-0.26, 2.24]**

Heterogeneity: Tau² = 0.74; Chi² = 9.94, df = 1 (P = 0.002); I² = 90%
Test for overall effect: Z = 1.56 (P = 0.12)

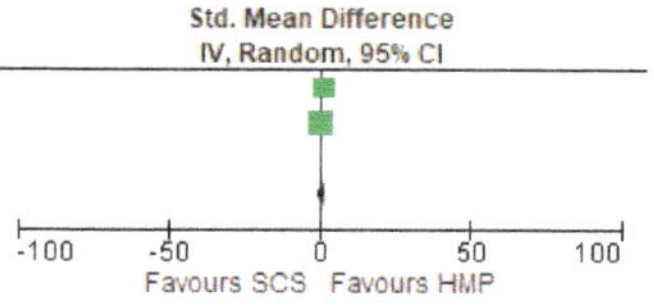

Figure 9. Estimated glomerular filtration rate (eGFR) in kidneys preserved via HMP and SCS; eGFR day 14.

Study or Subgroup	HMP Mean	HMP SD	HMP Total	SCS Mean	SCS SD	SCS Total	Weight	Std. Mean Difference IV, Random, 95% CI
Bellini 2019	40.6	4	20	36.6	3.4	20	43.1%	1.06 [0.39, 1.72]
Tedesco-Silva 2017	54.4	28.6	80	48.3	19.8	80	56.9%	0.25 [-0.06, 0.56]
Total (95% CI)			**100**			**100**	**100.0%**	**0.60 [-0.19, 1.38]**

Heterogeneity: Tau² = 0.26; Chi² = 4.66, df = 1 (P = 0.03); I² = 79%
Test for overall effect: Z = 1.49 (P = 0.14)

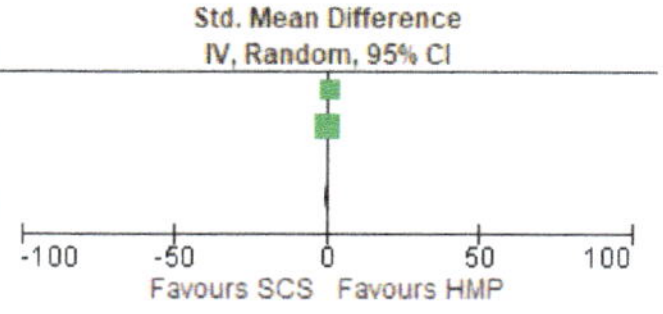

Figure 10. Estimated glomerular filtration rate (eGFR) in kidneys preserved via HMP and SCS; eGFR day 365.

3.10. Liver Transplant Outcomes

PNF, EAD, and AST serum levels, bilirubin serum levels, and the incidence of biliary strictures were meta-analysed.

3.11. Primary Non Function

In livers preserved both by HMP (Figure 11) and NMP (Figure 12), there was no significant difference in PNF compared to livers stored using SCS. The odds ratio comparing HMP to SCS was 0.36 95% CI 0.05 to 2.35, $p = 0.29$, and the odds ratio comparing NMP to SCS was 2.53 95% CI 0.10 to 62.70, $p = 0.67$.

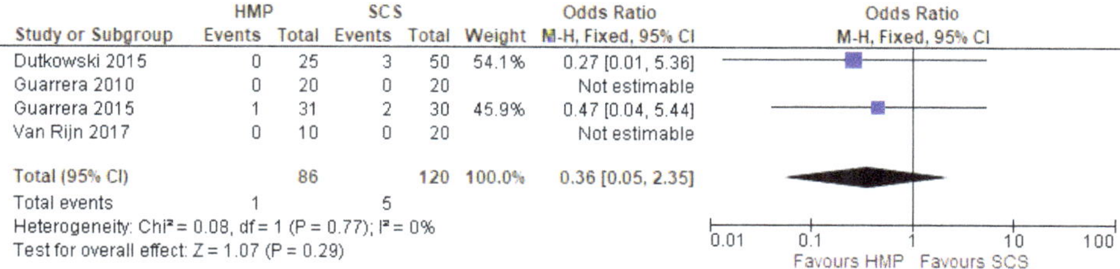

Figure 11. Primary nonfunction in livers preserved via HMP and SCS.

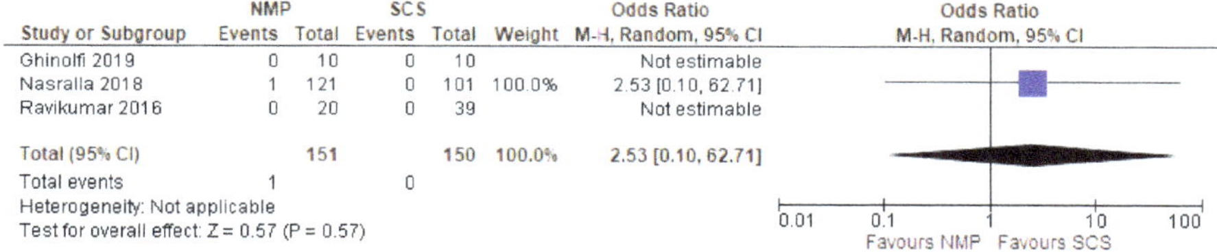

Figure 12. Primary nonfunction in livers preserved via NMP and SCS.

3.12. Early Allograft Dysfunction

Four studies [28–31] compared EAD prevalence in livers stored using HMP and SCS (206 patients). Overall, livers stored with HMP showed lower prevalence of EAD (OR: 0.36 95% CI 0.17 to 0.75, $p = 0.006$) (Figure 13). Similar results were reported by the three studies comparing EAD prevalence in livers stored using NMP and SCS (301 patients). Overall, livers stored with NMP also showed lower prevalence of EAD compared to SCS (OR: 0.36 95% CI 0.17 to 0.75, $p = 0.006$) (Figure 14).

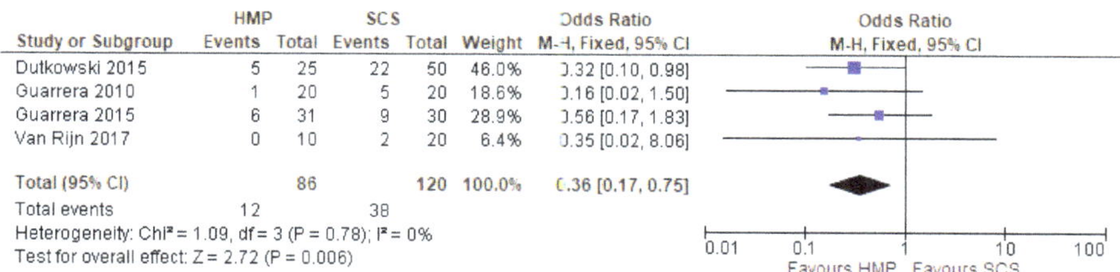

Figure 13. Early allograft dysfunction in livers preserved via HMP and SCS.

Figure 14. Early allograft dysfunction in livers preserved via NMP and SCS.

3.13. Serum AST

Two studies [28,29] (115 patients) comparing HMP to SCS demonstrated the superiority of HMP in reducing post-transplantation AST levels (SMD −0.59 95% CI −0.98 to −0.20, p = 0.003) (Figure 15). Similarly, four studies [32–35] that focused on comparing NMP to SCS demonstrated that livers preserved with NMP had significantly lower serum AST levels than SCS (OR: −0.63 95% CI −0.85 to −0.41, p < 0.00001) (Figure 16).

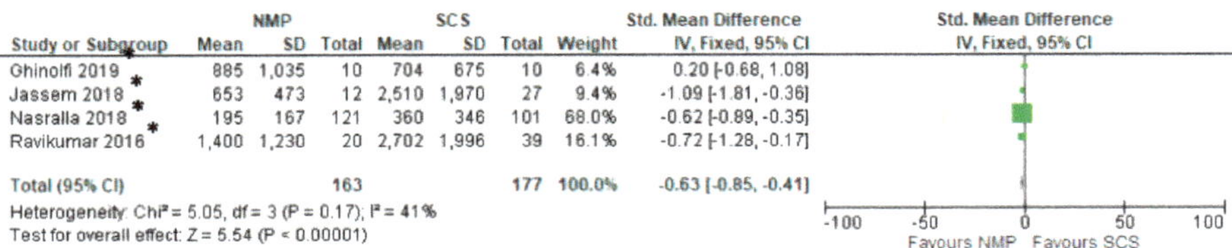

Figure 15. Peak serum AST in studies comparing HMP to SCS. In papers marked with "*", mean and standard deviation were calculated using the method described by Wan 2014 [5].

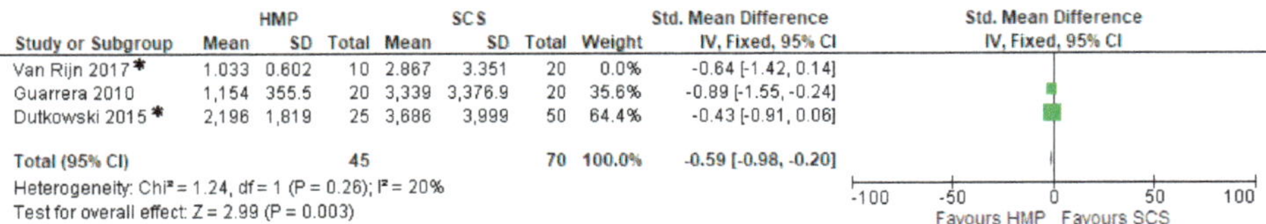

Figure 16. Peak serum AST in studies comparing NMP to SCS. In papers marked with "*", mean and standard deviation were calculated using the method described by Wan 2014 [5].

3.14. Serum Bilirubin

Results from Dutkowski [28], Guarrera [29], and van Rijn [31] (115 patients) demonstrated the overall significant decrease in post transplantation serum bilirubin (SMD: −0.59 95% CI −0.98 to −0.20, p = 0.003) in livers stored with HMP compared to SCS (Figure 17).

Study or Subgroup	HMP Mean	SD	Total	SCS Mean	SD	Total	Weight	Std. Mean Difference IV, Fixed, 95% CI
Van Rijn 2017 *	1.033	0.602	10	2.867	3.351	20	0.0%	-0.64 [-1.42, 0.14]
Guarrera 2010	1,154	355.5	20	3,339	3,376.9	20	35.6%	-0.89 [-1.55, -0.24]
Dutkowski 2015 *	2,196	1,819	25	3,686	3,999	50	64.4%	-0.43 [-0.91, 0.06]
Total (95% CI)			45			70	100.0%	-0.59 [-0.98, -0.20]

Heterogeneity: Chi² = 1.24, df = 1 (P = 0.26); I² = 20%
Test for overall effect: Z = 2.99 (P = 0.003)

Figure 17. One week post transplantation peak serum total bilirubin in studies comparing HMP to SCS. In papers marked with "*", mean and standard deviation were calculated using the method described by Wan 2014 [5].

Three studies [32,34,35] comparing NMP to SCS described total serum bilirubin one week post transplantation (181 patients), and demonstrated that there was no significant difference in bilirubin levels (SMD: −0.20 95% Ci −0.44 to 0.03, p = 0.09) (Figure 18).

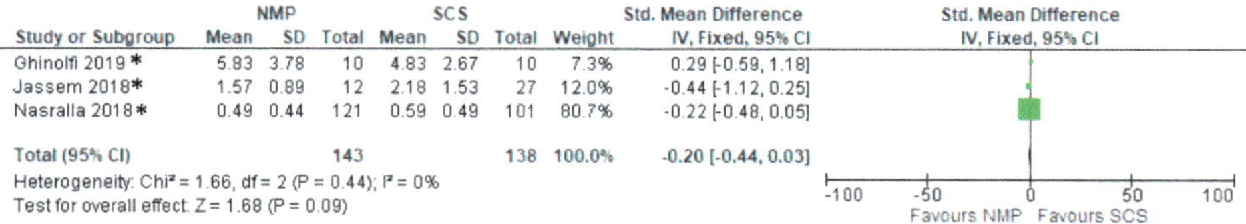

Figure 18. One week post transplantation peak serum total bilirubin in studies comparing NMP to SCS. In papers marked with "*", mean and standard deviation were calculated using the method described by Wan 2014 [5].

3.15. Biliary Strictures

Four studies [28–31] (Figure 19) comparing SCS to HMP in the preservation of livers (206 patients) demonstrated significant difference in incidence of post-transplantation strictures (OR: 2.59 95% CI 1.19 to 5.61, $p = 0.02$).

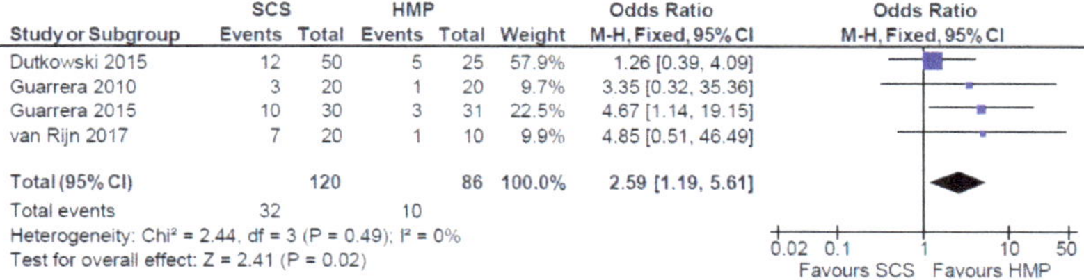

Figure 19. Post transplantation biliary stricture rates in studies comparing HMP to SCS.

4. Discussion

This meta-analysis assessed the impact of dynamic preservation techniques on the viability and incidence of reperfusion injury in kidney and liver versus the traditional static cold storage before transplantation. The results were further sub-analysed in relation to the different organs considered.

HMP demonstrated significantly lowered delayed graft function incidence in transplanted kidneys compared to SCS, but it, however, had no effect on its duration, although only four studies reported this parameter. Furthermore, HMP was associated with reduced PNF and prolonged one-year graft survival, demonstrating the importance of machine perfusion technology in the utilisation of graft from extended criteria donors. Overall, serum creatinine of the transplanted grafts was similar, although a difference in eGFR could be seen on day 7 post transplantation. In the long term, there was yet no difference in kidneys preserved via HMP and SCS. This might lead to the debate of whether the long-term function of an organ is intrinsically related to the quality of the organ itself (standard or extended criteria), whilst the immediate post-transplant function is directly dependant on the preservation technique. For this reason, emergent possibilities of reconditioning during preservation are considered to improve the quality of the organ and to possibly impact the long-term outcome. In that regard, nutrients, therapeutic gases, mesenchymal stromal cells, gene therapies, and nanoparticles could be delivered to effectively repair an extended criteria organ during the preservation period and prior to implantation. The use of oxygen might in particular contribute to the long-term outcome of the preserved parenchymal cells. It is in fact of note, as shown in in Figure 10, that a difference in the one year eGFR is in favour of HMP kidneys preserved with an oxygenated circuit. Additional oxygen may support the aerobic activity and contrast the injury process of the cells with a more prominent effect in the long term. Furthermore, the efficiency of MP in assessing organ quality with possible reconditioning and predicting transplant outcome are of great interest in modern transplant practice, with an emerging role of these novel technologies to be evaluated as a possible diagnostic tool.

Differently from the kidney, no difference in PNF was seen in livers preserved via HMP or NMP compared to SCS; in liver preservation both HMP and NMP have demonstrated superior outcomes when it comes to mitigating early allograft dysfunction and post transplantation AST levels compared to SCS, but only HMP was able to significantly decrease serum bilirubin and the incidence of biliary strictures, compared to SCS. In addition to this, the value of AST as an end point is controversial because there can be a release of AST in the perfusate during MP; therefore, a more reliable marker should be considered in future studies. These conflicting results might be related to the relatively small numbers of RCT with, therefore, no sufficient evidence to conclude a clear superiority of one modality compared to the other. What appears to be clear is that more clinical studies are needed for verification with homogeneous parameters to measure the outcomes of interest.

In conclusion, there is growing evidence that MP allows for the utilisation of marginal kidneys with lower primary and delayed graft function rates. There is also evidence of improved early allograft dysfunction after dynamic preservation for livers, but more studies are needed to prove the potential superiority of these novel technologies.

Author Contributions: M.I.B. designed the study, analysed the data and wrote the paper; M.N. performed the study, collected the data and wrote the paper; J.Y. performed the study and collected the data; V.P. designed the study, analysed the data and review the paper.

Conflicts of Interest: The authors declare no conflict of interest.

Abbreviations

AST	Aspartate transaminase
DGF	Delayed Graft Function
DBD	Donor after Brain Death
DCD	Donor after Cardiac Death
EAD	Early Allograft Dysfunction
eGFR	estimated Glomerular Filtration Rate
ECD	Expanded Criteria Donor
HMP	Hypothermic Machine Perfusion
HTK	Histidine-Tryptophan-Ketoglutarate
KPS-1	Kidney Perfusion Solution 1
MP	Machine Perfusion
OR	Odds Ratio
PNF	Primary Non-Function
RCT	Randomized Controlled Trial
SCS	Static Cold Storage
SMD	Standardised Mean Difference
SPS-1	Static Preservation Solution 1

References

1. Dube, G.K.; Brennan, C.; Husain, S.A.; Crew, R.J.; Chiles, M.C.; Cohen, D.J.; Mohan, S. Outcomes of kidney transplant from deceased donors with acute kidney injury and prolonged cold ischemia time a retrospective cohort study. *Transpl. Int.* **2019**, *32*, 646–657. [CrossRef] [PubMed]
2. Bellini, M.I.; D'Andrea, V. Organ preservation: Which temperature for which organ? *J. Int. Med Res.* **2019**, *47*, 2323–2325. [CrossRef] [PubMed]
3. Olthoff, K.M.; Kulik, L.; Samstein, B.; Kaminski, M.; Abecassis, M.; Emond, J.; Shaked, A.; Christie, J.D. Validation of a current definition of early allograft dysfunction in liver transplant recipients and analysis of risk factors. *Liver Transpl.* **2010**, *16*, 943–949. [CrossRef] [PubMed]
4. Tokodai, K.; Amada, N.; Kikuchi, H.; Haga, I.; Takayama, T.; Nakamura, A. Body fat percentage as a marker of new-onset diabetes mellitus after kidney transplantation. *Transpl. Proc.* **2013**, *45*, 1544–1547. [CrossRef] [PubMed]

5.   Wan, X.; Wang, W.Q.; Liu, J.M.; Tong, T.J. Estimating the Sample Mean and Standard Deviation from the Sample Size, Median, Range And/or Interquartile Range. *BMC Med. Res. Methodol.* **2014**, *14*, 135. [CrossRef] [PubMed]

6.   Amaduzzi, A.; Catena, F.; Montori, G.; Ravaioli, M.; Pinna, A. Hypothermic Machine Perfusion (HMP) versus Static Cold Storage (CS) in Kidney Allograft Preservation. Prospective Case-Control Trial: RO-077. *Transpl. Int.* **2011**, *24*, 151.

7.   Bellini, M.I.; Charalampidis, S.; Herbert, P.E.; Bonatsos, V.; Crane, J.; Muthusamy, A.; Dor, F.G.M.F.; Papalois, V. Cold Pulsatile Machine Perfusion versus Static Cold Storage in Kidney Transplantation: A Single Centre Experience. *BioMed Res. Int.* **2019**, *2019*, 7435248. [CrossRef]

8.   Dion, M.S.; McGregor, T.B.; McAlister, V.C.; Luke, P.P.; Sener, A. Hypothermic machine perfusion improves Doppler ultrasonography resistive indices and long-term allograft function after renal transplantation: A single-centre analysis. *BJU Int.* **2015**, *116*, 932–937. [CrossRef]

9.   Forde, J.C.; Shields, W.P.; Zimmermann, J.A.; Smyth, G.P.; Eng, M.; Power, R.E.; Mohan, P.; Hickey, D.P.; Little, D.M. Single Centre Experience of Hypothermic Continuous Machine Perfusion of Kidneys from Extended Criteria Deceased Heart-Beating Donors: 1826. *Transplant. J.* **2012**, *94*, 512. [CrossRef]

10. Forde, J.C.; Shields, W.P.; Azhar, M.; Daly, P.J.; Zimmermann, J.A.; Smyth, G.P.; Eng, M.P.; Power, R.E.; Mohan, P.; Hickey, D.P.; et al. Single centre experience of hypothermic machine perfusion of kidneys from extended criteria deceased heart-beating donors: A comparative study. *Ir. J. Med Sci.* **2016**, *185*, 121–125. [CrossRef]

11. Gallinat, A.; Amrillaeva, V.; Hoyer, D.; Kocabayoglu, P.; Treckmann, J.; Van Meel, M.; Samuel, U.; Minor, T.; Paul, A. End-Ischemic Hypothermic In-House Machine Perfusion improves 1-year graft survival in ECD Kidneys: O258. *Transpl. Int.* **2015**, *28*, 95.

12. Gallinat, A.; Moers, C.; Treckmann, J.; Smits, J.M.; Leuvenink, H.G.; Lefering, R.; Van Heurn, E.; Kirste, G.R.; Squifflet, J.P.; Rahmel, A.; et al. Machine perfusion versus cold storage for the preservation of kidneys from donors >/= 65 years allocated in the Eurotransplant Senior Programme. *Nephrol. Dial. Transplant.* **2012**, *27*, 4458–4463. [CrossRef] [PubMed]

13. Gallinat, A.; Amrillaeva, V.; Hoyer, D.P.; Kocabayoglu, P.; Benko, T.; Treckman, J.W.; Van Meel, M.; Samuel, U.; Minor, T.; Paul, A. Reconditioning by end-ischemic hypothermic in-house machine perfusion: A promising strategy to improve outcome in expanded criteria donors kidney transplantation. *Clin. Transplant.* **2017**, *31*. [CrossRef] [PubMed]

14. Guy, A.; McGrogan, D.; Inston, N.; Ready, A. Hypothermic machine perfusion permits extended cold ischemia times with improved early graft function. *Exp. Clin. Transplant.* **2015**, *13*, 130–137. [PubMed]

15. Jochmans, I.; Moers, C.; Smits, J.M.; Leuvenink, H.G.; Treckmann, J.; Paul, A.; Rahmel, A.; Squifflet, J.P.; Van Heurn, E.; Monbaliu, D.; et al. Machine perfusion versus cold storage for the preservation of kidneys donated after cardiac death: A multicenter, randomized, controlled trial. *Ann. Surg.* **2010**, *252*, 756–764. [CrossRef] [PubMed]

16. Kox, J.; Moers, C.; Monbaliu, D.; Strelniece, A.; Treckmann, J.; Jochmans, I.; Leuvenink, H.; Van Heurn, E.; Pirenne, J.; Paul, A.; et al. The benefits of hypothermic machine preservation and short cold ischemia times in deceased donor kidneys. *Transplantation* **2018**, *102*, 1344–1350. [CrossRef] [PubMed]

17. Kuo, H.T.; Huang, E.; Bunnapradist, S. Machine Perfusion Versus Cold Storage in Deceased Donor Kidney Transplantation, an Analysis of the OPTN/UNOS Database: Abstract# 633 Poster Board #-Session: P32-I. *Am. J. Transplant.* **2011**, *11*, 220.

18. Merion, R.M.; Oh, H.K.; Port, F.K.; Toledo-Pereyra, L.H.; Turcotte, J.G. A prospective controlled trial of cold-storage versus machine-perfusion preservation in cadaveric renal transplantation. *Transplantation* **1990**, *50*, 230–233. [CrossRef] [PubMed]

19. Moers, C.; Smits, J.M.; Maathuis, M.H.; Treckmann, J.; van Gelder, F.; Napieralski, B.P.; van kasterop-kutz, M.; van der heide, J.J.; Squifflet, J.P.; van heurn, E.; et al. Machine perfusion or cold storage in deceased-donor kidney transplantation. *New Engl. J. Med.* **2009**, *360*, 7–19. [CrossRef] [PubMed]

20. Moustafellos, P.; Hadjianastassiou, V.; Roy, D.; Muktadir, A.; Contractor, H.; Vaidya, A.; Friend, P.J. The influence of pulsatile preservation in kidney transplantation from non-heart-beating donors. *Transplant. Proc.* **2007**, *39*, 1323–1325. [CrossRef]

21. Paul, A.; Moers, C.; Smits, J.; Maathuis, H.; Van Der Heide, J.H.; Van Heurn, E.; Squifflet, J.P.; Pirenne, J.; Ploeg, R.; Treckmann, J. Machine Perfusion versus Cold Storage in Transplantation of Kidneys from older Deceased Donors: Results of a Prospective Randomized Multicentral Trial: 236. *Transplantation* **2008**, *86* (Suppl. 2S), 83. [CrossRef]

22. Plata-Munoz, J.; Muthusamy, A.; Elker, D.; Brockmann, J.; Sinha, S.; Vaidya, A.; Friend, P.; Fuggle, S. Beneficial Effect of Preservation by Machine Perfusion on Postoperative Outocme of Kidneys from Controlled Donors after Cardiac Death: 2325. *Transpl. J.* **2010**, *90*, 579. [CrossRef]

23. Sedigh, A.; Tufveson, G.; Backman, L.; Biglarnia, A.R.; Lorant, T. Initial experience with hypothermic machine perfusion of kidneys from deceased donors in the Uppsala region in Sweden. *Transpl. Proc.* **2013**, *45*, 1168–1171. [CrossRef] [PubMed]

24. Tedesco-Silva, H.; Mello Offerni, J.C.; Ayres Carneiro, V.; Ivani de Paula, M.; Neto, E.D.; Brambate Carvalhinho Lemos, F.; Requiao Moura, L.R.; Pacheco, E.; de Morais Cunha, M.F.; Francisco da Silva, E.; et al. Randomized Trial of Machine Perfusion Versus Cold Storage in Recipients of Deceased Donor Kidney Transplants With High Incidence of Delayed Graft Function. *Transpl. Direct* **2017**, *3*, e155. [CrossRef] [PubMed]

25. Wang, W.; Xie, D.; Hu, X.; Yin, H.; Liu, H.; Zhang, X. Effect of Hypothermic Machine Perfusion on the Preservation of Kidneys Donated After Cardiac Death: A Single-Center, Randomized, Controlled Trial. *Artif. Organs* **2017**, *41*, 753–758. [CrossRef] [PubMed]

26. Yao, L.; Zhou, H.; Wang, Y.; Wang, G.; Wang, W.; Chen, M.; Zhang, K.; Fu, Y. Hypothermic Machine Perfusion in DCD Kidney Transplantation: A Single Center Experience. *Urol. Int.* **2016**, *96*, 148–151. [CrossRef]

27. Yuan, X.; Zhou, J.; Chen, C.; Han, M.; Wang, X.; He, X. The Application of Machine Perfusion Preservation of Kidneys in Cardiac Death Donor Kidney Transplantation: Abstract# 1464. *Transplant* **2014**, *98*, 10.

28. Dutkowski, P.; Polak, W.G.; Muiesan, P.; Schlegel, A.; Verhoeven, C.J.; Scalera, I.; De Oliveirra, M.L.; Kron, P.; Clavien, P.A. First Comparison of Hypothermic Oxygenated PErfusion Versus Static Cold Storage of Human Donation After Cardiac Death Liver Transplants: An International-matched Case Analysis. *Ann. Surg.* **2015**, *262*, 764–770. [CrossRef]

29. Guarrera, J.V.; Henry, S.D.; Samstein, B.; Odeh-Ramadan, R.; Kinkhabwala, M.; Goldstein, M.J.; Ratner, L.E.; Renz, J.F.; Lee, H.T.; Brown, R.S.; et al. Hypothermic machine preservation in human liver transplantation: The first clinical series. *Am. J. Transpl.* **2010**, *10*, 372–381. [CrossRef]

30. Guarrera, J.V.; Henry, S.D.; Samstein, B.; Reznik, E.; Musat, C.; Lukose, T.I.; Ratner, L.E.; Brown, R.S., Jr.; Kato, T.; Emond, J.C. Hypothermic machine preservation facilitates successful transplantation of "orphan" extended criteria donor livers. *Am. J. Transpl.* **2015**, *15*, 161–169. [CrossRef]

31. van Rijn, R.; Karimian, N.; Matton, A.P.M.; Burlage, L.C.; Westerkamp, A.C.; van den Berg, A.P.; de Kleine, R.H.J.; de Bore, M.T.; Lisman, T.; Porte, R.J. Dual hypothermic oxygenated machine perfusion in liver transplants donated after circulatory death. *Br. J. Surg.* **2017**, *104*, 907–917. [CrossRef] [PubMed]

32. Nasralla, D.; Coussios, C.C.; Mergental, H.; Akhtar, M.Z.; Butler, A.J.; Ceresa, C.D.L.; Chiocchaia, V.; Dutton, S.J.; Garcia-Valdecasas, J.C.; Heaton, N.; et al. A randomized trial of normothermic preservation in liver transplantation. *Nature* **2018**, *557*, 50–56. [CrossRef] [PubMed]

33. Ravikumar, R.; Jassem, W.; Mergental, H.; Heaton, N.; Mirza, D.; Perera, M.T.; Quaglia, A.; Holroyd, D.; Vogel, T.; Coussios, C.C.; et al. Liver Transplantation After Ex Vivo Normothermic Machine Preservation: A Phase 1 (First-in-Man) Clinical Trial. *Am. J. Transpl.* **2016**, *16*, 1779–1787. [CrossRef] [PubMed]

34. Jassem, W.; Xystrakis, E.; Ghnewa, Y.G.; Yuksel, M.; Pop, O.; Martinez-Llordella, M.; Jabri, Y.; Huang, X.; Lozano, J.J.; Quaglia, A.; et al. Normothermic Machine Perfusion (NMP) Inhibits Proinflammatory Responses in the Liver and Promotes Regeneration. *Hepatology* **2018**, *70*, 682–695. [CrossRef] [PubMed]

35. Ghinolfi, D.; Rreka, E.; De Tata, V.; Franzini, M.; Pezzati, D.; Fierabracci, V.; Masini, M.; Cacciatoinsilla, A.; Bindi, M.L.; Marselli, L.; et al. Pilot, Open, Randomized, Prospective Trial for Normothermic Machine Perfusion Evaluation in Liver Transplantation From Older Donors. *Liver Transpl.* **2019**, *25*, 436–449. [CrossRef] [PubMed]

Journal of
Clinical Medicine

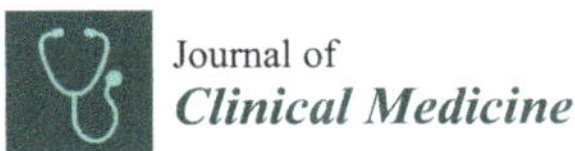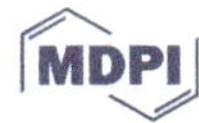

Article

Efficacy and Safety of Belatacept Treatment in Renal Allograft Recipients at High Cardiovascular Risk—A Single Center Experience

Hannes Neuwirt [1,*], Irmgard Leitner-Lechner [2], Julia Kerschbaum [1], Michael Ertl [1], Florian Pöggsteiner [1], Nicolas Pölt [1], Julius Matzler [1], Hannelore Sprenger-Mähr [3], Michael Rudnicki [1], Peter Schratzberger [1], Iris E. Eder [4] and Gert Mayer [1]

[1] Department of Internal Medicine IV-Nephrology and Hypertension, Medical University of Innsbruck, Anichstrasse 35, Innsbruck A-6020, Austria

[2] Department of Pharmacology, Section for Molecular and Cellular Pharmacology, Medical University of Innsbruck, Peter-Mayr-Strasse 1a, Innsbruck 6020, Austria

[3] Landeskrankenhaus Feldkirch, Department of Internal Medicine III—Nephrology, Carinagasse 47, Feldkirch 6800, Austria

[4] Department of Urology, Medical University of Innsbruck, Anichstrasse 35, Innsbruck A-6020, Austria

*   Correspondence: Hannes.Neuwirt@i-med.ac.at

Received: 2 July 2019; Accepted: 1 August 2019; Published: 3 August 2019

Abstract: Belatacept is an attractive option for immunosuppression after renal transplantation. Renal allograft function is superior when compared to calcineurin inhibitor (CNI) based therapy in "de novo" treated patients and it has also been proposed that individuals at high cardiovascular (CV) risk may benefit most. In this retrospective cohort study, we assessed the efficacy and safety of treating patients at high cardiovascular risk with Belatacept ($n = 34$, for 1194 observation months) when compared to a matched control group of 150 individuals under CNI immunosuppression (for 7309 months of observation). The estimated glomerular filtration rate (eGFR) increased for patients taking Belatacept but decreased during CNI-based therapy (+2.60 vs. -0.89 mL/min/1.73 m^2/year, $p = 0.006$). In a multivariate Cox regression model, Belatacept remained the only significant factor associated with the improvement of eGFR (HR 4.35, 95%CI 2.39–7.93). Belatacept treatment was not a significant risk factor for renal allograft rejection or graft loss. In terms of safety, the only significant risk factor for de novo cardiovascular events was a pre-existing cerebrovascular disease, but Belatacept was not associated with a significant risk reduction. Belatacept treatment was not associated with an increased risk of severe infections, cytomegalo virus (CMV) or BK-virus reactivation, malignancy or death in the multivariate Cox regression analysis. Belatacept is an efficient and safe option for patients after renal transplantation at high cardiovascular risk.

Keywords: kidney transplantation; Belatacept; cardiovascular high risk; outcome

---

1. Introduction

Calcineurin inhibitors (CNIs) are currently the standard immunosuppressive therapy after renal transplantation. Their introduction into clinical practice has improved short-term outcomes dramatically. Unfortunately, the rate of late allograft loss has not significantly improved [1] and it is generally accepted that CNI nephrotoxicity contributes to this problem. Thus, multiple studies have investigated the impact of CNI-free immunosuppression on renal allograft function and patient and graft survival. The use of mammalian target of rapamycin inhibitors (mTORi) is impeded by drop-out rates of up to 40% due to side effects [2] and furthermore is associated with higher allograft rejection rates [3].

Belatacept inhibits T-cell activation by blocking a co-stimulatory signal by binding to CD80/CD86 on antigen presenting cells [4]. It is currently approved for the de novo immunosuppression of renal allograft recipients in combination with mycophenolic acid and steroids. Studies have demonstrated an improved allograft survival over several years when compared to cyclosporine A-based immunosuppression [5,6]. Furthermore, a protocol for switching patients from CNIs to Belatacept has been published [7,8]. This conversion improved kidney function relative to the baseline and was safe concerning risk of death or transplant loss. Finally, it has been proposed that Belatacept-based regimens might have beneficial effects, especially in patients at high cardiovascular (CV) risk (reviewed by [9]). One mechanism might be a reduction of pulse wave velocity in patients treated with Belatacept compared to CNI-treated patients [10,11]. However, "real world" data on renal outcomes and especially safety in the latter individuals are sparse.

Thus, we conducted a retrospective cohort study in renal allograft recipients at high CV risk and compared the efficacy and safety of Belatacept treatment in 34 patients to the outcomes of 150 patients treated with CNI (mainly tacrolimus) based immunosuppression.

2. Materials and Methods

2.1. Patient Population

Belatacept has been used in 42 renal transplant recipients at our center since 2010 and in this retrospective cohort study, all patients at high cardiovascular risk (definition see below) have been included (n = 34). Eighteen patients were treated de novo and 16 were converted at a median of 1.6 months (interquartile range (IQR), 0.6–4.2 months) after transplantation, mainly due to biopsy confirmed or clinically suspected renal CNI toxicity. No patient in this group was returned to CNI therapy thereafter. As we were interested in studying the efficacy and safety in patients on either CNI or Belatacept therapy, the day of conversion was taken as the baseline in these individuals and all clinical endpoints were adjudicated to the Belatacept group. Due to the early conversion, we excluded the time on CNI from any calculation. The study was conducted in accordance with the Declaration of Helsinki, and the protocol was approved by the Ethics Committee of the Medical University Innsbruck (Project-ID: 1137/2019).

The median observation duration on Belatacept was 35 months, no patient was lost for follow-up and the total period on therapy analysed was 1194 months. All renal allograft recipients (n = 309) on CNI-based immunosuppression that received their transplant between 1 January, 2010 and 31 December, 2012 formed the control cohort. Of these, 150 also fulfilled the criteria for high cardiovascular risk. No patients were lost for follow-up, the median follow-up was 48 months and the total analysed period of months on therapy was 7309. High cardiovascular risk was defined by the presence of any significant pre-transplant coronary artery disease (CAD) confirmed on angiography, a history of myocardial infarction, peripheral artery disease (PAD) (cardiovascular disease) or stroke (cerebrovascular disease) or the presence of diabetes mellitus in combination with arterial hypertension.

2.2. Endpoints

Efficacy endpoints were renal allograft function as assessed by a change of eGFR on therapy, number of rejection episodes (either confirmed by biopsy or clinically based on an improvement of allograft function after anti-rejection therapy) or graft loss. The estimated glomerular filtration rate (eGFR) was calculated using the abbreviated MDRD formula. ΔeGFR was calculated by dividing the difference between eGFR at last follow-up and the baseline by the number of follow-up years. The safety endpoints were de novo cardiovascular events (new myocardial infarction, newly diagnosed CAD of any stage, newly diagnosed peripheral artery disease), severe infections (defined as infection leading to the admission of the patient to hospital), cytomegalo virus (CMV) reactivation (diagnosed by PCR with or without a clinical CMV infection), BKV reactivation (as determined by PCR in serum and/or urine), de novo malignancy and death. All efficacy and safety endpoints were identified using patients' records.

2.3. Statistics

The reported values represent either medians and interquartile ranges (IQR) or the number of patients and percentages of the respective cohort. Proportions were compared using the Chi^2 or Fisher exact tests. Non-parametric tests were used to compare continuous variables. The factors potentially associated with the eGFR, the eGFR-slope (eGFR), and efficacy and safety parameters were assessed using a Cox regression analysis. In particular, those factors were: Belatacept treatment, recipient age, male gender of the recipient, recipient BMI, a CMV high risk mismatch (D+/R-), the presence of diabetes mellitus or arterial hypertension, the presence of cerebrovascular or cardiovascular disease, the time on renal replacement therapy (RRT) before renal transplantation (RTx), number of previous RTx, number of HLA mismatches, intraoperative urine production (initial diuresis), number of post-operative (PO)—meaning after renal transplantation—hemodialysis sessions (HDs), the absence or presence of steroids at discharge, the presence of serum-creatinine at discharge, the absence or presence of steroids at the last follow-up, the extended criteria donor (ECD) organ, the male sex of the donor, and donor age. A history of rejection was also included, with an exception for the endpoint rejection episodes. Variables with a p-value < 0.05 in univariate analysis were included in the multivariate analysis, where again a p-value < 0.05 was considered statistically significant. The analysis was performed using SPSS Version 24.

3. Results

3.1. Baseline

Baseline data are shown in Table 1. Belatacept patients spent a shorter period of time on renal replacement therapy (RRT) before renal transplantation, were more likely to suffer from CV disease or hypertension and less likely to have diabetes mellitus compared to CNI patients. The baseline data were not significantly different between de novo and converted Belatacept patients, except for the higher proportion of male recipients in de novo patients (17/18 vs. 8/16, $p = 0.003$).

3.2. Renal Transplantation

Concerning renal transplantation (RTx, Table 2), the donor type was significantly different between CNI- and Belatacept-treated patients. This was primarily driven by a higher proportion of living donors and deceased donors that died due to circulatory reasons in the Belatacept group. The Belatacept patients received more organs from female donors and donors were older (61 vs 49.5 years) and had a higher BMI compared to CNI patients. The proportion of patients with intraoperative urine production (initial diuresis) was lower (76% vs. 95%) and the number of hemodialysis sessions (HDs) was significantly higher in Belatacept patients. Hence, renal allograft function at discharge, as assessed by serum creatinine (1.52 vs. 2.20 mg/ml, $p = 0.001$) and eGFR (MDRD) (44.5 vs. 28 mL/min/1.73 m^2, $p = 0.001$), was significantly worse in Belatacept patients.

3.3. Efficacy

The median follow-up (Table 3) was 1462 and 1054 days in CNI and Belatacept patients ($p = 0.084$), respectively. Belatacept was continued in all patients with a maintained graft function during follow-up (31/34). The number of patients on steroids at follow-up and the proportion of hypertensive patients were higher in the Belatacept group.

Table 1. Baseline data of control and Belatacept patients.

	Control (*n* = 150)		Belatacept (*n* = 34)		
	Median/*n*	IQR/(%)	Median/*n*	IQR/(%)	*p*
BMI [kg/m^2]	25.1	22.6–28.4	26.1	22.6–30.6	0.304
Male Sex *n* (%)	37	(24.67)	9	(26.47)	0.826
Age at time of RTx [years]	59.6	49.4–66.8	57.2	38.7–65.4	0.325
Time on RRT [months]	53.8	29.6–80.5	35.6	22.2–52.1	0.006 *
Primary Renal Disease *n* (%)					
Diabetic Nephropathy	51	(34.00)	5	(14.71)	0.031 *
Vascular Nephropathy	25	(16.67)	5	(14.71)	0.768
IgA Nephropathy	7	(4.67)	6	(17.65)	0.017 *
other Glomerulonephritis	18	(12.00)	2	(5.88)	0.377
ADPKD	12	(8.00)	5	(14.71)	0.321
other hereditary disease	2	(1.33)	0	(0.00)	1.000
ANCA Vasculitis	0	(0.00)	0	(0.00)	n.c.
Lupus nephropathy	2	(1.33)	0	(0.00)	1.000
chronic kidney disease NOS	33	(22.00)	11	(32.35)	0.209
Number of previous RTx *n* (%)					0.671
0	114	(76.00)	29	(85.29)	
1	24	(16.00)	4	(11.76)	
2	10	(6.67)	1	(2.94)	
3	1	(0.67)	0	(0.00)	
4	1	(0.67)	0	(0.00)	
Diabetes *n* (%)	85	(56.67)	11	(32.35)	0.009 *
Cerebrovascular disease *n* (%)	12	(8.00)	4	(11.76)	0.503
Cardiovascular disease *n* (%)	113	(75.33)	32	(94.12)	0.016 *
Arterial Hypertension *n* (%)	126	(84.00)	34	(100)	0.014 *

The median and interquartile range (IQR) are depicted except for nominal variables, where the number of patients (*n*) and percentages are shown. *p*-values < 0.05 are marked with an asterisk *. BMI: body mass index, RTx: renal transplantation, RRT: renal replacement therapy, ADPKD: autosomal dominant polycystic kidney disease, ANCA: antineutrophil cytoplasmic antibody, NOS: not otherwise specified, n.c.: not calculated.

Table 2. Data at the time of Renal Transplantation (RTx).

	Control (*n* = 150)		Belatacept (*n* = 34)		
	Median/*n*	IQR/(%)	Median/*n*	IQR/(%)	*p*
Donor Type *n* (%)					
Living donor	6	(4.00)	5	(14.71)	0.032 *
DD (CVA/SAB/SDH)	86	(57.33)	22	(64.71)	0.431
DD (trauma)	41	(27.33)	0	(0.00)	0.001 *
DD (circulatory)	6	(4.00)	5	(14.71)	0.032 *
DD (suicide)	7	(4.67)	2	(5.88)	0.673
DD (other)	4	(2.67)	0	(0.00)	1.000
ECD *n* (%)	65	(43.33)	18	(52.94)	0.309
Male Donor Sex *n* (%)	80	(53.33)	9	(26.47)	0.005 *
Donor Age [years]	49.5	37–66	61	51–68	0.003 *
Donor BMI [kg/m^2]	24.9	22.5–27.7	26.3	24.5–28.6	0.034 *
CMV mismatch *n* (%)					0.947
Donor-/Recipient-	20	(13.33)	5	(14.71)	
Donor-/Recipient+ or Donor+/Recipient+	100	(66.66)	22	(64.71)	
Donor+/Recipient-	30	(20.00)	7	(20.59)	
Number of HLA Mismatches	3	3–5	3	2–5	0.843
Initial Diuresis *n* (%)	143	(95.33)	26	(76.47)	<0.001 *
Number of PO HDs after RTx	0	0–2	1	0–5	0.015 *
On Steroids at discharge *n* (%)	141	(94.00)	34	(100.00)	0.214
S-Creatinine at discharge (mg/dL)	1.52	1.21–2.11	2.20	1.40–2.98	0.001 *
eGFR at discharge (MDRD) (mL/min/1.73 m^2)	44.5	30–9	28	22–51	0.001 *

Median and IQR are depicted except for nominal variables, where the number of patients (*n*) and percentages are shown. *p*-values < 0.05 are marked with an asterisk *. DD: deceased donor, CVA: cerebrovascular event, SAB: subarachnoidal bleeding, SDH: subdural hematoma, ECD: extended criteria donor, CMV mismatch: "–" means sero-negative, "+" means sero-positive, PO HDs: postoperative hemodialysis sessions, RTx: renal transplantation, S-Creatinine: serum creatinine.

Table 3. Data at last follow-up.

	Control ($n = 150$)		Belatacept ($n = 34$)		
	Median/n	IQR/(%)	Median/n	IQR/(%)	p
Follow-up [days]	1462	718–2115	1054	772–1363	0.084
IS-CNI/mTor/Bela n (%)					<0.001 *
none	14	9.33	3	8.82	
Tac	105	70.00	0	0.00	
CsA	25	16.67	0	0.00	
Bela	0	0.00	31	91.17	
mTORi	6	4.00	0	0	
IS-Antimetabolites n (%)					0.221
none	32	21.33	5	14.71	
Mycophenolate Mofetil (MMF)	75	50.00	19	55.88	
Mycophenolic acid (MPA)	16	10.67	7	20.59	
Azathioprine	25	16.67	2	5.88	
other	2	1.33	1	2.94	
IS-On steroids n (%)	71	47.33	28	82.35	<0.001 *
Serum Creatinine (mg/dL)	1.62	1.25–2.36	1.96	1.342.31	0.404
eGFR (MDRD) (mL/min/1.73m^2)	41	27–60	36.5	25–52	0.329
ΔeGFR (MDRD) (mL/min/1.73m^2/year)	−0.89	−6.05–3.02	2.6	−1.85–7.76	0.006*
Cerebrovascular disease n (%)	13	8.67	5	14.71	0.335
Cardiovascular disease n (%)	118	78.67	33	97.06	0.004 *
Arterial Hypertension n (%)	120	80.00	30	88.24	1.000

Median and IQR are depicted except for nominal variables, where the number of patients (n) and percentages are shown. p-values < 0.05 are marked with an asterisk *. Data on cerebro- and cardiovascular diseases show cumulative numbers of events at follow-up. De novo events are depicted in Table 5. IS-CNI/mTOR/Bela: immunosuppression concerning tacrolimus (Tac), cyclosporine A (CsA), Belatacept (Bela), mTOR inhibitors (mTORi). IS-Antimetabolites: immunosuppression concerning mycophenolate mofetil (MMF), mycophenolic acid (MPA), azathioprine (Aza).

Concerning efficacy, renal allograft function as assessed by serum creatinine/eGFR improved in Belatacept-treated patients and slightly worsened in CNI patients, yielding a non-significant difference between the groups at follow-up (in contrast to the time of discharge after RTx). ΔeGFR of the patients on Belatacept was positive compared to CNI patients (+2.60 vs. −0.89 mL/min/1.73 m^2/year, p = 0.006). The median ΔeGFR in the whole cohort (Belatacept plus CNI patients, n = 184) was + 0.35 mL/min/1.73 m^2 (Table 4). The only factor significantly associated with a ΔeGFR above the median in the multivariate model (adjusted for significant factors in the univariate analysis including Belatacept treatment, recipient BMI, number of postoperative HDs, the presence of serum-creatinine at discharge and donors' age) was Belatacept treatment (HR 4.35, 95%CI 2.387–7.926, p < 0.001, Table 4). Rejection episodes and graft loss were not significantly different between Belatacept and CNI patients (Table 5). Neither Belatacept nor any other parameter was a significant risk factor for rejection in the univariate Cox regression. Univariate correlated risk factors for graft loss were a higher recipient BMI (HR 1.126, 95%CI 1.038–1.222, p = 0.004), number of postoperative HDs (HR 1.178, 95%CI 1.041–1.333, p = 0.009) and higher serum-creatinine at discharge (HR 1.593, 95%CI 1.179–2.166, p =0.03). BMI (HR 1.116, 95%CI 1.003–1.242, p = 0.043) and number of postoperative HDs (HR 1.253, 95%CI 1.027–1.530, p = 0.027) remained significant after multivariate adjustments. Belatacept was not a risk factor for graft loss (HR 0.987, 95%CI 0.283–3.417, p = 0.980).

Table 4. Cox regression for eGFR better than the median (+0.35 mL/min/1.73 m^2/year) at last follow-up. We calculated univariate hazard ratios (HR) for risk factors. All significant univariate risk factors were used in the multivariate model. BMI: body mass index, RTx: renal transplantation, PO HD: postoperative hemodialysis session, ECD: extended criteria donor.

Factor	Univariate Analysis			Multivariate Analysis [1]		
	HR	95%-CI	*p*	HR	95%-CI	*p*
Belatacept	5.629	3.239–9.783	<0.001 *	4.350	2.387–7.926	<0.001 *
Recipient Age	1.012	0.994–1.030	0.184			
Male recipient Sex	1.435	0.863–2.388	0.164			
BMI	1.063	1.018–1.111	0.006*	1.024	0.979–1.072	0.300
Diabetes	0.799	0.524–1.218	0.297			
Cerebrovascular disease	1.365	0.704–2.646	0.357			
Cardiovascular disease	1.050	0.624–1.767	0.853			
Arterial hypertension	0.846	0.475–1.508	0.572			
Number of previous RTx	0.741	0.499–1.098	0.135			
HLA mismatch	0.649	0.416–1.011	0.056			
Initial Diuresis	0.502	0.200–1.260	0.142			
Number of PO HDs	1.117	1.051–1.187	<0.001 *	1.037	0.953–1.129	0.395
Steroid at discharge	2.424	0.760–7.731	0.134			
Creatinine at discharge	1.437	1.238–1.667	<0.001 *	1.218	0.885–1.675	0.226
ECD	1.357	0.891–2.066	0.154			
Male Donor Sex	1.131	0.742–1.725	0.566			
Donor Age	1.018	1.005–1.032	0.007 *	1.004	0.990–1.019	0.546

[1] adjusted for Belatacept treatment, BMI, number of postoperative (PO) hemodialysis sessions (HDs), eGFR at discharge and donor age. *p*-values < 0.05 are marked with an asterisk *.

Table 5. Efficacy and safety endpoints at last follow-up. *p*-values < 0.05 are marked with an asterisk *. CMV: cytomegalo virus, BKV: polyoma virus.

	CNI (*n* = 150)		Belatacept (*n* = 34)			
EFFICACY	*n*	%	*n*	%	*p*	Log-Rank
Rejection	13	8.7	4	11.8	0.524	0.295
Graft loss	17	11.3	3	8.8	1.000	0.980
SAFETY						
De novo CV events	5	3.33	1	2.94	1.000	0.550
Severe Infection	35	23.3	13	38.2	0.074	0.013*
Type of severe Infection					0.003 *	
none	115	76.7	21	61.8		
Diarrhea	1	0.7	3	8.8		
Urinary tract infection	15	10.0	6	17.6		
Pneumonia	15	10.0	1	2.9		
Sepsis	4	2.7	3	8.8		
Any CMV reactivation	60	40.0	16	47.1	0.450	0.932
BKV reactivation in serum	16	10.7	7	20.6	0.148	0.136
BKV reactivation in urine	37	24.7	10	29.4	0.567	0.718
Malignancy	2	1.3	0	0.0	1.000	0.650
Death	22	14.7	4	11.8	0.790	0.861
Cause of Death					0.921	
unknown	5	3.3	1	2.9		
Sepsis	7	4.7	2	5.9		
Cardiac	7	4.7	1	2.9		
Malignancy	2	1.3	0	0.0		
Stroke	1	0.7	0	0.0		

3.4. Safety

We found no difference between CNI- and Belatacept-treated patients concerning all safety endpoints, except for severe infection (Figure 1, Table 5).

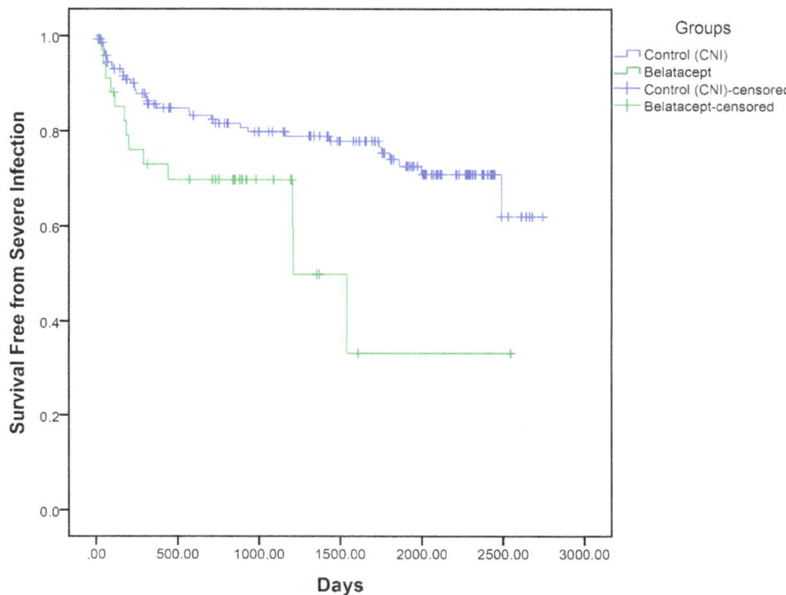

Figure 1. KM-Plot for severe infection (Log-Rank p = 0.013), defined as infection leading to the admission of the patient to hospital.

Concerning severe infections, defined as infections leading to the admission of the patient to hospital, we found more infections in the Belatacept group (38.2 vs. 23.3%, Log-Rank p = 0.013). The type of severe infection also differed between the groups, with a higher proportion of diarrhoea, urinary tract infections and sepsis, but fewer instances of pneumonia, in Belatacept-treated patients. In the univariate Cox regression analysis, Belatacept treatment, number of postoperative HDs, the presence of creatinine at discharge, ECD and donor age were significant risk factors for severe infections (Table 6), while the male sex of the recipient was a protective factor. In the multivariate analysis, no risk factor remained significant (including Belatacept), whereas the male sex of the recipient remained a significant protective factor for severe infection in our cohort. It is noteworthy that Belatacept was not a significant risk factor in any Cox regression analysis for all other safety endpoints. Risk factors for CMV reactivation were number of postoperative HDs (HR 1.123, 95%CI 1.050–1.201, p = 0.001) and the presence of serum-creatinine at discharge (HR 1.335, 95%CI 1.087–1.638, p = 0.006) of which none remained significant in a multivariate model. A risk factor for BKV reactivation in patients' plasma was treatment with steroids at follow-up (HR 3.358, 95%CI 1.246–9.051, p = 0.017) whereas the male sex of the donor was protective (HR 0.362, 95%CI 0.142–0.917, p = 0.032). The treatment with steroids at follow-up remained significant in the multivariate model (HR 2.850, 95%CI 1.042–7.796, p = 0.041). BKV reactivation in patients' urine was significantly correlated with recipient (HR 1.041, 95%CI 1.013–1.069, p = 0.004) and donor age (HR 1.020, 95%CI 1.001–1.038, p = 0.036), of which recipient age remained multivariately significant (HR 1.033, 95%CI 1.003–1.064, p = 0.029).

Table 6. Cox regression for severe infection. All the significant risk factors from the univariate Cox-Regression are shown and were included in the multivariate analysis. *p*-values < 0.05 are marked with an asterisk *.

Factor	Univariate Analysis			Multivariate Analysis [1]		
	HR	95%-CI	*p*	HR	95%-CI	*p*
Belatacept	2.236	1.163–4.301	0.016 *	1.363	0.659–2.819	0.403
Male recipient Sex	0.548	0.305–0.983	0.044 *	0.459	0.242–0.870	0.017 *
Number of PO HDs	1.156	1.062–1.259	0.001 *	1.057	0.939–1.189	0.358
Creatinine at discharge	1.602	1.255–2.044	<0.001 *	1.131	0.628–2.037	0.682
ECD	2.867	1.578–5.209	0.001 *	1.373	0.488–3.858	0.548
Donor Age	1.032	1.012–1.052	0.002 *	1.019	0.985–1.054	0.287

[1] adjusted for belatacept treatment, male recipient sex, number of post-operative (PO) hemodialysis sessions (HDs), creatinine ad discharge, extended criteria donor (ECD), donor age.

The only univariate risk factor for the safety endpoint de novo cardiovascular events was pre-existing cerebrovascular disease (HR 6.144, 95%CI 1.026–36.798, *p* = 0.047). All other parameters, and especially Belatacept (HR 1.938, 95%CI 0.214–17.591, *p* = 0.557), were not significant. Concerning malignancy, we found no significant factor in the univariate Cox regression. Univariate risk factors for death were recipient age (HR 1.044, 95%CI 1.006–1.083, *p* = 0.023), HLA mismatch (HR 2.27, 95%CI 1.011–5.099, *p* = 0.047) and the presence of creatinine at discharge (HR 1.350, 95%CI 1.018–1.791, *p* = 0.037). Recipient age was the only significant risk factor for death in multivariate Cox regression (HR 1.036, 95%CI 1.001–1.074, *p* = 0.046).

4. Discussion

We conducted a retrospective cohort study of renal allograft recipients at high cardiovascular risk either treated with a Belatacept- or CNI-based immunosuppressive regimen. eGFR improved with Belatacept treatment, but slightly decreased during CNI therapy and, in the multivariate analysis, Belatacept treatment was the only significant factor for the improvement of ΔeGFR. This is in line with the BENEFIT and BENEFIT-EXT studies, which also demonstrated an increase of GFR over a follow-up of seven years [12–14]. However, the CNI comparator cohort consisted of cyclosporine A-treated patients only, whereas our group was mainly treated with tacrolimus (68% of patients). Our recipients were of a similar age (56 years) to recipients in BENEFIT-EXT, but older compared to BENEFIT (43 years). Additionally, our CV high risk cohorts consisted of more diabetic patients (CNI group: 57%, Belatacept group: 32% vs. BENEFIT: 15%, BENEFIT-EXT: 16%) and had worse donor characteristics (living donors: CNI group 4%, Belatacept group 15% vs. BENEFIT 58%, BENEFIT-EXT not reported). Furthermore, the BENEFIT studies did not report the number of patients suffering from established cardiovascular disease, which was substantial in our Belatacept (94%) and CNI patients (75%). Nevertheless, and although Belatacept patients had inferior renal allograft function at the time of discharge after transplantation, serum creatinine levels and eGFR were similar at follow-up in this high CV risk cohort compared to CNI-treated patients. Bertrand et al. [15] and Le Meur et al. [16] reported similar results in 17 and 25 patients treated with Belatacept, because of vascular damage and CNI intolerance.

Belatacept was not associated with an increased risk of rejection in our patients. BENEFIT-EXT [17] reported a higher risk in Belatacept-treated patients, whereas BENEFIT [18] found no significant difference. However, our CNI cohort was mainly treated with tacrolimus, which is generally accepted to have a slightly higher immunosuppressive potential, rather than cyclosporine A as in the BENEFIT(-EXT) studies. Belatacept was not a risk factor for graft loss in our cohort (HR 0.987, 95%CI 0.283–3.417, *p* = 0.980), which is in line with the literature [17,18].

Concerning safety and in contrast to Florman et al. [13], we found that Belatacept treatment was associated with an increased incidence of severe infections in the univariate Cox regression. The most obvious differences were higher event rates of diarrhoea, urinary tract infection and sepsis. Sepsis as an endpoint has not been reported in any previous studies of Belatacept patients. In line with our data, gastroenteritis and urinary tract infections were numerically higher in the switch studies [7,8,19]. However, in the multivariate regression analysis, Belatacept treatment was not associated with an increase of this endpoint. One explanation for the higher incidence of gastroenteritis (diarrhoea) might be the more frequent use of mycophenlate in Belatacept patients (76.47 vs. 60.67%; 1.26–fold more), which is known to have such gastrointestinal side-effects. The reason for this is that physicians tend to prescribe the triple combination of mycophenolic acid, steroids and Belatacept, as only this regimen was approved for renal allograft recipients. However, it cannot be ruled out that some examples of mycophenolate-associated diarrhoea have been misdiagnosed as infectious diarrhoea, therefore increasing the proportion of diarrhoea in Belatacept patients compared to CNI patients, although the fold-change of diarrhoea (8.8 vs. 0.7%, 12.57-fold) substantially exceeds the use of mycophenlate in the Belatacept compared to the CNI group (1.26-fold, see above). Additionally, the proportion of mycophenolate-treated patients in the switch studies was almost identical between the groups (and higher compared to our data (approx. 94%)) [7,8,19].

In our cohort, Belatacept treatment was not a risk factor for CMV reactivation, malignancy or death. This is in line with the published data cited above. Additionally, Belatacept treatment was not a risk factor for BKV reactivations either in patients' serum or urine. Unfortunately, data on these endpoints were not reported in the BENEFIT and BENEFIT-EXT studies. Nevertheless, our data is in line with the phase II studies, which showed only slightly increased cumulative incidence rates (0.85 vs. 0 [19]) and events (4 vs. 0% [8] and 2 vs. 0% [7]) in Belatacept patients. Unfortunately, no statistics were calculated in these studies.

Published data suggest a beneficial impact of Belatacept on arterial stiffness and metabolic parameters (e.g., arterial hypertension and lipid profile) or post-transplant diabetes mellitus. The authors concluded that this could improve kidney transplant recipients' survival by reducing events related to those factors [9,17,18,20]. However, available data from the long-term outcomes of these studies do not show a significant difference in severely adverse events (including cardiac or vascular disorders) [12,14]. Concerning patients with high cardiovascular risk, the only study that has been published so far was a post-hoc analysis of patients with pre-existing diabetes of the BENEFIT and BENEFIT-EXT cohorts. Patient survival and renal function were numerically but not significantly higher in Belatacept patients at 12 months' follow-up and, unfortunately, cardiovascular events were not reported [8]. Hence, to the best of our knowledge, this is the first report on cardiovascular events in Belatacept compared to CNI-treated patients. We found no difference between Belatacept- and CNI-treated patients concerning de novo cardiovascular events with a cumulative follow-up of 1194 months in Belatacept (n = 35) and 7309 months in CNI patients (n = 150).

Our study has limitations. Firstly, this is a retrospective study, which by nature does not provide the same data quality as a prospective design. Secondly, the size of the study population is relatively small, as we included only 34 Belatacept patients and 150 CNI patients as a comparator. Thirdly, the baseline characteristics of time on RRT, primary renal disease, diabetes, cardiovascular disease and arterial hypertension were different between our two populations (Table 1) and it is possible that statistical methods were not able to correct appropriately for this issue. Fourthly, the median time of follow-up was longer in CNI patients (Belatacept: 1054 vs. CNI: 1462 days) but not statistically significant (p = 0.084). From our point of view, the duration of follow-up is still significant, although one might argue that a longer follow-up would have been beneficial, especially for the end point "cardiovascular event". However, the number of studies that have published data of renal allograft recipients on Belatacept-based immunosuppression is generally limited. In total, until the end of 2014, the data of 521 Belatacept patients, which were compared to CNI-treated controls, were published [21]. Recently, one study of 17 Belatacept patients matched to 18 control patients, and two studies of 25 and 6 cases that were converted from CNI to Belatacept without a control population, were published [15,16,22]. The randomized controlled trials BENEFIT [18], BENEFIT-EXT [17] and the switch study [8] originally reported one-year results of 181, 129 and 81 belatacept patients compared to a CNI-treated cohort of similar size. Hence, we believe that our cohort size and follow-up period is considerable and contributes information in a real world setting.

In conclusion, we believe that Belatacept is an efficient, beneficial and safe option for renal allograft recipients at high cardiovascular risk. In our cohort, Belatacept treatment was associated with a superior graft function compared to a CNI-treated cohort and was not a risk factor for renal allograft rejection, -loss, severe infection, CMV- or BKV-reactivation, malignancy or death.

Author Contributions: Conceptualization: H.N.; Data curation: H.N., I.L.-L., M.E., F.P., N.P., J.M., H.S.-M., M.R., P.S.; Formal analysis: H.N., M.E., F.P., N.P., J.M., M.R.; Methodology: H.N., J.K., G.M.; Project administration: H.N., G.M.; Software: H.N.; Supervision: H.N.; Validation: H.N., I.L.-L., M.R.; Writing-original draft: H.N., M.R., P.S., I.E.E., G.M.; Writing-review & editing: H.N., I.E.E., G.M.

Funding: This research received no external funding.

Conflicts of Interest: The authors declare no conflict of interest.

Abbreviations

BKV	polyoma virus
BMI	body mass index
CAD	coronary artery disease
CD	cluster of differentiation
CMV	cytomegalo virus
CNI	calcineurin inhibitor
CV	cardiovascular
CVA	cerebrovascular event
DD	deceased donor
ECD	extended criteria donor
eGFR	estimated glomerular filtration rate
HD	hemodialysis
HLA	human leukocyte antigen
HR	hazard ratio
IQR	interquartile range
mTORi	mammalian target of rapamycin inhibitor
PAD	peripheral artery disease
PCR	polymerase chain reaction
PO	post-operative after renal transplantation
RRT	renal replacement therapy
RTx	renal transplantation
SAB	subarachnoideal bleeding
SDH	subdural hematoma
95%CI	95% confidence interval

References

1. Lamb, K.E.; Lodhi, S.; Meier-Kriesche, H.U. Long-term renal allograft survival in the United States: A critical reappraisal. *Am. J. Transplant.* **2011**, *11*, 450–462. [CrossRef] [PubMed]
2. Stallone, G.; Infante, B.; Grandaliano, G.; Gesualdo, L. Management of side effects of sirolimus therapy. *Transplantation* **2009**, *87* (Suppl. 8), S23–S26. [CrossRef]
3. Ekberg, H.; Tedesco-Silva, H.; Demirbas, A.; Vítko, S.; Nashan, B.; Gürkan, A.; Margreiter, R.; Hugo, C.; Grinyó, J.M.; Frei, U.; et al. Reduced exposure to calcineurin inhibitors in renal transplantation. *N. Engl. J. Med.* **2007**, *357*, 2562–2575. [CrossRef] [PubMed]
4. Latek, R.; Fleener, C.; Lamian, V.; Kulbokas, E., 3rd; Davis, P.M.; Suchard, S.J.; Curran, M.; Vincenti, F.; Townsend, R. Assessment of belatacept-mediated costimulation blockade through evaluation of CD80/86-receptor saturation. *Transplantation* **2009**, *87*, 926–933. [CrossRef] [PubMed]

5. Vincenti, F.; Larsen, C.P.; Alberu, J.; Bresnahan, B.; Garcia, V.D.; Kothari, J.; Lang, P.; Urrea, E.M.; Massari, P.; Mondragon-Ramirez, G.; et al. Three-year outcomes from BENEFIT: A randomized: Active-controlled: Parallel-group study in adult kidney transplant recipients. *Am. J. Transplant.* **2012**, *12*, 210–217. [CrossRef] [PubMed]

6. Vincenti, F.; Rostaing, L.; Grinyo, J.; Rice, K.; Steinberg, S.; Gaite, L.; Moal, M.C.; Mondragon-Ramirez, G.A.; Kothari, J.; Polinsky, M.S.; et al. Belatacept and long-term outcomes in kidney transplantation. *N. Engl. J. Med.* **2016**, *374*, 333–343. [CrossRef] [PubMed]

7. Grinyo, J.; Alberu, J.; Contieri, F.L.; Manfro, R.C.; Mondragon, G.; Nainan, G.; Rial Mdel, C.; Steinberg, S.; Vincenti, F.; Dong, Y.; et al. Improvement in renal function in kidney transplant recipients switched from cyclosporine or tacrolimus to belatacept: 2-year results from the long-term extension of a phase II study. *Transpl. Int.* **2012**, *25*, 1059–1064. [CrossRef] [PubMed]

8. Rostaing, L.; Massari, P.; Garcia, V.D.; Mancilla-Urrea, E.; Nainan, G.; del Carmen Rial, M.; Steinberg, S.; Vincenti, F.; Shi, R.; Di Russo, G.; et al. Switching from calcineurin inhibitor-based regimens to a belatacept-based regimen in renal transplant recipients: A randomized phase II study. *Clin. J. Am. Soc. Nephrol.* **2011**, *6*, 430–439. [CrossRef]

9. Melilli, E.; Manonelles, A.; Montero, N.; Grinyo, J.; Martinez-Castelao, A.; Bestard, O.; Cruzado, J. Impact of immunosuppressive therapy on arterial stiffness in kidney transplantation: Are all treatments the same? *Clin. Kidney J.* **2018**, *11*, 413–421. [CrossRef]

10. Melilli, E.; Bestard-Matamoros, O.; Manonelles-Montero, A.; Sala-Bassa, N.; Mast, R.; Grinyo-Boira, J.M.; Cruzado, J.M. Arterial stiffness in kidney transplantation: A single center case-control study comparing belatacept versus calcineurin inhibitor immunosuppressive based regimen. *Nefrologia* **2015**, *35*, 58–65. [CrossRef]

11. Seibert, F.S.; Steltzer, J.; Melilli, E.; Grannas, G.; Pagonas, N.; Bauer, F.; Zidek, W.; Grinyo, J.; Westhoff, T.H. Differential impact of belatacept and cyclosporine A on central aortic blood pressure and arterial stiffness after renal transplantation. *Clin. Transplant.* **2014**, *28*, 1004–1009. [CrossRef] [PubMed]

12. Durrbach, A.; Pestana, J.M.; Florman, S.; Del Carmen Rial, M.; Rostaing, L.; Kuypers, D.; Matas, A.; Wekerle, T.; Polinsky, M.; Meier-Kriesche, H.U.; et al. Long-term outcomes in belatacept- versus cyclosporine-treated recipients of extended criteria donor kidneys: Final results from benefit-ext: A phase III randomized study. *Am. J. Transplant.* **2016**, *16*, 3192–3201. [CrossRef] [PubMed]

13. Florman, S.; Becker, T.; Bresnahan, B.; Chevaile-Ramos, A.; Carvalho, D.; Grannas, G.; Muehlbacher, F.; O'Connell, P.J.; Meier-Kriesche, H.U.; Larsen, C.P. Efficacy and safety outcomes of extended criteria donor kidneys by subtype: Subgroup analysis of BENEFIT-EXT at 7 years after transplant. *Am. J. Transplant.* **2017**, *17*, 180–190. [CrossRef] [PubMed]

14. Rostaing, L.; Vincenti, F.; Grinyo, J.; Rice, K.M.; Bresnahan, B.; Steinberg, S.; Gang, S.; Gaite, L.E.; Moal, M.C.; Mondragon-Ramirez, G.A.; et al. Long-term belatacept exposure maintains efficacy and safety at 5 years: Results from the long-term extension of the BENEFIT study. *Am. J. Transplant.* **2013**, *13*, 2875–2883. [CrossRef] [PubMed]

15. Bertrand, D.; Cheddani, L.; Etienne, I.; Francois, A.; Hanoy, M.; Laurent, C.; Lebourg, L.; Le Roy, F.; Lelandais, L.; Loron, M.C.; et al. Belatacept rescue therapy in kidney transplant recipients with vascular lesions: A case control study. *Am. J. Transplant.* **2017**, *17*, 2937–2944. [CrossRef] [PubMed]

16. Le Meur, Y.; Aulagnon, F.; Bertrand, D.; Heng, A.E.; Lavaud, S.; Caillard, S.; Longuet, H.; Sberro-Soussan, R.; Doucet, L.; Grall, A.; et al. Effect of an early switch to belatacept among calcineurin inhibitor-intolerant graft recipients of kidneys from extended-criteria donors. *Am. J. Transplant.* **2016**, *16*, 2181–2186. [CrossRef]

17. Durrbach, A.; Pestana, J.M.; Pearson, T.; Vincenti, F.; Garcia, V.D.; Campistol, J.; Rial Mdel, C.; Florman, S.; Block, A.; Di Russo, G.; et al. A phase III study of belatacept versus cyclosporine in kidney transplants from extended criteria donors (BENEFIT-EXT study). *Am. J. Transplant.* **2010**, *10*, 547–557. [CrossRef] [PubMed]

18. Vincenti, F.; Charpentier, B.; Vanrenterghem, Y.; Rostaing, L.; Bresnahan, B.; Darji, P.; Massari, P.; Mondragon-Ramirez, G.A.; Agarwal, M.; Di Russo, G.; et al. A phase III study of belatacept-based immunosuppression regimens versus cyclosporine in renal transplant recipients (BENEFIT study). *Am. J. Transplant.* **2010**, *10*, 535–546. [CrossRef]

19. Grinyo, J.M.; Del Carmen Rial, M.; Alberu, J.; Steinberg, S.M.; Manfro, R.C.; Nainan, G.; Vincenti, F.; Jones-Burton, C.; Kamar, N. Safety and efficacy outcomes 3 years after switching to belatacept from a calcineurin inhibitor in kidney transplant recipients: Results from a phase 2 randomized trial. *Am. J. Kidney Dis.* **2017**, *69*, 587–594. [CrossRef]
20. Wissing, K.M.; Pipeleers, L. Obesity: Metabolic syndrome and diabetes mellitus after renal transplantation: Prevention and treatment. *Transplant. Rev. (Orlando)* **2014**, *28*, 37–46. [CrossRef]
21. Masson, P.; Henderson, L.; Chapman, J.R.; Craig, J.C.; Webster, A.C. Belatacept for kidney transplant recipients. *Cochrane Database Syst Rev* **2014**. [CrossRef] [PubMed]
22. Gupta, G.; Regmi, A.; Kumar, D.; Posner, S.; Posner, M.P.; Sharma, A.; Cotterell, A.; Bhati, C.S.; Kimball, P.; Massey, H.D.; et al. Safe conversion from tacrolimus to belatacept in high immunologic risk kidney transplant recipients with allograft dysfunction. *Am. J. Transplant.* **2015**, *15*, 2726–2731. [CrossRef] [PubMed]

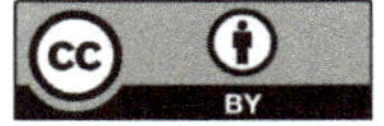

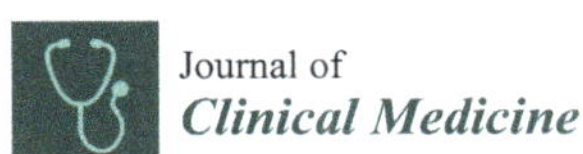
Journal of
Clinical Medicine

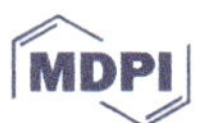

Article

Analysis of the Effects of Day-Time vs. Night-Time Surgery on Renal Transplant Patient Outcomes

Nesrin Sugünes [1], Anna Bichmann [2], Nadine Biernath [1], Robert Peters [1], Klemens Budde [3], Lutz Liefeldt [3], Thorsten Schlomm [1] and Frank Friedersdorff [1,*]

[1] Department of Urology, Charité-Universitätsmedizin Berlin, Corporate Member of Freie Universität Berlin, Humboldt-Universität zu Berlin, and Berlin Institute of Health, Charitéplatz 1, 10117 Berlin, Germany
[2] Department of Anesthesiology and Operative Intensive Care Medicine, Charité-Universitätsmedizin Berlin, Corporate Member of Freie Universität Berlin, Humboldt-Universität zu Berlin, and Berlin Institute of Health, Charitéplatz 1, 10117 Berlin, Germany
[3] Department of Nephrology, Charité-Universitätsmedizin Berlin, Corporate Member of Freie Universität Berlin, Humboldt-Universität zu Berlin, and Berlin Institute of Health, 10117 Berlin, Germany
*   Correspondence: frank.friedersdorff@charite.de

Received: 30 June 2019; Accepted: 12 July 2019; Published: 18 July 2019

Abstract: Sleep deprivation and disruption of the circadian rhythms could impair individual surgical performance and decision making. For this purpose, this study identified potential confounding factors on surgical renal transplant patient outcomes during day and night. Our retrospective cohort study of 215 adult renal cadaver transplant recipients, of which 132 recipients were allocated in the "day-time" group and 83 recipients in the "night-time" group, primarily stratified the patients into two cohorts, depending on the start time. Within a 24 h operational system, "day-time" was considered as being from 8 a.m. to 8 p.m. and "night-time" from 8 p.m. to 8 a.m.. Primary outcomes examined patient and graft survival after three months and one year. Secondary outcomes included the presence of acute rejection (AR) and delayed graft function (DGF), as well as the rate of postoperative complications. In log-rank testing, "day-time" surgery was associated with a significantly higher risk of patient death ($p = 0.003$), whereas long-term graft survival was unaffected by the operative time of day. The mean cold ischemia time (CIT), which was 12.4 ± 5.3 h in the "night-time" group, was significantly longer compared to 10.7 ± 3.6 for those during the day ($p = 0.01$). We observed that "night-time" kidney recipients experienced more wound complications. From our single-centre data, we conclude that night-time kidney transplantation does not increase the risk of adverse events or predispose the patient to a worse outcome. Nevertheless, further research is required to explore the effect of fatigue on nocturnal surgical performance.

Keywords: night-time renal transplantation; graft survival; patient survival/outcome; surgical complications

---

1. Introduction

Kidney transplant outcomes have improved in recent years through novel technical approaches and immunosuppressive therapy [1–4]. There is still a deleterious impact of surgical complications on graft and patient survival [5,6]. Several risk factors of surgical complications have been identified, including donor and recipient characteristics, organ recovery and surgical implantation techniques [7]. Recipients with a prolonged cold ischemia time (CIT) have a greater risk for delayed graft function (DGF) and diminished long-term allograft survival [8]. To reduce CIT, surgery is initiated at any time of the day to preserve the organ quality. Further risk factors which are detrimental for patient outcome are human factors, including physical and mental fatigue and sleep deprivation, which are known to affect communication, attention and situational awareness, as well as psychomotor function [9,10].

It has been hypothesized that sleep deprivation reduces the performance of surgeons by affecting cognitive and fine motor skills [11,12]. In a technically demanding field, such as renal transplantation, meticulous preparation and excellent suturing techniques are required to prevent vascular and urologic complications [7]. The impact of physician fatigue on the medical error rate and clinical outcomes has been actively researched [13–15]. A number of studies demonstrated that operative outcomes were not related to sleep deprivation [16–18], whereas others link mental fatigue to surgical complication rates after general procedures [19]; and mortality after liver transplants [20]. To our knowledge, the literature regarding the impact of night-time surgery on outcomes after kidney transplantation is underrepresented and recent studies have reported conflicting results [21–24]. For this purpose, we conducted a retrospective cohort study to examine the association between the time of day of transplantation surgery (night-time vs. day-time) on surgical renal transplant patient outcomes. The primary outcomes examined were patient and graft survival after three months and one year. Secondary outcomes included the presence of acute rejection (AR) and DGF and other postoperative complications. We hypothesize, that renal transplantation surgery performed during the night-time would have inferior outcomes compared to those performed during the day.

2. Methods

We performed a retrospective cohort study of all adult patients undergoing cadaver renal transplantation at Charité University Hospital Campus Mitte, between 01.01.2011 and 31.12.14. Data on kidney transplantation and operative variables, as well as follow-up data, were obtained retrospectively from internal SAP (System, Anwendung, Produkte) and national TBase (Kidney Transplant Information System) electronic databases. The entire analysis was in adherence with correct scientific research work terms of the Charité Medical University of Berlin including full anonymization of patient data ('Good Scientific Practice', version 29/03/18).

2.1. Study Population

Transplants were stratified by the operative time of day. "Day-time" surgery was defined as surgery that started between 8:00 a.m. and 8:00 p.m. and "night-time" surgery was defined as surgery that started between 8:00 p.m. and 8:00 a.m. Twelve surgeons performed all the transplantations using standard surgical techniques. Kidneys were placed either in the right or left iliac fossa via an extraperitoneal approach. The renal graft vessels were anastomosed end-to-side to the recipient external or common iliac vessels. In all cases, except for one patient with urinary diversions (ileal conduit), a standard Lich–Gregoir ureteroneocystostomy was performed. A double-J ureteral stent was systematically inserted and removed six weeks later, followed by a urethral catheter for ten days postoperatively. All recipients received intravenous prophylactic antibiotics at the time of transplant. Graft function was monitored by Doppler ultrasound scanning, serum creatinine level and urine output measurements. The routine immunosuppression protocol that was initiated consisted of a triple regimen, including calcineurin inhibitors or a mammalian target of rapamycin inhibitors, mycophenolate mofetil (MMF), and steroids.

2.2. Data Collection

Patient and donor demographics and clinical data were collected by chart review. The parameters evaluated in this study were, recipient characteristics of age, gender, body mass index (BMI), comorbidities (hypertension, diabetes mellitus, cardiovascular disease, stroke and peripheral vascular disease), previous abdominal surgery, causation of end-stage renal disease, previous transplantation, duration of pre-transplant dialysis, and human leukocyte antigen (HLA) mismatches. The donor features were age, gender, BMI, site of donor kidney, number of graft arteries and the presence of graft vessels atherosclerosis. Perioperative factors included the surgeon's experience (consultant, resident), cold and warm ischemia time (WIT), and incidence of intraoperative complications. CIT was defined as the time between the start of cold perfusion and removal of the renal allograft from ice. Warm ischemia time was defined as the time between the placement of the renal allograft into the iliac fossa of the recipient until revascularization of the kidney occurred.

2.3. Outcome Measures

The primary outcomes examined were patient and graft survival after three months and one year, respectively. Secondary outcomes included the presence of AR and DGF, as well as the rate of postoperative complications. Postoperative complications were examined for the first three months after surgery and defined according to the Clavien–Dindo classification system [20].

2.4. Statistical Analysis

Univariate comparisons were performed using the Chi-Square test or Fisher exact test for categorical variables. Continuous variables were tested with the non-paired Student t-test and the Mann–Whitney-U test for data with non-normal distribution. Categorical variables were displayed as n (%) and continuous variables mean ± standard deviation (SD); and nonparametric distribution as median (minimum-maximum). Patient and allograft survival rates were estimated using the Kaplan–Meier method and comparisons of survival rates were performed using the log-rank test. For all statistical measures, a p-value below 0.05 was considered statistically significant. Statistical analyses were performed using SPSS software (SPSS Inc., version 25, Armonk, NY, USA).

3. Results

The baseline characteristics and operative parameters in the two groups stratified according to the time surgery was performed are presented in Table 1. The two groups were similar with respect to most of the baseline characteristics, except for the higher distribution of male donors for the "day-time" group ($p = 0.05$). The mean CIT was 12.4 ± 5.3 h in the "night-time" group compared with 10.7 ± 3.6 for the "day-time" cohort ($p = 0.01$). The total operative time from skin incision to wound closure was similar in kidney transplants performed at all times. Considering the surgical expertise, 76.5% of "day-time" procedures were performed by a consultant compared to 72.3% during the "night-time" ($p = 0.49$). A total of six intraoperative surgical complications occurred in the overall cohort of 215 recipients (2.8%): renal artery stenosis ($n = 2$), renal vein injury ($n = 2$), renal vein thrombosis ($n = 1$) and iatrogenic bladder perforation ($n = 1$), which were immediately treated. The difference in incidence of intraoperative surgical complication was statistically insignificant with 3.8% ($n = 5$) during the day and 1.2% ($n = 1$) during the night ($p = 0.34$). We observed a higher incidence of DGF nocturnal operations with 54.2% compared to 47.7% in the "day-time" group ($p = 0.35$). The incidence of AR was 25% for "night-time" compared to 22% for "day-time" allograft recipients ($p = 0.57$). Table 2 shows patient outcomes.

Table 1. Recipient and donor characteristics and operative details. Results are presented as mean and standard deviations or as absolute and relative frequencies; h—hours; min—minutes; ESRD—end-stage renal disease; * statistically significant.

Donor Characteristics	All ($n = 215$)	8:00 a.m.–8:00 p.m. ($n = 132$)	8:00 p.m.–8:00 a.m. ($n = 83$)	p-Value
Age (years)	54.2 ± 14.8	55.2 ± 15.1	52.5 ± 14.3	0.19
Male gender	114 (53.0%)	77 (58.3%)	37 (44.6%)	0.05
BMI (kg/m^2)	25.8 ± 4.4	25.8 ± 4.2	25.8 ± 4.8	0.88
Right kidney side	107 (49.8%)	66 (50.0%)	41 (49.4%)	0.93
Multiple renal arteries (%)	45 (20.9%)	28 (21.2%)	17 (20.5%)	0.90
Atherosclerosis of graft vessels	128 (59.5%)	77 (58.3%)	51 (61.4%)	0.65
Recipient Characteristics				
Age (years)	53.3 ± 14.7	54.6 ± 14.6	51.1 ±14.7	0.12
Age > 65 years	64 (29.8%)	44 (33.3%)	20 (24.1%)	0.15

Table 1. *Cont.*

Donor Characteristics	All (n = 215)	8:00 a.m.–8:00 p.m. (n = 132)	8:00 p.m.–8:00 a.m. (n = 83)	p-Value
Male gender	120 (55.8%)	78 (59.1%)	42 (50.6%)	0.22
BMI (kg/m^2)	25.8 ± 4.4	26.2 ± 4.4	25.2 ± 4.5	0.12
Cause of ESRD				
Glomerulonephritis	85 (39.5%)	52 (39.4%)	33 (39.8%)	
Hypertension/renovascular	41 (19.1%)	25 (18.9%)	16 (19.3%)	
Polycystic kidney disease	31 (14.4%)	20 (15.2%)	11 (13.3%)	
Diabetes mellitus	16 (7.4%)	10 (7.6%)	6 (7.2%)	
Interstitial nephritis	8 (3.7%)	5 (3.8%)	3 (3.6%)	
System diseases	8 (3.7%)	4 (3.0%)	4 (4.8%)	
Reflux nephropathy	6 (2.8%)	3 (2.3%)	3 (3.6%)	
Congenital uropathy	4 (1.9%)	2 (1.5%)	2 (2.4%)	
Other	12 (5.6%)	8 (6.1%)	4 (4.8%)	
Unknown	4 (1.9%)	3 (2.3%)	1 (1.2%)	
Re-transplantation	29 (13.5%)	17 (12.9%)	12 (14.5%)	0.74
Duration on dialysis (days)	2304 ± 1155	2331 ± 1145.5	2261 ± 1174.6	0.67
Mean HLA-mismatches	2.5 ± 1.5	2.5 ± 1.5	2.5 ± 1.5	0.95
Co-Morbidities				
Diabetes mellitus	44 (20.5%)	29 (22.0%)	15 (18.1%)	0.49
Hypertension	184 (85.6%)	110 (83.3%)	74 (89.2%)	0.24 *
Pre-transplant cardiovascular disease	47 (21.9%)	33 (25.0%)	14 (16.9%)	0.16
Stroke	18 (8.4%)	11 (8.3%)	7 (8.4%)	0.98
Peripheral vascular disease	21 (9.8%)	7 (5.3%)	14 (16.9%)	0.05
Pre-transplant abdominal surgery	84 (39.1%)	56 (42.4%)	28 (33.7%)	0.20
Operation Characteristics				
Total operative time (min)	203 ± 46.3	203.5 ± 44.4	202.3 ± 49.6	0.85
Warm ischemia time (min)	51.2 ± 12.3	51.4 ± 12.1	50.8 ± 12.6	0.74
Cold ischemia time (h)	11.4 ± 4.5	10.7 ± 3.6	12.4 ± 5.3	0.01 *
Consultant	161 (74.9%)	101 (76.5%)	60 (72.3%)	0.49
Intraoperative complication	6 (2.8%)	5 (3.8%)	1 (1.2%)	0.34

Table 2. Graft and recipient outcome, * statistically significant.

	All (n = 215)	8:00 a.m.–8:00 p.m. (n = 132)	8:00 p.m.–8:00 a.m. (n = 83)	p-Value
Overall patient survival				0.017 *
At 3 months	212 (98.6%)	129 (97.7%)	83 (100%)	
At 1 year	206 (95.8%)	123 (93.2%)	83 (100%)	
Death censored graft survival				0.907
At 3 months	207 (96.3%)	126 (95.5%)	81 (97.6%)	
At 1 year	202 (93.9%)	123 (93.2%)	79 (95.2%)	
Delayed graft function	108 (50.2%)	63 (47.7%)	45 (54.2%)	0.350
Acute rejection rate	50 (23.3%)	29 (22%)	21 (25.3%)	0.570
Serum creatinine (mg/dL) after transplantation median (range)				
1 week (n = 213)	4.4 (0.93–14.51)	4.4 (0.93–12.99)	4.4 (1.06–14.51)	0.730
4 weeks (n = 212)	1.72 (0.68–17.0)	1.74 (0.68–17.0)	1.71 (0.80–7.16)	0.710
24 weeks (n = 205)	1.45 (0.59–4.42)	1.45 (0.59–4.42)	1.45 (0.71–3.35)	0.660
60 weeks (n = 200)	1.38 (0.46–4.71)	1.39 (0.46–4.71)	1.34 (0.67–2.49)	0.270
Follow-up (months)	49.2 ± 14.6	47.1 ± 15.6	52.50 ± 12.4	0.008 *

3.1. Patient and Graft Survival

The Kaplan–Meier survival curves for patient survival (Figure 1a) and death-censored allograft survival (Figure 1a) by status are shown in Figure 1. In log-rank testing, "day-time" operation was associated with a significantly higher risk of patient death (log-rank test 5.65; $p = 0.017$). During the first 12 months after surgery, a total of nine deaths occurred in the overall sample of 215 kidney transplants recipients (4.18%). No death occurred in the "night-time" kidney group within one year of transplantation, whereas two of the 132 "day-time" renal recipients died with a functioning transplant (one case of coronary heart disease, and one of malignancy) and seven patients died after returning to dialysis (all cases due to bacterial sepsis). Kaplan–Meier analyses demonstrated no statistically significant differences for death-censored graft survival (Figure 1b) between the "night-time" and "day-time" recipient cohorts (log-rank test 0.014; $p = 0.907$).

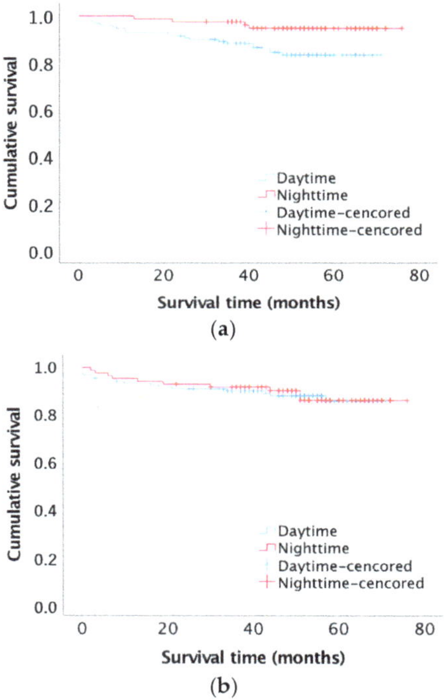

Figure 1. (**a**) Kaplan–Meier survival curve for patient survival after "day-time" and "night-time" renal transplantation (log-rank test 5.65; $p = 0.017$); (**b**) Kaplan–Meier survival curve for death censored graft survival of patients after "day-time" and "night-time" renal transplantation (log-rank test 0.014; $p = 0.907$).

3.2. Early Graft Failure

During the first three months post-operation, graft failure was noticed in seven out of 132 "day-time" allograft recipients (5.3%), and in two out of 83 (2.4%) "night-time" transplant recipients ($p = 0.49$). In the "day-time" cohort, the most common cause of graft failure was primary non-function ($n = 3$), whereas recurrent disease, sepsis and death with functioning graft were noticed in the other cases, respectively. One "day-time" renal transplant recipient suffered an invasive fungal infection, which produced an allograft vessels aneurysm leading to graft loss. From the "night-time" group, two recipients (2.4%) lost the graft during the first three months after transplantation, due to AR and graft infection.

3.3. Postoperative Complications

One or more postoperative complications occurred in 74 out of the 132 "day-time" renal transplant recipients (56%) compared to 41 of the 83 "night-time" allograft recipients (49%) during the first three months post-operation ($p = 0.34$). Each category of complication assessed by the Clavien–Dindo grading system was analysed separately against the two-time groups, of which no category was significantly different (Table 3). In particular, "night-time" and "day-time" renal recipients did not differ significantly in the incidence of postoperative complications requiring medical or surgical reintervention (Clavien–Dindo Grade IIIa/b). Table 4 shows the number of operations that were performed within each time period and the incidence of surgical complications. The most common surgical complications in both groups included haemorrhagic events requiring blood transfusions or surgical intervention (17.2%), lymphoceles (10.7%), seromas (9.7%), and wound dehiscence (7%). A statistically insignificant higher incidence of wound complications among "night-time" kidney recipients was observed. The incidence of urologic complications was higher for the "day-time" surgery, which was also statistically insignificant. Among the 12 patients with urological complications, nine (6.8%) occurred within the "day-time" group and three (3.6%) during the "night-time" group. Five patients (2.3%) were treated with interventional procedures and two (0.7%) received surgical intervention under general anaesthesia. Ureteric necrosis occurred in one "day-time" renal recipient, which was treated with ureteric re-implantation. The incidence of vascular complications within three months post-transplantation was, respectively, 4.5% for "day-time" and 2.4% for "night-time" surgery. In four cases (1.9%), an early secondary surgical intervention was required for vascular complications. Renal artery stenosis occurred in 0.9% of all recipients. Renal artery aneurysm and renal vein thrombosis occurred equally at the rate of 0.5%.

Table 3. Postoperative complications with Clavien–Dindo Classification. Results are presented as absolute and relative frequencies. * If more than one occurred per case, according to patient records, the complication with the highest degree was selected (Minor I+II, Major complications IIIa-IVb, Mortality V).

	All ($n = 215$)	8:00 a.m.–8:00 p.m. ($n = 132$)	8:00 p.m.–8:00 a.m. ($n = 83$)	p-Value
Complications (all grades)	115 (46.5%)	58 (43.9%)	42 (50.6%)	0.340
Grade of complication *				
I	25 (11.6%)	17 (12.9%)	8 (9.6%)	0.470
II	39 (18.1%)	24 (18.2%)	15 (18.1%)	0.984
IIIa	15 (7.0%)	11 (8.3%)	4 (4.8%)	0.325
IIIb	28 (13.0%)	16 (12.0%)	12 (14.5%)	0.620
IVa	3 (1.4%)	3 (2.3%)	0 (0%)	0.286
IVb	4 1.9%)	2 (1.5%)	2 (2.4%)	0.640
V	1 (0.5%)	1 (0.8%)	0 (0%)	1.000

Table 4. Incidence of surgical complications. Incidence is expressed as percentages (%) of total number (n) of patients.

Surgical Complications	All ($n = 215$)	8:00 a.m.–8:00 p.m. ($n = 132$)	8:00 p.m.–8:00 a.m. ($n = 83$)	p-Value
Vascular				
Renal artery stenosis	2 (0.9%)	1 (0.8%)	1 (1.2%)	1.0
Renal vein thrombosis	1 (0.5%)	1 (0.8%)	0	1.0
Iliac artery thrombosis	1 (0.5%)	1 (0.8%)	0	1.0
Renal artery aneurysm	1 (0.5%)	1 (0.8%)	0	1.0
Renal anastomotic leak	1 (0.5%)	0	1 (1.2%)	0.39
Renal pole infarct	1 (0.5%)	1 (0.8%)	0	1.0
Coeliac Trunk stenosis	1 (0.5%)	1 (0.8%)	0	1.0

Table 4. *Cont.*

Surgical Complications	All (*n* = 215)	8:00 a.m.–8:00 p.m. (*n* = 132)	8:00 p.m.–8:00 a.m. (*n* = 83)	*p*-Value
Haemorrhagic				
Haematoma	31 (14%)	20 (15.2%)	11 (13.3%)	0.70
Haemorrhage	6 (2.8%)	3 (2.3%)	3 (3.6%)	0.56
Urological				
Urinary leak	3 (1.4%)	2 (1.5%)	1 (1.2%)	1.0
Urethral necrosis	1 (0.5%)	1 (0.8%)	0	1.0
Urethral stent complication	1 (0.5%)	1 (0.8%)	0	1.0
Urethral stricture	2 (0.9%)	1 (0.8%)	1 (1.2%)	1.0
Bladder outflow obstruction/Blood clot retention	4 (1.9%)	4 (3.0%)	0	0.16
Wound related				
Lymphocele	23 (10.7%)	13 (9.8%)	10 (12%)	0.53
Seroma	17 (7.9%)	9 (6.8%)	8 (9.6%)	0.46
Wound dehiscence	15 (7%)	9 (6.8%)	6 (7.3%)	0.89
Impaired wound healing	3 (1.4%)	0	3 (3.6%)	0.06
Wound infection	3 (1.4%)	3 (2.3%)	0	0.29

4. Discussion

Over the past decade, increased understanding of the effects of shift work and sleep deprivation on neurocognitive functions and physicians health has been established [25]. A single-center study by Rothschild et al. suggested that surgical outcomes were compromised if surgeons had less than six hours of sleep per shift [19]. Traffinder et al. reported that fatigued surgeons made 20% more errors and took 14% longer to perform laparoscopic tasks [26]. On the other hand, studies have demonstrated that outcomes of surgical procedures may not be adversely affected by fatigue or disruption of the normal circadian rhythm [16–18]. Five studies with limited numbers of transplants have previously assessed this issue by focusing on the impact of night-time surgery on graft outcome or complications in patients undergoing renal transplantation [21–24]. Only one single-center study, performed by Fechner et al., demonstrated that night-time surgery carries a higher risk of adverse events and poorer outcomes, particularly driven by higher rates of vascular complications [21]. Kienzel et al. reported that, if transplantations were postponed until the next morning, the increase in CIT would decrease the long-term survival [22]. Seow et al. did not observe an adverse effect of night-time surgery on patient outcomes but highlighted surgical clinical expertise to be a crucial factor for surgical complications [23]. Several limitations need to be considered in the interpretation of the contradictory results. Most studies published to date reported great variability in the methodology and outcome measures. In addition, the definition and understanding of sleep deprivation varied widely among previous investigators. Mentioned studies are frequently single-center and reported the results of a small groups of surgeons, which limits the generalizability. In the present study, we did not find any significant impact of night-time kidney transplant surgery on outcomes including three-month and one-year patient or allograft survival, postoperative complications, DGF or AR in the first year. Our analysis revealed a variable incidence of complications among the different time groups and we could not determine any consistent trend. While the incidence of vascular, haemorrhagic and urological complications was greatest in the "day-time" operative group, wound complications occurred more often among recipients of "night-time" transplants without statistical significance. The mean CIT was slightly longer among those who underwent night-time transplant operations compared to the "day-time" cohort. We observed diminished patient survival among "day-time" renal transplant recipients compared to "night-time" allograft recipients, whereas long-term graft survival was unaffected by the time of day. With no significant difference in baseline characteristics, except for the slighter higher distribution of male donors in the "day-time" cohort, the reasons for this observation are still unclear.

We have controlled for a majority of the clinically meaningful variables available to us in this data set, but it is possible that yet unidentified biologic factors could account for the difference in patient survival between the "night-time" and "day-time" cohorts. With this in mind, there is an urgent need for research in order to clarify the biological consequences of sleep disturbance and fatigue among renal transplant patients. The influence of circadian rhythmicity on physiologic functions related to renal cells, including blood pressure control and homeostasis regulation, is a well-studied phenomenon [27–30]. Evidence suggests that reduced sleep duration and disturbed circadian rhythms may increase sympathetic nervous system stimulation, increase blood pressure, and impair metabolic regulation [31–33]. Thus, misalignment of intrinsic circadian rhythms with environmental time may contribute to poor kidney functioning and renal injury among kidney transplant recipients and donors. Future study is required to clarify this issue. There may be several possible explanations for the lack of 'night-time effect' on outcomes after renal transplantation in this study. Recent studies have demonstrated that there is inter-individual variability in vulnerability to cognitive deficits from sleep loss and the ability to sustain effective neurocognitive performance [34,35], suggesting a reason why there were no differences between the "day-time" and "night-time" cohorts in our study. Van Dongen et al. reported differences in endogenous regulatory processes among individuals, which may affect their tolerance for shift work and cognitive performance during work shifts [36]. Performance adaption across successive shifts has been observed [37,38]. Leff et al. suggested improvement in technical procedural skills across remaining night shifts may be due to ongoing learning or adaption to chronic fatigue [37]. When considering the impact of nocturnal shift work on surgical performance, it is essential to also consider the effects of societal and environmental forces that may contribute to the biological consequences of circadian misalignment. It is known, that there is a detrimental effect of noise inside the operating room on the performance of surgeons and anaesthesiologists [39]. The exposure to excessive operating room noise and distractions during the main day-time business hours may impair cognitive skills. Other factors influencing the performance of a surgeon, such as leadership and communication may be at least as important as technical skills and the number of hours slept [40]. In addition, the use of caffeine and periods of short naps may mitigate the potential risks associated with sleep deprivation [41]. A study of this nature has some limitations, primarily through its retrospective design. The small overall number of patients and individual complications in our cohort might weaken the conclusions of our pilot-study and limits the power to detect differences. To assess severity, we additionally categorised all postoperative complications using the Clavien–Dindo classification system. Although this system has been proven to be reproducible and applicable with minimal interobserver variability, it has some limitations [42]. Data regarding a surgeon's subjective perception of fatigue, resting time and quantification of sleep deprivation were not available and could not be included in the analysis. It is further possible, that transplant surgeons perform day-time procedures beginning at 8 am after being 'on-call' overnight. With that in mind, one may argue whether the classification based on time group selections assumes that day-time surgeons are well rested, and perform better than night-time surgeons regardless of their overall workload. We cannot lose sight of other potential variables such as the effect of procurement-related organ lesions on renal transplant outcome. Data concerning surgeons' fitness before procurement were not available. Further investigation is needed aiming to record errors during organ procurement related to surgeons' fatigue.

5. Concluding Remarks and Future Directions

To date, there are very few reports on the effect of night-time surgery on renal transplant outcomes. We, therefore, believe that the initial results from this pilot-study are a welcome addition to the urological literature and provide encouragement for further analysis. We concluded that night- time kidney surgery does not carry a higher risk of adverse events and poorer outcome among patients undergoing renal transplantation. Consequently, kidney transplantation should be immediately performed regardless of the time of the day, with the known adverse effects of prolonged CIT. However, in order to fully assess the effects of sleep deprivation and circadian rhythm disturbance on surgical performance in kidney transplantation, prospective research involving larger cohorts is needed. Therefore, among other things, a transparent evidence-based assessment of the level of fatigue, shift intensity and sleep quality in medicine, especially in the field of surgery, is required. Moreover, systems-based interventions, as well as individual coping strategies and experiences that mitigate the effects of fatigue and disruption of the circadian rhythms, should be taken into consideration. In addition, there is a need for future research focusing on the impact of sleep displacement and circadian misalignment on renal functioning among recipients and donors in the field of kidney transplantation.

Author Contributions: F.F., K.B. and L.L. designed the study; N.S. analyzed the data and wrote the manuscript; A.B., R.P., T.S. and N.B. drafted and revised the paper; all authors approved the final version of the manuscript.

Acknowledgments: We acknowledge support from the German Research Foundation (DFG) and the Open Access Publication Fund of Charité–Universitätsmedizin Berlin.

Conflicts of Interest: The authors have no conflict of interest to disclose.

References

1. Hariharan, S.; Johnson, C.P.; Bresnahan, B.A.; Taranto, S.E.; McIntosh, M.J.; Stablein, D. Improved graft survival after renal transplantation in the United States, 1988 to 1996. *N. Engl. J. Med.* **2000**, *342*, 605–612. [CrossRef] [PubMed]

2. Halloran, P.F. Immunosuppressive drugs for kidney transplantation. *N. Engl. J. Med.* **2004**, *351*, 2715–2729. [CrossRef] [PubMed]

3. Brockschmidt, C.; Huber, N.; Paschke, S.; Hartmann, B.; Henne-Bruns, D.; Wittau, M. Minimal access kidney transplant: A novel technique to reduce surgical tissue trauma. *Exp. Clin. Transplant.* **2012**, *10*, 319–324. [CrossRef] [PubMed]

4. Bessede, T.; Droupy, S.; Hammoudi, Y.; Bedretdinova, D.; Durrbach, A.; Charpentier, B.; Benoit, G. Surgical prevention and management of vascular complications of kidney transplantation. *Transpl. Int.* **2012**, *25*, 994–1001. [CrossRef] [PubMed]

5. Osman, Y.; Shokeir, A.; Ali-el-Dein, B.; Tantawy, M.; Wafa, E.W.; el-Dein, A.B.; Ghoneim, M.A. Vascular complications after live donor renal transplantation: Study of risk factors and effects on graft and patient survival. *J. Urol.* **2003**, *169*, 859–862. [CrossRef] [PubMed]

6. Phelan, P.J.; O'Kelly, P.; Tarazi, M.; Tarazi, N.; Salehmohamed, M.R.; Little, D.M.; Magee, C.; Conlon, P.J. Renal allograft loss in the first post-operative month: Causes and consequences. *Clin. Transplant.* **2012**, *26*, 544–549. [CrossRef]

7. Humar, A.; Matas, A.J. Surgical complications after kidney transplantation. *Semin. Dial.* **2005**, *18*, 505–510. [CrossRef]

8. Debout, A.; Foucher, Y.; Trébern-Launay, K.; Legendre, C.; Kreis, H.; Mourad, G.; Garrigue, V.; Morelon, E.; Buron, F.; Rostaing, L.; et al. Each additional hour of cold ischemia time significantly increases the risk of graft failure and mortality following renal transplantation. *Kidney Int.* **2015**, *87*, 343–349. [CrossRef]

9. Olson, E.J.; Drage, L.A.; Auger, R.R. Sleep deprivation, physician performance, and patient safety. *Chest* **2009**, *136*, 1389–1396. [CrossRef]

10. Lockley, S.W.; Barger, L.K.; Ayas, N.T.; Rothschild, J.M.; Czeisler, C.A.; Landrigan, C.P.; Harvard Work Hours, Health and Safety Group. Effects of health care provider work hours and sleep deprivation on safety and performance. *Jt. Comm. J. Qual. Patient Saf.* **2007**, *33* (Suppl. 11), 7–18. [CrossRef]

11. Eastridge, B.J.; Hamilton, E.C.; O'Keefe, G.E.; Rege, R.V.; Valentine, R.J.; Jones, D.J.; Tesfay, S.; Thal, E.R. Effect of sleep deprivation on the performance of simulated laparoscopic surgical skill. *Am. J. Surg.* **2003**, *186*, 169–174. [CrossRef]

12. Gerdes, J.; Kahol, K.; Smith, M.; Leyba, M.J.; Ferrara, J.J. Jack Barney award: The effect of fatigue on cognitive and psychomotor skills of trauma residents and attending surgeons. *Am. J. Surg.* **2008**, *196*, 813–819, discussion 819–820. [CrossRef]

13. Peskun, C.; Walmsley, D.; Waddell, J.; Schemitsch, E. Effect of surgeon fatigue on hip and knee arthroplasty. *Can. J. Surg.* **2012**, *55*, 81–86. [CrossRef]

14. Kelz, R.R.; Freeman, K.M.; Hosokawa, P.W.; Asch, D.A.; Spitz, F.R.; Moskowitz, M.; Henderson, W.G.; Mitchell, M.E.; Itani, K.M. Time of day is associated with postoperative morbidity: An analysis of the national surgical quality improvement program data. *Ann. Surg.* **2008**, *247*, 544–552. [CrossRef]

15. Egol, K.A.; Tolisano, A.M.; Spratt, K.F.; Koval, K.J. Mortality rates following trauma: The difference is night and day. *J. Emerg. Trauma Shock* **2011**, *4*, 178–183.

16. Schieman, C.; MacLean, A.R.; Buie, W.D.; Rudmik, L.R.; Ghali, W.A.; Dixon, E. Does surgeon fatigue influence outcomes after anterior resection for rectal cancer? *Am. J. Surg.* **2008**, *195*, 684–687, discussion 687–688. [CrossRef]

17. Yaghoubian, A.; Kaji, A.H.; Ishaque, B.; Park, J.; Rosing, D.K.; Lee, S.; Stabile, B.E.; de Virgilio, C. Acute care surgery performed by sleep deprived residents: Are outcomes affected? *J. Surg. Res.* **2010**, *163*, 192–196. [CrossRef]

18. Ellman, P.I.; Kron, I.L.; Alvis, J.S.; Tache-Leon, C.; Maxey, T.S.; Reece, T.B.; Peeler, B.B.; Kern, J.A.; Tribble, C.G. Acute sleep deprivation in the thoracic surgical resident does not affect operative outcomes. *Ann. Thorac. Surg.* **2005**, *80*, 60–64, discussion 64–65. [CrossRef]

19. Rothschild, J.M.; Keohane, C.A.; Rogers, S.; Gardner, R.; Lipsitz, S.R.; Salzberg, C.A.; Yu, T.; Yoon, C.S.; Williams, D.H.; Wien, M.F.; et al. Risks of complications by attending physicians after performing nighttime procedures. *JAMA* **2009**, *302*, 1565–1572. [CrossRef]

20. Lonze, B.E.; Parsikia, A.; Feyssa, E.L.; Khanmoradi, K.; Araya, V.R.; Zaki, R.F.; Segev, D.L.; Ortiz, J.A. Operative start times and complications after liver transplantation. *Am. J. Transplant.* **2010**, *10*, 1842–1849. [CrossRef]

21. Fechner, G.; Pezold, C.; Hauser, S.; Gerhardt, T.; Muller, S.C. Kidney's nightshift, kidney's nightmare? Comparison of daylight and nighttime kidney transplantation: Impact on complications and graft survival. *Transplant. Proc.* **2008**, *40*, 1341–1344. [CrossRef]

22. Kienzl-Wagner, K.; Schneiderbauer, S.; Bosmuller, C.; Schneeberger, S.; Pratschke, J.; Ollinger, R. Nighttime procedures are not associated with adverse outcomes in kidney transplantation. *Transpl. Int.* **2013**, *26*, 879–885. [CrossRef]

23. Seow, Y.Y.; Alkari, B.; Dyer, P.; Riad, H. Cold ischemia time, surgeon, time of day, and surgical complications. *Transplantation* **2004**, *77*, 1386–1389. [CrossRef]

24. Brunschot, D.M.; Hoitsma, A.J.; van der Jagt, M.F.; d'Ancona, F.C.; Donders, R.A.; van Laarhoven, C.J.; Hilbrands, L.B.; Warle, M.C. Nighttime kidney transplantation is associated with less pure technical graft failure. *World J. Urol.* **2016**, *34*, 955–961. [CrossRef]

25. Van Dongen, H.P.; Maislin, G.; Mullington, J.M.; Dinges, D.F. The cumulative cost of additional wakefulness: Dose-response effects on neurobehavioral functions and sleep physiology from chronic sleep restriction and total sleep deprivation. *Sleep* **2003**, *26*, 117–126. [CrossRef]

26. Taffinder, N.J.; McManus, I.C.; Gul, Y.; Russell, R.C.; Darzi, A. Effect of sleep deprivation on surgeons' dexterity on laparoscopy simulator. *Lancet* **1998**, *352*, 1191. [CrossRef]

27. Zuber, A.M.; Centeno, G.; Pradervand, S.; Nikolaeva, S.; Maquelin, L.; Cardinaux, L.; Bonny, O.; Firsov, D. Molecular clock is involved in predictive circadian adjustment of renal function. *Proc. Natl. Acad. Sci. USA* **2009**, *106*, 16523–16528. [CrossRef]

28. Myung, J.; Wu, M.Y.; Lee, C.Y.; Rahim, A.R.; Truong, V.H.; Wu, D.; Piggins, H.D.; Wu, M.S. The Kidney Clock Contributes to Timekeeping by the Master Circadian Clock. *Int. J. Mol. Sci.* **2019**, *20*, 2765. [CrossRef]

29. Tokonami, N.; Mordasini, D.; Pradervand, S.; Centeno, G.; Jouffe, C.; Maillard, M.; Bonny, O.; Gachon, F.; Gomez, R.A.; Sequeira-Lopez, M.L.; et al. Local renal circadian clocks control fluid-electrolyte homeostasis and BP. *J. Am. Soc. Nephrol.* **2014**, *25*, 1430–1439. [CrossRef]

30. Gumz, M.L. Tick tock: Time to recognize the kidney clock. *J. Am. Soc. Nephrol.* **2014**, *25*, 1369–1371. [CrossRef]

31. Spiegel, K.; Leproult, R.; Van Cauter, E. Impact of sleep debt on metabolic and endocrine function. *Lancet* **1999**, *354*, 1435–1439. [CrossRef]

32. Sayk, F.; Teckentrup, C.; Becker, C.; Heutling, D.; Wellhöner, P.; Lehnert, H.; Dodt, C. Effects of selective slow-wave sleep deprivation on nocturnal blood pressure dipping and daytime blood pressure regulation. *Am. J. Physiol. Regul. Integr. Comp. Physiol.* **2010**, *298*, R191–R197. [CrossRef]

33. Spiegel, K.; Tasali, E.; Leproult, R.; Van Cauter, E. Effects of poor and short sleep on glucose metabolism and obesity risk. *Nat. Rev. Endocrinol.* **2009**, *5*, 253–261. [CrossRef]

34. Van Dongen, H.P.; Bender, A.M.; Dinges, D.F. Systematic individual differences in sleep homeostatic and circadian rhythm contributions to neurobehavioral impairment during sleep deprivation. *Accid. Anal. Prev.* **2012**, *45*, 11–16. [CrossRef]
35. Chee, M.W.; Tan, J.C. Lapsing when sleep deprived: Neural activation characteristics of resistant and vulnerable individuals. *Neuroimage* **2010**, *51*, 835–843. [CrossRef]
36. Van Dongen, H.P. Shift work and inter-individual differences in sleep and sleepiness. *Chronobiol. Int.* **2006**, *23*, 1139–1147. [CrossRef]
37. Leff, D.R.; Aggarwal, R.; Rana, M.; Nakhjavani, B.; Purkayastha, S.; Khullar, V.; Darzi, A.W. Laparoscopic skills suffer on the first shift of sequential night shifts: Program directors beware and residents prepare. *Ann. Surg.* **2008**, *247*, 530–539. [CrossRef]
38. Lamond, N.; Dorrian, J.; Roach, G.D.; McCulloch, K.; Holmes, A.L.; Burgess, H.J.; Fletcher, A.; Dawson, D. The impact of a week of simulated night work on sleep, circadian phase, and performance. *Occup. Environ. Med.* **2003**, *60*, e13. [CrossRef]
39. Katz, J.D. Noise in the operating room. *Anesthesiology* **2014**, *121*, 894–898. [CrossRef]
40. Moorthy, K.; Munz, Y.; Forrest, D.; Pandey, V.; Undre, S.; Vincent, C.; Darzi, A. Surgical crisis management skills training and assessment: A simulation[corrected]-based approach to enhancing operating room performance. *Ann. Surg.* **2006**, *244*, 139–147. [CrossRef]
41. Aggarwal, R.; Mishra, A.; Crochet, P.; Sirimanna, P.; Darzi, A. Effect of caffeine and taurine on simulated laparoscopy performed following sleep deprivation. *Br. J. Surg.* **2011**, *98*, 1666–1672. [CrossRef] [PubMed]
42. Yoon, P.D.; Chalasani, V.; Woo, H.H. Use of Clavien-Dindo classification in reporting and grading complications after urological surgical procedures: Analysis of 2010 to 2012. *J. Urol.* **2013**, *190*, 1271–1274. [CrossRef]

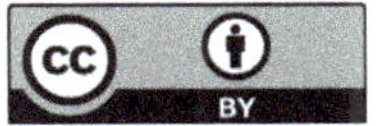

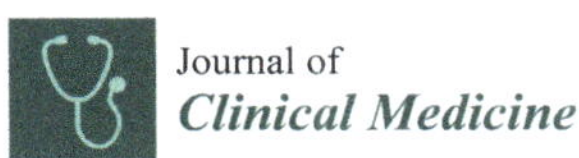

Journal of
Clinical Medicine

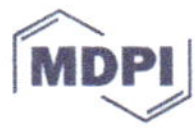

Article

CD45RC Expression of Circulating CD8$^+$ T Cells Predicts Acute Allograft Rejection: A Cohort Study of 128 Kidney Transplant Patients

Marie Lemerle [1], Anne-Sophie Garnier [1], Martin Planchais [1], Benoit Brilland [1], Yves Delneste [2,3], Jean-François Subra [1,2], Odile Blanchet [4], Simon Blanchard [2], Anne Croue [5], Agnès Duveau [1] and Jean-François Augusto [1,2,*]

[1] Service de Néphrologie-Dialyse-Transplantation, CHU Angers, 49000 Angers, France
[2] CRCINA, INSERM, Université de Nantes, Université d'Angers, 49100 Angers, France
[3] Service d'Immunologie et d'Allergologie, CHU Angers, 49000 Angers, France
[4] Centre de ressources biologiques, BB-0033-00038, Université d'Angers, CHU d'Angers, 49000 Angers, France
[5] Département de Pathologie Cellulaire et Tissulaire, CHU d'Angers, 49000 Angers, France
[*] Correspondence: jfaugusto@chu-angers.fr; Tel.: +33-(0)-241-355-063; Fax: +33-(0)-241-354-892

Received: 22 June 2019; Accepted: 29 July 2019; Published: 1 August 2019

Abstract: Predictive biomarkers of acute rejection (AR) are lacking. Pre-transplant expression of CD45RC on blood CD8$^+$ T cells has been shown to predict AR in kidney transplant (KT) patients. The objective of the present study was to study CD45RC expression in a large cohort of KT recipients exposed to modern immunosuppressive regimens. CD45RC expression on T cells was analyzed in 128 KT patients, where 31 patients developed AR, of which 24 were found to be T-cell mediated (TCMR). Pre-transplant CD4$^+$ and CD8$^+$ CR45RC^{high} T cell proportions were significantly higher in patients with AR. The frequency of CD45RC^{high} T cells was significantly associated with age at transplantation but was not significantly different according to gender, history of transplantation, pre-transplant immunization, and de novo donor specific anti-Human Leucocyte Antigen (HLA) antibody. Survival-free AR was significantly better in patients with CD8$^+$ CD45RC^{high} T cells below 58.4% (p = 0.0005), but not different according to CD4$^+$ T cells (p = 0.073). According to multivariate analysis, CD8$^+$ CD45RC^{high} T cells above 58.4% increased the risk of AR 4-fold (HR 3.96, p = 0.003). Thus, pre-transplant CD45RC expression on CD8$^+$ T cells predicted AR, mainly TCMR, in KT patients under modern immunosuppressive therapies. We suggest that CD45RC expression should be evaluated in a prospective study to validate its usefulness to quantify the pre-transplant risk of AR.

Keywords: kidney transplantation; acute rejection; lymphocyte; CD45RC

1. Introduction

Significant progress has been made over the past few years in the immunological and histological fields, allowing for better differentiation and to refine the diagnosis and prognosis of T cell-mediated rejection (TCMR) and of antibody-mediated rejection (ABMR) in kidney transplant patients [1]. While both rejection types may develop concomitantly, TCMR mainly occurs within the first year post-transplant, while ABMR usually develops later in the course and is associated with the presence of preformed or de novo donor-specific anti-Human Leucocyte Antigen (HLA) antibodies (DSA) [1,2]. Although modern immunosuppressive regimens efficiently prevent allograft rejection in most patients, acute rejection (AR) episodes still occur in some patients and are associated with premature graft loss and morbidity [1–3].

Several risk factors of AR have been identified in previous studies including young age, female gender, black race, and immunological characteristics (HLA mismatch, pre-transplant or de novo

DSA) [4]. However, despite being indicative at the population level, when considered at the individual level, most of these factors do not allow for the accurate stratification of AR risk, especially in "low immunological risk patients," which represents most kidney transplant candidates. The identification of patients with higher versus lower AR risk among low immunological risk patients would theoretically allow one to tailor the immunosuppressive regimen according to the AR risk and thus to decrease post-transplant morbidity [5,6].

The risk of allograft rejection relies on graft-, environmental-, and host-related factors [1]. However, the molecular mechanisms underlining the development of alloreactivity are far from being fully understood [7]. An illustrative example of the inter-individual variability of AR risk is represented by operationally tolerant patients, defined as solid allograft recipients that do not develop allograft rejection despite immunosuppressive treatment discontinuation [7]. Thanks to intrinsic immunological factors, and probably also acquired factors, these patients are unable to mount an efficient alloreactive response.

The identification of biomarkers reflecting the level of tolerance emerges as a major goal in solid organ transplantation. This would allow one to tailor the immunosuppressive regimens, especially in low immunological risk kidney transplant candidates. Given that $CD4^+$ and $CD8^+$ T cell subsets have an essential role in the development of alloimmune response, defining T cell subpopulations with higher and lower alloimmune properties may constitute an interesting approach.

CD45 is a transmembrane protein tyrosine phosphatase heavily expressed on T cells and critical for signal transduction by regulating kinases of the Src-family [8,9]. Four CD45 isoforms (RO, RA, RB, RC), resulting from an alternative splicing of three exons, are expressed in humans [9]. The CD45RC isoform is highly expressed on human naive T cells with a bimodal and a trimodal pattern on $CD4^+$ T cells (high and low expression) and CD8+ T cells (low, intermediate, and high) [10,11]. These patterns of expression define CD45RC T cell subsets with different cytokine profiles. Interestingly, the expression of CD45RC on T cells is highly variable between individuals and is genetically determined [10–12].

We demonstrated in a previous work that the level of CD45RC expression at the surface of blood $CD8^+$ T cells before kidney transplantation was associated with the risk of AR after transplantation [10,13]. This study was conducted on a cohort of 89 kidney transplant recipients transplanted between 1999 and 2004, and we observed that a pre-transplant proportion of $CD8^+$ $CD45RC^{high}$ T cells above 54.7% conferred a 6-fold increased risk of developing AR after 4.8 years of follow-up [10]. The aim of the present study was thus to confirm this observation in a prospective cohort of kidney transplant patients treated with current immunosuppressive regimens.

2. Material and Methods

2.1. Study Design and Aim

This is a monocentric cohort study that included patients transplanted in the University Hospital of Angers between 2007 and 2015. During the period of the study, after giving their written consent, patients were offered the chance to participate to a biocollection ("Collection Néphrologie et voies urinaires"). Samples were collected before kidney transplantation and stored at the dedicated department ("Centre de Ressources Biologiques BB-0033-00038"). All patients that gave their written consent to the study were included. The primary aim of the study was to analyze the value of CD45RC expression on T cells for AR prediction. The study was approved by the Medical Ethics Committee of Angers University Hospital (2009/10).

2.2. Immunosuppressive Regimens

The immunosuppressive treatment was not imposed by the study and was based on the assessment of immunological risk according to clinical practice in our department as detailed hereafter. Low immunological risk patients, defined as first time kidney transplant recipients and with PRA < 20%, received two injections of Basiliximab (Simulect; Novartis Pharma, Basel, Switzerland), while higher immunological risk recipients (previous transplantation, PRA > 20%) were more likely to receive antithymocyte globulines (ATG; Thymoglobuline; Genzyme, Lyon, France) during the first 3 to 7 days post-transplant. ATG was also used for induction in donors with cardiac arrest before brain death, in non-heart-beating donors, and when delayed graft function was anticipated by clinician. Moreover, between 2010 and 2013, no induction therapy was performed in patients aged >70 years old. All patients received a single methylprednisolone bolus of 500 mg followed by prednisone (1 mg/kg/day) with a progressive tapering and discontinuation at the end of month 5 post-transplant, unless there was an occurrence of AR. A maintenance immunosuppressive regimen relied mainly on mycophenolate mofetil or mycophenolic acid and tacrolimus.

2.3. Data Collection and Definitions

Characteristics of the study population were collected prospectively via the systematic screening of patients' medical records. All clinical events and biological data were retained until last follow-up: anthropometric data, nature of original kidney disease, and graft donor characteristics. Diagnosis of acute rejection (AR) episodes was based on conventional clinical and laboratory criteria and confirmed using a histological examination of a graft biopsy (according to the last Banff Classification) [14]. AR diagnosis was based on clinical and laboratory criteria (clinically diagnosed AR) when the graft biopsy was non-contributive or contra-indicated.

2.4. Sample Collection

Peripheral blood mononuclear cells (PBMC) of kidney transplant candidates were prospectively harvested before transplantation and stored in liquid nitrogen. Patients with samples showing PBMC viability below 80% were excluded from the analysis.

After giving their written consent, fresh samples of end-stage renal disease (ESRD) patients and heathy individuals (HD) were used to monitor the proliferation capacities of CD45RC T cells.

2.5. Antibodies and Flow Cytometry Analysis

The following conjugated antibodies were used to characterize CD45RC T cell subpopulations: CD3-VioGreen (REA613), CD4-PerCP-Vio700 (REA623), CD8-PE-Vio770 (REA734), from Milteny Biotec, Bergisch-Gladbach, Germany; CD45RA-APC (HI100) from BD Biosciences, San Jose, CA, USA; and CD45RC-FITC (MT2) from IQ Product, Houston, TX, USA. Cell viability was systematically assessed (LIVE/DEAD Fixable Near-IR Dead Cell Stain kit; Fischer Scientific, Pittsburgh, PA, USA). Briefly, 10^6 cells were incubated with the viability dye according to the manufacturer's recommendations before incubation with the antibodies. Data were collected using a FACS-Canto II (BD Biosciences) cytometer and analyzed using the FlowJo software, Ashland, OR, USA. The expression of CD45RC is bimodal on $CD4^+$ T cells, some cells expressing low levels of CD45RC ($CD45RC^{low}$), and others expressing high levels ($CD45RC^{high}$). On $CD8^+$ T cells, expression of CD45RC is trimodal, the first fraction of cells expressing low levels ($CD45RC^{low}$), the second fraction expressing intermediate levels ($CD45RC^{Int}$), and the last fraction expressing high levels of CD45RC ($CD45RC^{high}$). Figure S1 illustrates the gating strategy.

2.6. CD45RC$^+$ T Cell Purification and T Cell Proliferation Analyses

CD45RC T cells were sorted from freshly isolated PBMC of end-stage renal disease (ESRD) patients and age/sex matched healthy donors (HD) using a FACS-Aria cytometer, BD Bioscience, San Jose, CA, USA. Briefly, after a gradient centrifugation, 2×10^7 PBMCs were stained using a Cell Trace Violet proliferation kit (Thermofischer, San Jose, CA, USA) for proliferation assessment and then stained using CD4-BV421 (L3T4, BD Biosciences), CD8-PE-Vio770 (REA734, Miltenyi Biotec), and CD45RC-FITC (MT2, IQ Product). $CD45RC^{high}$ and $CD45RC^{low}$ subpopulations were sorted among $CD4^+$ and $CD8^+$ T cells. Purity was always routinely above 95%. Then, 5×10^4 T cells were cultured at 37 °C in RPMI 1640 medium (containing 8% fetal calf serum) in 96-well round-bottomed microplates (Becton Dickinson, Franklin Lakes, NJ, USA), with or without a 1 µg/mL plate-bound anti-CD3

(Beckman-Coulter, Brea, CA, USA) and 0.5 µg/mL soluble anti-CD28 (Beckman-Coulter). After 72 h of culture, cells were harvested and proliferation was assessed using flow cytometry (FACS-Canto II; BD Biosciences).

2.7. Statistical Analysis

Data were expressed as a median with minimum to maximum values for continuous variables and absolute count with percentage for categorical variables. Categorical and continuous data were analyzed with χ^2 or Fischer's exact test and Mann–Whitney U tests, respectively. The Wilcoxon matched-pairs rank test was used to compare the proliferative capacities of T cells. The predictive values of the CD45RC subset frequency for the first AR episode were analyzed using receiver operating characteristics (ROC) curves. Subsequently, cut-off values were determined by using the Youden index. The Kaplan–Meyer method was used to analyze AR-free survivals according to predetermined cut-off values of CD45RC subset frequencies. A log-rank test was used to compare survival curves. Correlations were analyzed using Spearman's rank correlation test. Multivariate cox models were used to analyze the association between CD45RC subset frequencies and AR. Results are reported as hazard ratio (HR) with 95% CIs. All *p*-values were two-sided and a *p*-value lower than 0.05 was considered statistically significant. Statistical analysis was performed using Graphpad Prism® version 7 (San Diego, CA, USA) and SPSS® software version 22.0 (IBM, Armonk, NY, USA).

3. Results

3.1. Characteristics of the Population

Between January 1, 2007, and December 31, 2015, 396 patients underwent kidney transplantation in Angers University hospital. Among them, 292 patients had blood samples collected and stored in a biocollection before transplantation, and 140 gave their written consent to participate in the present study. Among these 140 patients, samples from 12 patients were excluded because of technical errors ($n = 6$) or poor blood cell viability ($n = 6$). Thus, 128 patients were included and finally analyzed (Figure 1, flowchart).

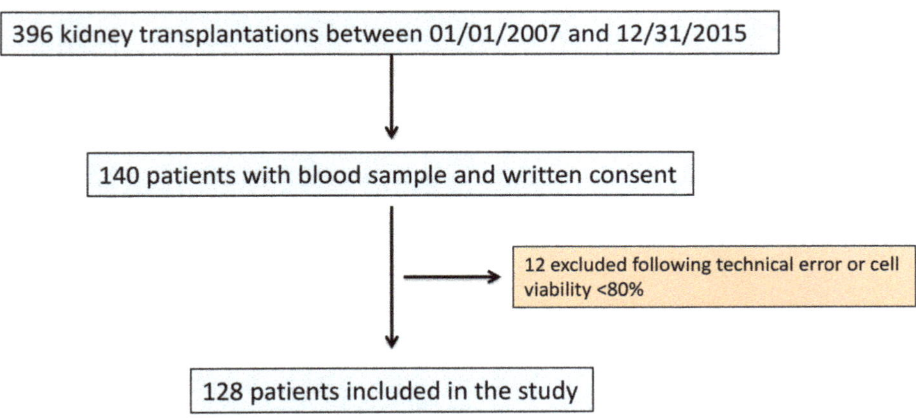

Figure 1. Flowchart of the study.

The population was predominantly composed of males, with a median age of 50.2 years. The main cause of ESRD was autosomal dominant polycystic kidney disease and patients were first-time transplanted in 90% of cases. Based on PRA, 69.5% were non-sensitized before transplantation, while 6.25% of patients had a PRA > 20%. Basiliximab was used predominantly for induction in 56.3% of patients and most patients received tacrolimus with mycophenolate mofetil as a maintenance regimen. These data are detailed in Table 1.

Table 1. Baseline characteristics of the population. Results are presented as a median with minimum to maximum value ranges for continuous variables and absolute count and percentage for categorical variables.

	All Patients ($n = 128$)
Baseline Characteristics	
Sex (M/F)	80/48
Age (years)	50.2 (18.0–79.2)
Weigh (kg)	71.0 (41.0–115.0)
BMI (kg/m^2)	25.0 (17.3–40.2)
Original nephropathy, *n* (%)	
ADPKD	33 (25.8)
IgA nephropathy	17 (13.3)
Other GN	13 (10.2)
TIN/urologic	13 (10.2)
Vascular nephropathy/diabetic GN	13 (10.2)
Vasculitis	3 (2.3)
Lupus nephritis	5 (3.9)
Undetermined nephropathy	18 (14.1)
Others	13 (10.2)
History of transplantation	
Pre-transplant dialysis, n (%)	92 (71.9)
Previous kidney transplantation, n (%)	13 (10.2)
Donor age, years	50.0 (3.0–87.0)
Cold ischemia time (hours)	16.6 (2.0–35.4)
HLA mismatch	
HLA A&B&DR	4.0 (0–6)
HLA A&B	3.0 (0–4)
HLA DR	1.0 (0–2)
Sensitization, *n* (%)	
Nonsensitized at transplantation	89 (69.5)
PRA < 10%	30 (23.4)
PRA 10–20%	1 (0.8)
PRA > 20%	8 (6.2)
Immunosuppressive regimens	
Induction therapy	
None, *n* (%)	6 (4.7)
Basiliximab, *n* (%)	72 (56.3)
Antithymocyte globulins, *n* (%)	50 (39.1)
Maintenance regimen	
Tac-based, *n* (%)	102 (79.6)
Cyclosporin-based, *n* (%)	26 (20.3)
MMF or MPA, *n* (%)	127 (99.2)

ADPKD, autosomic dominant polycystic kidney disease; BMI, body mass index; GN, glomerulonephritis; HLA, human leukocyte antigens; MMF, mycophenolate mofetil; MPA, mycophenolic acid; PRA, Panel Reactive Antibody; Tac, tacrolimus; TIN, tubulo-interstitial nephropathy.

3.2. Acute Rejection Episodes

The mean follow-up of the cohort was 3.82 ± 2.22 years. During the follow-up, AR occurred in 31 patients (24.2%) at a mean delay of 0.73 ± 1.24 years post-transplant. When considering only the first AR episode, 28 were histologically-proven and 3 were diagnosed based on clinical and biological criteria. Among the histologically-proven AR cases, 24 were TCMR, and 6 being borderlines. The four other AR episodes were ABMR in one case and mixed AR (TCMR and ABMR) in the three other cases.

At one-year post-transplant, mean serum creatinine was 141.4 ± 75.2 µmol/L and mean glomerular filtration rate (GFR) was 53.2 ± 21.8 mL/min/1.73 m^2. DSA developed in 15 patients (11.7%) during follow-up. These data are reported in Table 2.

Table 2. Acute rejection episodes. Results are presented as a median with minimum to maximum value ranges for continuous variables and absolute count and percentage for categorical variables.

Mean Follow-Up (Years)	3.82 ± 2.22 (0.02–8.53)
Acute Rejection	
Number of patients, *n* (%)	31 (24.2)
Mean delay to first AR (years)	0.73 ± 1.24 (0.02–4.83)
Histologically proven, *n* (%)	28 (90.3)
TCMR	24 (85.7)
Borderline	6 (25.0)
Grade IA	9 (37.5)
Grade IB	8 (33.3)
Grade IIA	1 (4.2)
AMR	1 (3.6)
Mixed AR	3 (10.7)
Non histologically proved AR	3 (9.7)
More than one AR episode	9 (7.0)
DSA, *n* (%)	15 (11.7)
Class I	4 (26.7)
Class II	11 (73.3)
Year 1 Post-Transplant Biological Results	
Serum creatinine (µmol/L) *	141.4 ± 75.2 (60.0–716)
GFR (mL/min/1.73 m^2) *	53.2 ± 21.8 (7.3–123)
Proteinuria/Creatininuria (g/g) *	0.25 ± 0.69 (0–5.78)

* In patients followed at the indicated time; AR, acute rejection; DSA, donor specific antibodies; GFR, glomerular filtration rate; disorder; TCMR, T-cell-mediated rejection; AMR, antibody-mediated rejection.

Patients that experienced AR received more frequently Basiliximab as induction therapy as compared to patients that did not experienced AR, who received more-frequent ATG (p = 0.035). Baseline characteristics, including age and pre-transplant immunization, were not significantly different between groups. These data are reported in Table 3. When borderline ARs were excluded, no significant differences were observed between patients with and without AR (Table S1).

Table 3. Univariate analysis of factors associated with acute rejection occurrence. Comparisons between groups were done using the Mann–Whitney U test for continuous variables and X^2 or Fisher exact tests for categorical variables. Continuous variables are expressed as a median with minimum to maximum values and categorical variables are expressed as their absolute count and percentage. Acute rejection groups were compared to the No AR group. Significant p-values appear in bold.

	No AR ($n = 97$)	AR ($n = 31$)	p	BPAR ($n = 28$)	p	Excluding Bor AR ($n = 22$)	p
Baseline Characteristics							
Sex (M/F)	62/35	18/13	0.558	16/12	0.514	12/10	0.413
Age (years)	50.3 (18.0–79.2)	48.2 (23.3–66.5)	0.301	48.8 (23.3–66.5)	0.368	45.5 (23.3–66.5)	0.206
No pretransplant immunization, n (%)	64 (66.0)	25 (80.6)	0.123	23 (82.1)	0.160	18 (81.8)	0.203
PRA > 20%, n (%)	7 (7.2)	1 (3.2)	0.679	1 (3.6)	0.682	1 (4.5)	1.000
History of Transplantation							
Previous kidney transplantation, n (%)	11 (11.3)	2 (6.5)	0.733	2 (7.1)	0.731	2 (9.1)	1.000
Pre-transplant dialysis, n (%)	77 (72.2)	22 (71.0)	0.897	20 (71.4)	0,939	15 (68.2)	0.709
Donor age, years	51.0 (3.0–87.0)	47.0 (36.0–80.0)	0.799	48 (36.0–80.0)	0.769	43 (37.0–68.0)	0.494
Cold ischemia time (hours)	17.0 (2.0–35.4)	15.6 (2.0–32.2)	0.434	15.5 (2.0–32.2)	0.299	15.5 (2.0–32.2)	0.359
HLA mismatch (ABDR), n	4.0 (0–6)	4.0 (0–6)	0.733	4.0 (0–6)	0.495	4.0 (0–6)	0.750
Delayed graft function, n (%)	22 (22.7)	6 (19.4)	0.658	5 (17.9)	0.551	4 (18.2)	0.779
De novo DSA, n (%)	12 (12.4)	3 (9.7)	1.000	3 (10.7)	1.000	3 (13.6)	1.000
Immunosuppressive Regimens							
Induction (none/Basiliximab/ATG), n (%)	4 (4.1)/49 (50.5)/44 (45.4)	2 (6.5)/23 (74.2)/6 (19.3)	**0.035**	2(7.1)/21(75.0)/5(17.9)	**0.031**	1(4.6)/16(72.7)/5(22.7)	0.145
Tacrolimus-based regimen, n (%)	78 (80.4)	23 (74.2)	0.393	22 (78.6)	0.752	16 (72.7)	0.370

AR, acute rejection; BPAR, biopsy proven acute rejection; Bor AR, borderline AR.

3.3. Proliferative Capacities of CD45RC T Cells

The proliferative properties of CD45RC T cells have been studied only in HD [10,11]. Thus, we analyzed the proliferative properties of subpopulations in ESRD patients as compared to age and sex-matched HD. As shown in Figure 2, proliferative properties of CD45RC T cells were not different between ESRD patients and HD, suggesting that their immune function was maintained in ESRD.

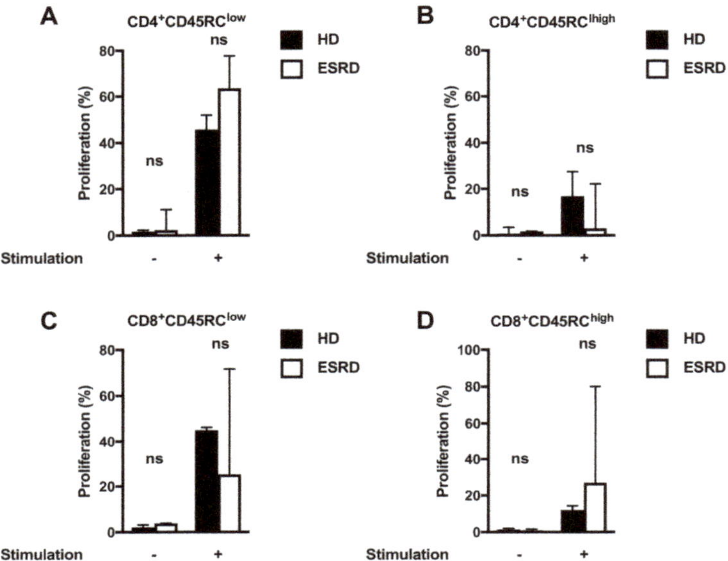

Figure 2. Analysis of proliferative capacities of CD45RC^{low} and CD45RC^{high} T cells in ESRD patients and HD. After 72 h, the proliferation of activated CD4$^+$CD45RC^{low} (**A**), CD4$^+$CD45RC^{high} (**B**), CD8$^+$CD45RC^{low} (**C**), and CD8$^+$CD45RC^{high} (**D**) T cell subsets of ESRD patients (black bars) and HD (white bars) was analyzed. The experiment reported results of four ESRD patients and four age and matched HD. Error bars show the median with a 95% CI. Comparisons were done using the Wilcoxon matched-pairs rank test. ns, non-significant. CI, Confidence Interval; ESRD: end-stage renal disease; HD: heathy individuals.

3.4. Association between CD45RC Expression on T Cells and Acute Rejection

We first analyzed the association of CD45RC expression on T cells with patient's characteristics. As shown in Figure 3, the level of CD45RC expression on CD4$^+$ and CD8$^+$ T cells were not significantly different according to gender, the number of previous transplantations, the level of pre-transplant immunization, or de novo DSA development. As previously reported in healthy subjects [10,11], CD45RC expression on CD4$^+$ and CD8$^+$ T cells was correlated with age ($p = 0.047$ and $p = 0.0002$, respectively).

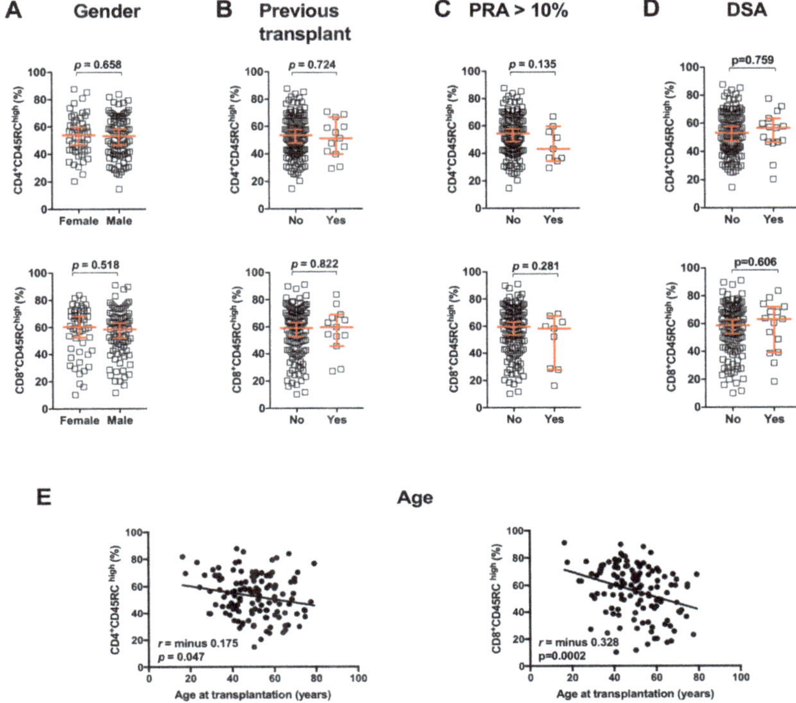

Figure 3. Proportion of CD45RC^{high} and CD45RC^{low} CD4+ and CD8+ T cells according to gender (**A**), previous transplantation (**B**), pre-transplant PRA (**C**), de novo DSA occurrence (**D**), and age at transplantation (**E**). For A–D, comparisons were done using the Mann–Whitney U test and error bars show median with a 95% CI. For E, correlation analysis was done using the Spearman test. CI, Confidence Interval; PRA, Panel Reactive Antibody.

We next analyzed the frequency of CD45RC T cell subsets according to the occurrence of AR (Table 4). In line with our previous observations [10], patients who experienced AR had a higher proportion of CD4$^+$ and CD8$^+$ CD45RC^{high} compared to patients that did not develop AR. The difference between groups remained significant regardless of whether all AR episodes were considered, when analysis was restricted to biopsy-proven ARs, or when borderline AR episodes were excluded. Moreover, the absolute number of both CD4$^+$ and CD8$^+$ CD45RC^{high} cells was significantly greater in patients that experienced AR ($p = 0.0101$ and 0.0073, respectively; Figure S2).

Table 4. Frequency of CD4$^+$ and CD8$^+$ CD45RC subsets according to AR occurrence. Comparisons were done using the Mann–Whitney U test. Significant *p*-values appear in bold.

Acute Rejection (all)	Yes *n* = 31	No *n* = 97	*p*
CD4$^+$CD45RC ^{high}	58.4 ± 13.7	51.2 ± 15.7	**0.023**
CD8$^+$CD45RC ^{high}	62.5 ± 13.3	53.6 ± 19.3	**0.019**
CD8$^+$CD45RC ^{int}	20.1 ± 7.7	23.2 ± 9.3	0.096
CD8$^+$CD45RC ^{low}	17.9 ± 9.8	23.7 ± 14.2	**0.035**
Biopsy-Proven AR *	Yes *n* = 28	No *n* = 97	*p*
CD4$^+$CD45RC ^{high}	59.2 ± 13.3	51.2 ± 15.7	**0.016**
CD8$^+$CD45RC ^{high}	62.3 ± 13.0	53.6 ± 18.0	**0.010**
CD8$^+$CD45RC ^{int}	20.1 ± 7.9	23.2 ± 9.3	0.117
CD8$^+$CD45RC ^{low}	18.0 ± 10.3	23.7 ± 14.2	**0.049**
Acute Rejection (excluding borderline AR) **	Yes *n* = 22	No *n* = 97	*p*
CD4$^+$CD45RC ^{high}	60.0 ± 13.4	51.2 ± 15.7	**0.016**
CD8$^+$CD45RC ^{high}	64.4 ± 12.2	53.6 ± 19.3	**0.014**
CD8$^+$CD45RC ^{int}	19.7 ± 8.1	23.2 ± 9.3	0.110
CD8$^+$CD45RC ^{low}	16.4 ± 7.9	23.7 ± 14.2	**0.020**

* Patients with clinical diagnosed AR without biopsy were excluded. ** Patients with biopsy-proven AR excluding patients with borderline AR. CD45RC subsets were determined as specified in the Materials and Method section. High, high expression; Low, low expression; Int, intermediate expression.

3.5. Value of CD45RC Expression on T Cell for Acute Rejection Prediction

We next analyzed the best thresholds of CD4$^+$ and CD8$^+$ CD45RC^{high} T cell frequencies for AR prediction. Using ROC curve analysis, we could determine 45.4% and 58.4% as the best thresholds of CD4$^+$ and CD8$^+$ CD45RC^{high} frequencies for AR prediction, respectively (Figure 4A). Using these thresholds, we observed that AR-free survival was significantly greater in patients with a CD8$^+$ CD45RC^{high} T cell frequency below 58.4% (p = 0.0005), while AR-free survival was not significantly different according to CD4$^+$ CD45RC^{high} T cell frequencies (p = 0.073) (Figure 4, upper and lower panel). Thus, CD8$^+$ CD45RC^{high} T cell frequency allows one to better differentiate patients at risk of AR, as compared to CD4$^+$ CD45RC^{high} T cells. The sensitivity, the specificity, and the positive predictive and negative predictive values of CD8$^+$ CD45RC^{high} T cell frequency above 58.4% for ARs were 80.6%, 55.7%, 36.8%, and 90%, respectively. These results are illustrated in Figure 4C. We did not observe any correlation between TCMR severity and the proportion of CD8$^+$ CD45RC^{high} T cells (Figure S3).

We finally analyzed the risk factors of AR in a cox model analysis (Table 5). We successively considered all ARs (including those clinically diagnosed), ARs excluding borderline cases, and biopsy-proven ARs. A CD8$^+$ CD45RC^{high} T cell frequency above 58.4% was significantly associated with AR after adjustment on type of induction. The CD8$^+$ CD45RC^{high} T cell frequency and ATG as an induction treatment were both associated with AR (all, including borderline) and biopsy-proven AR. When borderline ARs were excluded, ATG was no longer significantly associated with AR occurrence.

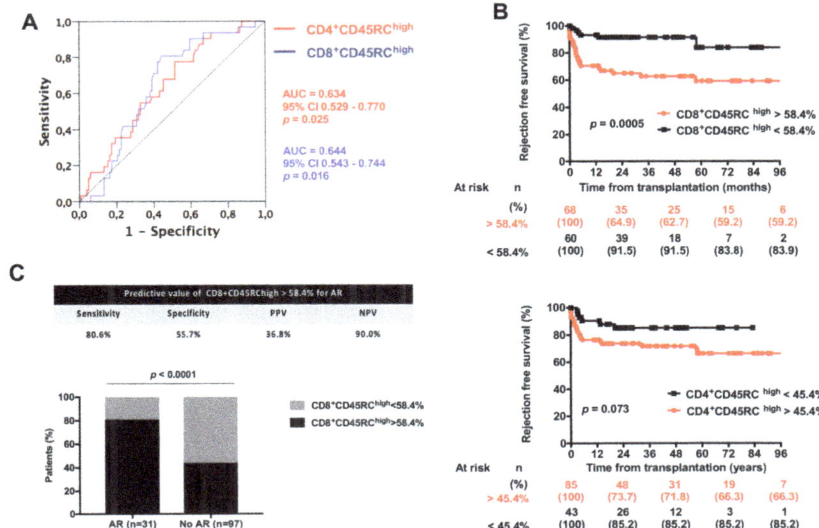

Figure 4. Predictive value of CD4$^+$ and CD8$^+$ CD45RC T cell subsets. (**A**) ROC curve analysis of CD4$^+$ and CD8$^+$ CD45RC^{high} T cell subsets for AR prediction. (**B**) Rejection-free survival of patients according to CD8$^+$ (upper panel) and CD4$^+$ CD45RC^{high} T cell proportions. Comparison between survivals was done using a log-rank test. (**C**) predictive values of CD8$^+$ CD45RC^{high} T cell above 58.4% for AR prediction. AUC: Area Under Curve.

Table 5. Multivariate cox analysis of factors associated with acute rejection occurrence. Significant *p*-values appear in bold.

	Multivariate Cox Models	HR	95% CI	*p*
All ARs	CD8$^+$CD45RC^{high} (>58.4%)	4.04	1.65–9.88	**0.002**
	Induction (ATG)	0.39	0.16–0.94	**0.037**
ARs excluding borderlines *	CD8$^+$CD45RC^{high} (>58.4%)	4.42	1.49–13.1	**0.007**
	Induction (ATG)	0.46	0.17–1.25	0.130
Biopsy-proven ARs **	CD8$^+$CD45RC^{high} (>58.4%)	3.59	1.45–8.89	**0.006**
	Induction (ATG)	0.35	0.13–0.93	**0.035**

* Patients with a biopsy–proven AR excluding patients with a borderline AR. ** Patients with a clinically diagnosed AR without biopsy were excluded.

4. Discussion

In the present work, we confirmed that the CD8$^+$ CD45RC^{high} T cell subset was associated with an increased risk of AR. We could determine that patients with a proportion of CD8$^+$ CD45RC^{high} T cell frequency above 58.4% had a 4-fold increased risk of AR. Thus, these results are in line with our previous work [10,13] and confirm the interest of CD45RC expression on T cells to assess the immunological risk of candidates to kidney transplantation.

As compared to our previous work [10,13], in the present study, patients were treated with current immunosuppressive strategies. Indeed, most patients received Basiliximab as an induction regimen and tacrolimus maintenance, while ATG and tacrolimus monotherapy after 6 months post-transplant was the most commonly used regimen in our previous study. Another important difference is that patients considered at high immunological risk were included in the present study. Although, pre-transplant sensitized patients represented a minority of the study population, we suggest that CD45RC expression may also help determine the AR risk in this specific population. Interestingly, CD45RC expression was not significantly different between patients with or without previous kidney transplantation or who were sensitized before kidney transplantation, which suggests that previous exposure to immunosuppressive drugs may not affect CD45RC expression on T cells. As previously reported, CD45RC expression was negatively associated with age, and correlation was greater for the CD8[+] T cell subset [10,11]. A genetic control of CD45RC on T cells has been demonstrated in rats [12,15]; however, its regulation in humans remains largely unknown.

AR incidence, including borderline AR, in our study was 24.2% after a mean follow-up of almost 4 years. As expected, most AR episodes were TCMR, with ABMR being implicated in only four AR episodes. This observation is in line with recent reports [3,16] showing the predominant occurrence of TCMR as compared to ABMR in the first few years of transplantation. Most AR episodes occurred within the first few years following kidney transplantation, which is also in line with published data [17,18]. Thus, CD45RC expression mainly allows one to assess the risk of TCMR, which represented the majority of ARs in the cohort. Interestingly, we did not observe any difference in CD45RC[high] T cell subset frequency according to subsequent DSA development, which suggests that CD45RC status does not allow one to assess the risk of ABMR. TCMR still represents a significant cause of morbidity in the era of ABMR, the latter being the main cause of late graft lost [19]. Moreover, several recent reports suggested that the occurrence of TCMR is independently linked to subsequent interstitial fibrosis development [20] and probably an increased risk of ABMR development by exposing HLA antigens within kidney [18,21,22]. Thus, these data suggest that decreasing the rate of TCMR, including sub-clinical TCMR, could allow one to improve the long-term graft outcome and decrease the risk of ABMR. This reinforces the need to better delineate patients at high TCMR risk to prevent it by adjusting the immunosuppressive regimen.

Interestingly, not only CD45RC proportion was associated with AR occurrence, but also the absolute count of CD45RC[high] CD4[+] and especially CD8[+] T cells. In vitro, CD45RC[high] CD8[+] T cells from HD mainly produced interferon gamma a key cytokine in TCMR, and poor levels of regulatory cytokines [10]. Whether, the ESRD milieu affects the cytokine profile of CD45RC T cell subsets remains to be fully analyzed. However, we show here that CD45RC T cell subsets from ESRD patients had a similar proliferative capacity as compared to those of HD. This suggests that the immune functions of CD45RC T cell subsets were preserved in a uremic context.

We could determine in the present study that 58.4% was the best threshold of CD8[+] CD45RC[high] T cells for AR prediction. In our previous work, the best threshold was determined at 54.7% [10]. Finally, moving the cut-off to this value would result in minimal changes in the predictive value of CD8[+] CD45RC[high] T cells in the present study. The very closed cut-off values as determined in the two works, conducted in two different populations with different immunosuppressive regimens, reinforces the strength of this biomarker.

The present study has several limitations. First, only 32% of patients transplanted during the period were included and we could not exclude a selection bias. Next, AR diagnosis was based on for-cause biopsies and not protocol biopsies. Thus, the value of CD45RC expression for subclinical rejection remains to be investigated. Moreover, given the relatively short follow-up, we were not able to analyze the relationship between pre-transplant CD45RC expression and the risk of ABMR, which occurred in only four patients in the present study.

In conclusion, the present study confirmed and extended the data on CD45RC that has appeared as a promising biomarker to assess the risk of AR before transplantation. This work confirmed that the pre-transplant proportion of CD8[+] CD45RC[high] T cells is associated with a 4-fold increased risk of AR, mainly TCMR. Thus, CD45RC could be used to help define the immunological risk and the level of immunosuppressive regimen before kidney transplantation. However, the value of CD45RC expression on T cells should be evaluated in a multicenter prospective cohort study with protocol biopsies to confirm its usefulness and to study its predictive value for subclinical AR.

Supplementary Materials: The following are available online at http://www.mdpi.com/2077-0383/8/8/1147/s1. Figure S1. Representative experiment showing the cytometry gating strategy. Figure S2. Absolute number of CD4$^+$ and CD8$^+$ CDR45RC^{high} T cells according to AR occurrence. Figure S3. Correlation between CD8$^+$ CD45RC^{high} T cell proportion and the severity of TCMR. The correlation was analyzed using Spearman's test. Table S1: Univariate analysis of factors associated with acute rejection occurrence. Patients with borderline AR were excluded from the analysis.

Author Contributions: Conceptualization, J.-F.A., A.D., and J.-F.S.; Methodology, J.-F.A., A.D., and J.-F.S.; Validation, J.-F.A.; Formal Analysis, M.L., S.B., A.-S.G., and B.B.; Investigation, M.L., A.-S.G., and J.-F.A.; Resources, O.B.; Data Curation, O.B.; Writing—Original Draft Preparation, M.L., M.P., and A.-S.G.; Writing—Review and Editing, J.-F.A., J.-F.S., O.B., Y.D., A.D., and A.C.; Supervision, J.-F.A. and J.-F.S.; Project Administration, J.-F.A.

Acknowledgments: We acknowledge Ms Jolivot Denise and the members of "La Maison de la Recherche" of the University Hospital of Angers for the help they provided in this project.

Conflicts of Interest: The authors declare no conflict of interest.

Abbreviations

ABMR	antibody-mediated rejection
AR	acute rejection
ATG	anti-thymocytes globulins
DSA	Donor specific anti-HLA antibodies
HD	healthy donors
PRA	panel reactive antibody
PBMC	plasma blood mononuclear cells
ROC	receiver operating curve
TCMR	T-cell-mediated rejection

References

1. Nankivell, B.J.; Alexander, S.I. Rejection of the kidney allograft. *N. Engl. J. Med.* **2010**, *363*, 1451–1462. [CrossRef] [PubMed]

2. Loupy, A.; Lefaucheur, C. Antibody-mediated rejection of solid-organ allografts. *N. Engl. J. Med.* **2018**, *379*, 1150–1160. [CrossRef] [PubMed]

3. Bouatou, Y.; Viglietti, D.; Pievani, D.; Louis, K.; Duong Van Huyen, J.P.; Rabant, M.; Aubert, O.; Taupin, J.L.; Glotz, D.; Legendre, C.; et al. Response to treatment and long-term outcomes in kidney transplant recipients with acute t cell-mediated rejection. *Am. J. Transplant.* **2019**. [CrossRef] [PubMed]

4. Lebranchu, Y.; Baan, C.; Biancone, L.; Legendre, C.; Morales, J.M.; Naesens, M.; Thomusch, O.; Friend, P. Pretransplant identification of acute rejection risk following kidney transplantation. *Transplant. Int.* **2014**, *27*, 129–138. [CrossRef] [PubMed]

5. Cantarovich, D.; Vistoli, F.; Soulillou, J.P. Immunosuppression minimization in kidney transplantation. *Front. Biosci.* **2008**, *13*, 1413–1432. [CrossRef] [PubMed]

6. Pascual, M.; Theruvath, T.; Kawai, T.; Tolkoff-Rubin, N.; Cosimi, A.B. Strategies to improve long-term outcomes after renal transplantation. *N. Engl. J. Med.* **2002**, *346*, 580–590. [CrossRef] [PubMed]

7. Londono, M.C.; Danger, R.; Giral, M.; Soulillou, J.P.; Sanchez-Fueyo, A.; Brouard, S. A need for biomarkers of operational tolerance in liver and kidney transplantation. *Am. J. Transplant.* **2012**, *12*, 1370–1377. [CrossRef]

8. Clark, M.C.; Baum, L.G. T cells modulate glycans on cd43 and cd45 during development and activation, signal regulation, and survival. *Ann. N. Y. Acad. Sci.* **2012**, *1253*, 58–67. [CrossRef]

9. Hermiston, M.L.; Xu, Z.; Weiss, A. Cd45: A critical regulator of signaling thresholds in immune cells. *Annu. Rev. Immunol.* **2003**, *21*, 107–137. [CrossRef]

10. Ordonez, L.; Bernard, I.; Chabod, M.; Augusto, J.F.; Lauwers-Cances, V.; Cristini, C.; Cuturi, M.C.; Subra, J.F.; Saoudi, A. A higher risk of acute rejection of human kidney allografts can be predicted from the level of cd45rc expressed by the recipients' cd8 t cells. *PLoS ONE* **2013**, *8*, e69791. [CrossRef]

11. Ordonez, L.; Bernard, I.; L'Faqihi-Olive, F.E.; Tervaert, J.W.; Damoiseaux, J.; Saoudi, A. Cd45rc isoform expression identifies functionally distinct t cell subsets differentially distributed between healthy individuals and aav patients. *PLoS ONE* **2009**, *4*, e5287. [CrossRef] [PubMed]

12. Subra, J.F.; Cautain, B.; Xystrakis, E.; Mas, M.; Lagrange, D.; Van Der Heijden, H.; Van De Gaar, M.J.; Druet, P.; Fournie, G.J.; Saoudi, A.; et al. The balance between cd45rchigh and cd45rclow cd4 t cells in rats is intrinsic to bone marrow-derived cells and is genetically controlled. *J. Immunol.* **2001**, *166*, 2944–2952. [CrossRef] [PubMed]

13. Garnier, A.S.; Planchais, M.; Riou, J.; Jacquemin, C.; Ordonez, L.; Saint-Andre, J.P.; Croue, A.; Saoudi, A.; Delneste, Y.; Devys, A.; et al. Pre-transplant cd45rc expression on blood t cells differentiates patients with cancer and rejection after kidney transplantation. *PLoS ONE* **2019**, *14*, e0214321. [CrossRef] [PubMed]

14. Haas, M.; Sis, B.; Racusen, L.C.; Solez, K.; Glotz, D.; Colvin, R.B.; Castro, M.C.; David, D.S.; David-Neto, E.; Bagnasco, S.M.; et al. Banff 2013 meeting report: Inclusion of c4d-negative antibody-mediated rejection and antibody-associated arterial lesions. *Am. J. Transplant.* **2014**, *14*, 272–283. [CrossRef] [PubMed]

15. Xystrakis, E.; Cavailles, P.; Dejean, A.S.; Cautain, B.; Colacios, C.; Lagrange, D.; van de Gaar, M.J.; Bernard, I.; Gonzalez-Dunia, D.; Damoiseaux, J.; et al. Functional and genetic analysis of two cd8 t cell subsets defined by the level of cd45rc expression in the rat. *J. Immunol.* **2004**, *173*, 3140–3147. [CrossRef] [PubMed]

16. Sellares, J.; De Freitas, D.G.; Mengel, M.; Reeve, J.; Einecke, G.; Sis, B.; Hidalgo, L.G.; Famulski, K.; Matas, A.; Halloran, P.F. Understanding the causes of kidney transplant failure: The dominant role of antibody-mediated rejection and nonadherence. *Am. J. Transplant.* **2012**, *12*, 388–399. [CrossRef] [PubMed]

17. Halloran, P.F.; Chang, J.; Famulski, K.; Hidalgo, L.G.; Salazar, I.D.; Merino Lopez, M.; Matas, A.; Picton, M.; De Freitas, D.; Bromberg, J.; et al. Disappearance of t cell-mediated rejection despite continued antibody-mediated rejection in late kidney transplant recipients. *J. Am. Soc. Nephrol.* **2015**, *26*, 1711–1720. [CrossRef]

18. Randhawa, P. T-cell-mediated rejection of the kidney in the era of donor-specific antibodies: Diagnostic challenges and clinical significance. *Curr. Opin. Organ Transplant.* **2015**, *20*, 325–332. [CrossRef]

19. Krisl, J.C.; Alloway, R.R.; Shield, A.R.; Govil, A.; Mogilishetty, G.; Cardi, M.; Diwan, T.; Abu Jawdeh, B.G.; Girnita, A.; Witte, D.; et al. Acute rejection clinically defined phenotypes correlate with long-term renal allograft survival. *Transplantation* **2015**, *99*, 2167–2173. [CrossRef]

20. Lefaucheur, C.; Gosset, C.; Rabant, M.; Viglietti, D.; Verine, J.; Aubert, O.; Louis, K.; Glotz, D.; Legendre, C.; Duong Van Huyen, J.P.; et al. T cell-mediated rejection is a major determinant of inflammation in scarred areas in kidney allografts. *Am. J. Transplant.* **2018**, *18*, 377–390. [CrossRef]

21. Wiebe, C.; Gibson, I.W.; Blydt-Hansen, T.D.; Karpinski, M.; Ho, J.; Storsley, L.J.; Goldberg, A.; Birk, P.E.; Rush, D.N.; Nickerson, P.W. Evolution and clinical pathologic correlations of de novo donor-specific hla antibody post kidney transplant. *Am. J. Transplant.* **2012**, *12*, 1157–1167. [CrossRef]

22. Moreso, F.; Carrera, M.; Goma, M.; Hueso, M.; Sellares, J.; Martorell, J.; Grinyo, J.M.; Seron, D. Early subclinical rejection as a risk factor for late chronic humoral rejection. *Transplantation* **2012**, *93*, 41–46. [CrossRef]

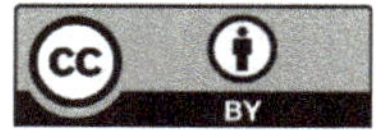

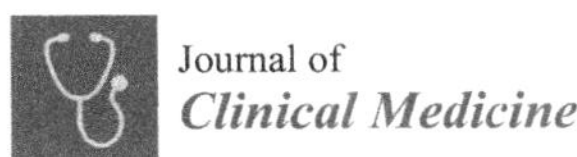 Journal of
Clinical Medicine

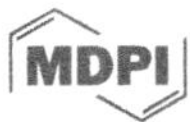

Article

Exposure to Hyperchloremia Is Associated with Poor Early Recovery of Kidney Graft Function after Living-Donor Kidney Transplantation: A Propensity Score-Matching Analysis

Jin Go [1], Sun-Cheol Park [2], Sang-Seob Yun [2], Jiyeon Ku [3], Jaesik Park [4], Jung-Woo Shim [4], Hyung Mook Lee [4], Yong-Suk Kim [4], Young Eun Moon [4], Sang Hyun Hong [4] and Min Suk Chae [4,*]

[1] Department of Surgery, Division of Vascular and Transplant Surgery, Mediplex Sejong Hospital, Incheon 21080, Korea
[2] Department of Surgery, Division of Vascular and Transplant Surgery, Seoul St. Mary's Hospital, College of Medicine, The Catholic University of Korea, Seoul 06591, Korea
[3] Department of Anesthesiology and Pain Medicine, Bucheon St. Mary's Hospital, College of Medicine, The Catholic University of Korea, Seoul 06591, Korea
[4] Department of Anesthesiology and Pain Medicine, Seoul St. Mary's Hospital, College of Medicine, The Catholic University of Korea, 222, Banpo-daero, Seocho-gu, Seoul 06591, Korea
* Correspondence: shscms@gmail.com; Tel.: +82-2-2258-6150; Fax: +82-2-537-1951

Received: 8 June 2019; Accepted: 1 July 2019; Published: 2 July 2019

Abstract: The effects of hyperchloremia on kidney grafts have not been investigated in patients undergoing living-donor kidney transplantation (LDKT). In this study, data from 200 adult patients undergoing elective LDKT between January 2016 and December 2017 were analyzed after propensity score (PS) matching. The patients were allocated to hyperchloremia and non-hyperchloremia groups according to the occurrence of hyperchloremia (i.e., $\geq$110 mEq/L) immediately after surgery. Poor early graft recovery was defined as estimated glomerular filtration rate (eGFR) < 60 mL/min/1.73 m^2 during the first 48 hours after surgery. After PS matching, no significant differences in perioperative recipient or donor graft parameters were observed between groups. Although the total amount of crystalloid fluid infused during surgery did not differ between groups, the proportions of main crystalloid fluid type used (i.e., 0.9% normal saline vs. Plasma Solution-A) did. The eGFR increased gradually during postoperative day (POD) 2 in both groups. However, the proportion of patients with eGFR > 60 mL/min/1.73 m^2 on POD 2 was higher in the non-hyperchloremia group than in the hyperchloremia group. In this PS-adjusted analysis, hyperchloremia was significantly associated with poor graft recovery on POD 2. In conclusion, exposure to hyperchloremia may have a negative impact on early graft recovery in LDKT.

Keywords: hyperchloremia; kidney graft dysfunction; living donor kidney transplantation

---

1. Introduction

Acute kidney injury (AKI) is a common complication that increases the risk of poor graft outcome in patients undergoing kidney transplantation (KT). Kidney grafts seem to be vulnerable to poor early function recovery because of various types of acute perioperative damage, such as ischemia-reperfusion injury, immunological insult, medication toxicity, and surgical stress [1]. In living-donor kidney transplantation (LDKT), better graft quality and patient condition result in better early graft function compared with deceased-donor KT. However, the reported incidence of poor early graft function after

LDKT is 10–20%, and this early graft dysfunction is closely related closely to an increased risk of long-term graft failure [2,3].

Chloride is a major anion in extracellular fluid and an essential element for plasma tonicity. Chloride plays a role in maintaining aspects of homeostasis, such as acid balance, muscular activation, and immunological response [4]. Hyperchloremia is a potential risk factor for AKI in critically ill patients admitted to the intensive care unit (ICU) [5–8]. In patients undergoing noncardiac surgery, the perioperative development of hyperchloremia was reported to be independently associated with morbidity and mortality risks [9]. These harmful effects of hyperchloremia have largely been investigated in the context of chloride-rich solution resuscitation, which has been found to have a detrimental impact on kidney function [10,11]. However, the relationship between hyperchloremia and AKI has been investigated only in native (i.e., not transplanted) kidneys, in the context of clinical conditions such as sepsis, subarachnoid hemorrhage, and abdominal surgery [5–8,12].

To date, the effects of hyperchloremia on kidney grafts have not been investigated in patients undergoing LDKT. We investigated the association between hyperchloremia and early graft function recovery. In addition, postoperative outcomes, such as the requirement for renal replacement therapy (RRT), graft rejection, and mortality, were investigated according to the occurrence of hyperchloremia.

2. Patients and Methods

2.1. Ethical Considerations

This study was approved by the Institutional Review Board and Ethics Committee of Seoul St. Mary's Hospital (KC19RESI0088) and was performed in accordance with the Declaration of Helsinki. The requirement for informed consent was waived due to the retrospective study design.

2.2. Study Population

The study population consisted of 330 adult patients (i.e., age $\geq$ 19 years) who underwent elective LDKT at Seoul St. Mary's Hospital between January 2016 and December 2017. Pediatric patients (i.e., age < 19 years), those undergoing deceased-donor or ABO-incompatible KT, patients undergoing multiorgan transplantation including the kidney, and those undergoing re-transplantation were excluded from the study because these patients require various and complex immunosuppression regimens or surgical technique application [13–17]. Patients with defective or missing recipient and donor graft data were also excluded. Based on the exclusion criteria, 29 patients were not included in the study. In total, 301 patients were initially enrolled and their data were included in propensity score (PS)-matching analysis; data from 200 matched patients were included in the final analysis.

2.3. Living Donor Kidney Transplantation

The surgical technique for LDKT involved an initial hockey-stick (i.e., pararectal inverted J-shaped curvilinear) incision and exposure of the right pelvic fossa. After back table preparation of the graft, end-to-side anastomoses between the recipient external iliac artery/vein and the graft renal artery/vein were performed using Prolene 6.0 resorbable monofilament (Ethicon, Somerville, NJ, USA). Subsequently, ureteroneocystostomy was performed with insertion of a double-J stent (INLAY ureteral stent; Bard Medical, Covington, GA, USA) using the Lich-Grègoir technique [18,19]. After careful hemostasis and re-assessment of the vascular anastomosis and renal pedicle area, closed drains were placed and the wound was closed.

Balanced anesthesia was applied using 1–2 mg/kg propofol (Fresenius Kabi, Bad Homburg, Germany) and 0.6 mg/kg rocuronium (Merck Sharp & Dohme Corp., Kenilworth, NJ, USA), and maintained using 2.0–6.0% desflurane (Baxter, Deerfield, IL, USA) with medical air/oxygen and continuous remifentanil (Hanlim Pharmaceutical Co., Ltd., Seoul, Republic of Korea) infusion at a rate of 0.1–0.5 µg/kg/min, as appropriate. The maintenance of appropriate hypnotic depth between 40 and 50 was ensured with a Bispectral Index™ instrument (Medtronic, Minneapolis, MN, USA). Central venous pressure (CVP) was monitored using a central venous catheter (Arrow, Morrisville, NC, USA) inserted before surgery. The optimal hemodynamic status was adjusted to a mean arterial pressure of ≥65 mmHg with infusion of dopamine (Reyon Pharm. Co., Ltd., Seoul, Republic of Korea) at a rate of 5–10 µg/kg/min. Mannitol (Daihan Pharm. Co., Ltd., Seoul, Republic of Korea) was used at doses of 20–50 g to promote urine flow [20]. However, we did not regularly cannulate and/or puncture a radial artery for continuous monitoring of blood pressure or arterial blood gas analysis (ABGA), to avoid arterial injury. We only measured ABGA when oxygen saturation was below 90% using pulse oximetry.

For intraoperative fluid therapy, an isotonic crystalloid fluid (0.9% normal saline (Daihan Pharm Co., Ltd.) or Plasma Solution-A (CJ Healthcare, Seoul, Republic of Korea)) was selected at the discretion of the attending anesthesiologist. The 0.9% normal saline (i.e., chloride-liberal fluid) included sodium chloride (9 g/L; 154 mEq/L sodium; and 154 mEq/L chloride). Plasma Solution-A (i.e., chloride-restrictive fluid) included magnesium chloride (0.3 g/L; 0 37 g/L potassium chloride, 3.68 g/L sodium acetate, 5.26 g/L sodium chloride, and 5.02 g/L sodium gluconate (140 mEq/L sodium, 98 mEq/L chloride, 5 mEq/L potassium, and 3 mEq/L magnesium)). Baseline isotonic crystalloid infusion was based on the estimated fluid maintenance requirements, calculated from the patient's weight and anticipated tissue trauma [21]. Additional fluid boluses were administered to reach a target CVP of 10–15 mmHg or hydration volume of 50–100 mL/kg, to ensure sufficient flow for the maintenance of adequate kidney graft perfusion and to replace the amount of urine output after graft reperfusion [22].

In the immunosuppressive regimen (Table 1), the induction drug was based on interleukin-2 receptor antagonist (i.e., Basiliximab) and T lymphocyte-depleting rabbit-derived anti-thymocyte globulin (i.e., thymoglobulin), and drug maintenance was based on a calcineurin inhibitor (i.e., tacrolimus), mycophenolate mofetil, and steroids. Steroid pulse therapy and/or thymoglobulin rescue therapy were applied in cases of graft rejection.

Table 1. Immunosuppressive regimen in living donor kidney transplantation.

	Maintain Immune Therapy		
Induction Therapy	Basiliximab	**20 mg IV. at Surgical Day and POD 4**	
	Thymoglobulin	1.25 mg/kg IV at surgical day and during POD 4	
Maintenance therapy	Tacrolimus	0.06 mg/kg on 2 day before surgery 0.05 mg/kg on 1 day before surgery	Dosage control under serum level after surgery
	Mycophenolate	MMF 750 mg/MYF 540 mg p.o. q.d. and raise bid after surgery	Under 50 kg patient MMF 500 mg/MYF 360 mg p.o. bid
	Steroids	Prednisone 125 mg IV qid and reduce until 60 mg tid	p.o. change until 10 mg p.o. bid for prednisolone
	Immune Therapy for Graft Rejection		
Steroid pulse therapy		Prednisone 500 mg IV/day	Cessation of IV within 5 days and switch to p.o. medication
Thymoglobulin rescue therapy		1.25 mg/kg IV for 5 days	

Abbreviations: POD, postoperative day; MMF; mycophenolate mofetil, MYF; mycophenolate sodium, IV; intravenous, p.o.; per oral; q.d., quaque die (every day); bid, bis in die (twice a day); qid, quarter in die (four times a day).

2.4. Measurement of Serum Chloride Levels

The baseline chloride level was estimated between the day after dialysis and the preoperative period, and serial chloride levels were measured 1 day before surgery, immediately after surgery, and on postoperative days (PODs) 1 and 2. The chloride level was analyzed by indirect potentiometry (Clinical Analyzer 7600; Hitachi, Tokyo, Japan).

The patients were divided according to the presence or absence of hyperchloremia (defined as ≥110 mEq/L [6,23]) immediately after surgery into the hyperchloremia group and the non-hyperchloremia group, respectively.

2.5. Definition of Poor Early Recovery of Kidney Graft Function

Kidney graft function was quantified based on the estimated glomerular filtration rate (eGFR), calculated using the Modification of Diet in Renal Disease formula: eGFR = 175 × standardized serum chloride$^{-1.154}$ × age$^{-0.203}$ × 1.212 (if black) × 0.742 (if female) [24]. The baseline eGFR was estimated between the day after dialysis and the preoperative period, and serial eGFRs were measured immediately after surgery and on PODs 1 and 2. Based on the eGFR, the degree of graft function was classified as chronic kidney disease (CKD) stage I (i.e., normal kidney function and eGFR ≥ 90 mL/min/1.73 m^2), stage II (i.e., mild loss of kidney function and eGFR 60–89 mL/min/1.73 m^2), stage IIIa (i.e., mild to moderate loss of kidney function and eGFR 45–59 mL/min/1.73 m^2), stage IIIb (i.e., moderate to severe loss of kidney function and eGFR 30–44 mL/min/1.73 m^2), stage IV (i.e., severe loss of kidney function and eGFR 15–29 mL/min/1.73 m^2), or stage V (i.e., kidney failure and eGFR < 15 mL/min/1.73 m^2) [25].

In the present study, poor early recovery of kidney graft function, defined as eGFR < 60 mL/min/1.73 m^2 during the first 48 hours after surgery [26], was the primary outcome.

2.6. Clinical Variables

Preoperative and intraoperative recipient and donor graft factors in the non-hyperchloremia and hyperchloremia groups were assessed by PS matching analysis. Preoperative recipient factors included age, sex, body mass index (BMI), comorbidities (i.e., diabetes mellitus (DM) and hypertension), dialysis history and duration, and laboratory variables (i.e., white blood cell count, platelet count, and hemoglobin, sodium, chloride, potassium, albumin, creatinine, and glucose concentrations). Intraoperative factors included the operation time, averages of vital signs (i.e., systolic and diastolic blood pressures, heart rate, CVP, and body temperature), and total amounts of crystalloid infusion, urine output, and blood loss. Donor graft factors included age, sex, BMI, graft weight, total graft ischemic time, and human leukocyte antigen level.

Postoperative clinical factors included RRT requirement, biopsy-proven graft rejection [27], and patient mortality during the follow-up period.

2.7. Statistical Analysis

The normality of continuous data was assessed using the Shapiro-Wilk test. Continuous data are expressed as medians and interquartile ranges, and categorical data are expressed as numbers and proportions. PS matching analysis was applied to reduce the impact of potential confounding factors on intergroup differences based on hyperchloremia [28,29]. PSs were derived to match patients at a 1:1 ratio using greedy matching algorithms without replacement. Perioperative recipient and donor graft factors were compared using the Mann–Whitney U test and χ^2 test or Fisher's exact test, as appropriate. Wilcoxon's signed-rank sum test and McNemar's test were used for analysis of the pair-matched data. Postoperative changes in the proportions of patients with kidney graft function classified as eGFR $\geq$ 60 vs. 30–59 vs. < 30 mL/min/1.73 m^2 were analyzed using Cochran's Q test with the McNemar post hoc test. The association of hyperchloremia with poor early recovery of kidney graft function was evaluated by multivariable logistic regression analysis with PS adjustment. The values are presented as odds ratios with 95% confidence intervals. All tests were two sided, and $p < 0.05$ was taken to indicate statistical significance. All statistical analyses were performed using R software version 2.10.1 (R Foundation for Statistical Computing, Vienna, Austria) and SPSS for Windows (ver. 24.0; SPSS Inc., Chicago, IL, USA).

3. Results

3.1. Demographic Characteristics of Patients Undergoing LDKT

The total study population of 301 patients comprised 188 (62.5%) males and 113 (35.5%) females with an average age of 49 $\pm$ 11 years and average BMI of 23.1 $\pm$ 3.5 kg/m^2. The incidences of DM and hypertension were 28.6% (n = 86) and 58.1% (n = 175), respectively. Dialysis was performed in 220 (73.1%) patients for an average duration of 30 $\pm$ 53 months. The average eGFR was 7.6 $\pm$ 3.5 mL/min/1.73 m^2. A total of 295 (98.0%) patients had CKD stage V (i.e., eGFR <15 mL/min/1.73 m^2), five (1.7%) patients had CKD stage IV (i.e., eGFR 15–29 mL/min/1.73 m^2), and one (0.03%) patient had CKD stage IIIb (i.e., eGFR 30–44 mL/min/1.73 m^2).

3.2. Comparison of Perioperative Factors before and after PS Matching

Before PS matching, there were significant differences between groups in preoperative findings (i.e., dialysis duration, sodium and glucose levels), intraoperative findings (i.e., average diastolic blood pressure and total amount of hemorrhage), and donor graft parameters (i.e., total graft ischemic time; Table 2). After PS matching, there were no significant differences in perioperative recipient or donor graft parameters between groups.

Table 2. Comparison of clinical perioperative factors between the non-hyperchloremia and hyperchloremia groups before and after propensity score matching analysis.

Group	Before PS Matching				After PS Matching			
	No Hyperchloremia	Hyperchloremia	p	SD	No Hyperchloremia	Hyperchloremia	p	SD
n	201	100			100	100		
Recipient parameter								
Preoperative finding								
Age (years)	50 (42–56)	53 (42–58)	0.087	0.118	52 (46–59)	53 (42–58)	0.850	−0.040
Sex (male)	121 (60.2%)	67 (67.0%)	0.251	−0.144	68 (68.0%)	67 (67.0%)	0.880	0.021
Body mass index (kg/m^2)	22.7 (20.7–25.2)	23.1 (21.2–25.2)	0.398	0.131	23.2 (21.1–25.6)	23.1 (21.2–25.2)	0.910	0.040
Comorbidity								
Diabetes mellitus	60 (29.9%)	26 (26.0%)	0.486	−0.087	29 (29.0%)	26 (26.0%)	0.635	−0.068
Hypertension	123 (61.2%)	52 (52.0%)	0.128	−0.183	53 (53.0%)	52 (52.0%)	0.887	−0.020
Dialysis history	141 (70.1%)	79 (79.0%)	0.103	0.216	76 (76.0%)	79 (79.0%)	0.611	0.073
Dialysis duration (month)	2.0 (0.0–30.0)	6.0 (1.0–57.0)	0.008	0.238	3.0 (0.0–37.5)	6.0 (1.0–57.0)	0.171	0.170
Laboratory analysis								
WBC count (x 10^9/L)	6.7 (5.1–8.8)	6.3 (4.7–8.1)	0.090	−0.238	6.6 (4.8–7.7)	6.3 (4.7–8.1)	0.581	−0.081
Hemoglobin (g/dL)	10.7 (9.5–12.0)	10.9 (9.9–11.9)	0.333	0.145	10.7 (9.5–12.0)	10.9 (9.9–11.9)	0.433	0.121
Platelet count (x 10^9/L)	178.0 (146.0–225.5)	183.0 (139.0–231.0)	0.874	−0.009	181.0 (149.0–236.8)	183.0 (139.0–231.0)	0.815	−0.016
Sodium (mEq/L)	137.0 (135.0–139.0)	138.0 (135.3–139.0)	0.018	0.175	137.0 (135.0–139.0)	138.0 (135.3–139.0)	0.094	0.127
Chloride (mEq/L)	98.0 (95.0–101.0)	98.0 (95.0–102.0)	0.387	0.173	98.0 (95.0–101.0)	98.0 (95.0–102.0)	0.698	0.115
Potassium (mEq/L)	4.8 (4.2–5.4)	4.7 (4.2–5.2)	0.400	−0.037	4.8 (4.2–5.4)	4.7 (4.2–5.2)	0.534	0.060
Albumin (g/dL)	4.0 (3.6–4.3)	4.0 (3.7–4.2)	0.553	0.106	3.9 (3.6–4.3)	4.0 (3.7–4.2)	0.383	0.087
Creatinine (mg/dL)	7.8 (6.2–9.9)	7.7 (6.3–10.4)	0.715	0.064	7.7 (6.2–9.5)	7.7 (6.3–10.4)	0.737	0.044
Glucose (mg/dL)	152.0 (126.5–189.0)	140.0 (100.8–171.3)	0.011	0.069	149.0 (121.5–190.8)	140.0 (100.8–171.3)	0.050	−0.034
Intraoperative finding								
Surgery time (min)	260 (222–295)	275 (230–309)	0.085	0.195	265 (235–302)	275 (230–309)	0.735	0.001
Average of vital sign								
SBP (mmHg)	125 (117–134)	123 (114–132)	0.186	−0.149	125 (115–131)	123 (114–132)	0.870	0.011
DBP (mmHg)	73 (65–79)	69 (63–77)	0.029	−0.274	71 (63–77)	69 (63–77)	0.525	−0.061
Heart rate (beats/min)	81 (73–89)	80 (71–86)	0.372	−0.039	80 (71–88)	80 (71–86)	0.855	0.012
CVP (mmHg)	10 (8–12)	10 (8–12)	0.174	0.186	10 (8–12)	10 (8–12)	0.991	0.026
Body temperature (°C)	36.3 (36.1–36.5)	36.3 (36.0–36.5)	0.482	−0.067	36.3 (36.1–36.5)	36.3 (36.0–36.5)	0.660	−0.030
Total crystalloid infusion (mL)	2900 (2200–3600)	3100 (2500–4100)	0.066	0.221	3190 (2500–3838)	3100 (2500–4100)	0.990	−0.014
Urine output (mL)	400 (200–700)	350 (100–700)	0.180	−0.131	375 (193–626)	350 (100–700)	0.777	−0.032
Blood loss (mL)	150 (100–250)	200 (150–300)	0.004	0.221	200 (100–300)	200 (150–300)	0.096	0.075

Table 2. *Cont.*

	Before PS Matching				After PS Matching			
Group	No Hyperchloremia	Hyperchloremia	*p*	SD	No Hyperchloremia	Hyperchloremia	*p*	SD
n	201	100			100	100		
Donor-graft parameter								
Age (years)	47 (35–54)	50 (36–56)	0.233	0.111	47 (34–53)	50 (36–56)	0.157	0.162
Sex (male)	103 (51.2%)	47 (47.0%)	0.488	0.085	47 (47.0%)	47 (47.0%)	1.000	0.000
Body mass index (kg/m^2)	23.7 (21.6–25.9)	23.1 (21.8–25.1)	0.276	−0.197	23.3 (21.0–25.4)	23.1 (21.8–25.1)	0.664	−0.006
Graft weight (g)	184.0 (160.0–216.0)	180.0 (160.5–212.0)	0.398	−0.172	178.0 (158.0–203.5)	180.0 (160.5–212.0)	0.374	0.090
Total graft ischemic time (min)	58 (43–85)	68 (51–126)	0.006	0.265	64 (45–109)	68 (51–126)	0.200	0.113
Human leukocyte antigen analysis								
PRA (positive)								
Class I	63 (31.3%)	36 (36.0%)	0.418	0.097	32 (32.0%)	36 (36.0%)	0.550	0.083
Class II	44 (21.9%)	31 (31.0%)	0.085	0.196	29 (29.0%)	31 (31.0%)	0.758	0.043
DSA (positive)								
Class I	41 (20.4%)	17 (17.0%)	0.481	−0.090	17 (17.0%)	17 (17.0%)	1.000	0.000
Class II	34 (16.9%)	24 (24.0%)	0.142	0.165	23 (23.0%)	24 (24.0%)	0.868	0.023
FCXM (positive)								
T-cell	2 (1.0%)	1 (1.0%)	1.000	0.000	1 (1.0%)	1 (1.0%)	1.000	0.000
B-cell	36 (17.9%)	20 (20.0%)	0.661	0.052	20 (20.0%)	20 (20.0%)	1.000	0.000

Abbreviations: WBC, white blood cell; SBP, systolic blood pressure; DBP, diastolic blood pressure; CVP, central venous pressure; PRA, panel reactive antibody; DSA, donor-specific antibody; FCXM, flow cytometric cross-match. Note: Values are expressed as the median (interquartile range) and number (proportion).

3.3. Comparison of Main Crystalloid Fluid Infusion during Surgery and Electrolyte Values Immediately after Surgery in PS-Matched Patients

The total amount of crystalloid fluid infused during surgery did not differ between groups. However, the proportions of main crystalloid fluid type used (i.e., 0.9% normal saline vs. Plasma Solution-A) differed between the groups (Table 3). With regard to electrolyte values immediately after surgery, serum sodium and potassium levels were similar in the two groups, but the serum chloride level was higher and the change in chloride level was greater in the hyperchloremia group.

Table 3. Comparison of main crystalloid fluid during surgery and electrolyte values immediately after surgery between propensity score-matched non-hyperchloremia and hyperchloremia groups.

Group	No Hyperchloremia	Hyperchloremia	p
n	100	100	
Total crystalloid fluid infusion (mL)	3190 (2500–3838)	3100 (2500–4100)	0.990
0.9% normal saline (%)	2.1 (1.7–2.6)	97.7 (95.8–98.4)	<0.001
Plasma Solution-A (%)	97.8 (96.8–98.2)	2.2 (1.6–3.9)	<0.001
Electrolyte values			
Chloride (mEq/L)	107.0 (103.0–108.8)	112.0 (111.0–114.0)	<0.001
[‡]Δ[Cl$^-$] (mEq/L)	8.0 (2.0–12.0)	15.0 (11.0–17.8)	<0.001
Sodium (mEq/L)	140.0 (137.0–142.0)	140.0 (138.0–142.0)	0.783
Potassium (mEq/L)	4.3 (4.0–4.6)	4.4 (4.0–4.9)	0.124

[‡]Δ[Cl$^-$] is defined as the difference in serum chloride between preoperative day and immediately after surgery. Note: Values are expressed as the median and interquartile range.

3.4. Serial Changes in eGFR until POD 2 in PS-Matched Patients

The eGFR, as an indicator of kidney graft function, increased gradually until POD 2 in both groups (Table 4). However, the proportion of patients with eGFR > 60 mL/min/1.73 m^2 increased significantly from immediately after surgery to PODs 1 and 2 in the non-hyperchloremia group (Table 5). On POD 2, the proportion of patients with eGFR > 60 mL/min/1.73 m^2 was larger and the proportion of patients with eGFR < 30 mL/min/1.73 m^2 was smaller in the non-hyperchloremia group than in the hyperchloremia group.

Table 4. Serial changes in estimated glomerular filtration rate during postoperative day 2 between propensity score-matched non-hyperchloremia and hyperchloremia groups.

Group	No Hyperchloremia	Hyperchloremia	p
n	100	100	
eGFR (mL/min/1.73 m^2)			
Immediately after surgery	21.5 (9.3–34.3)	17.5 (8.1–29.6)	0.151
Postoperative day 1	54.3 (23.2–77.3)[†††]	43.2 (13.5–70.4)[†††]	0.134
Postoperative day 2	66.7 (33.8–85.7)[†††,§§§]	53.4 (21.3–71.7)[†††,§§§]	0.058

Abbreviation: eGFR, estimated glomerular filtration rate; [†††]$p < 0.001$ compared to the level immediately after surgery in each group; [§§§]$p < 0.001$ compared to the level on postoperative day 1 in each group. Note: Values are expressed as the median and interquartile range.

Table 5. Comparison of kidney graft function according to estimated glomerular filtration rate during postoperative day 2 between propensity score-matched non-hyperchloremia and hyperchloremia groups.

Group	No Hyperchloremia	Hyperchloremia	*p*
n	100	100	
eGFR ≥ 60 mL/min/1.73 m^2			
Immediately after surgery	6 (6.0%)	2 (2.0%)	0.279
Postoperative day 1	44 (44.0%)[†††]	30 (30.0%)[†††]	0.040
Postoperative day 2	58 (58.0%)[†††,§§§]	38 (38.0%)[†††]	0.005
eGFR 59–30 mL/min/1.73 m^2			
Immediately after surgery	25 (25.0%)	23 (23.0%)	0.741
Postoperative day 1	28 (28.0%)	32 (32.0%)	0.537
Postoperative day 2	23 (23.0%)	30 (30.0%)	0.262
eGFR < 30 mL/min/1.73 m^2			
Immediately after surgery	69 (69.0%)	75 (75.0%)	0.345
Postoperative day 1	28 (28.0%)[†††]	38 (38.0%)[†††]	0.133
Postoperative day 2	19 (19.0%)[†††,§§]	32 (32.0%)[†††]	0.035

Abbreviation: eGFR, estimated glomerular filtration rate; [†††]$p < 0.001$ compared to the level immediately after surgery in each group, [§§]$p < 0.01$ compared to the level on postoperative day 1 in each group, [§§§]$p < 0.001$ compared to the level on postoperative day 1 in each group. Note: Values are expressed as number and proportion.

3.5. Association of Hyperchloremia with Kidney Graft Function (i.e., eGFR ≤ 60 mL/min/1.73 m^2) on POD 2

Hyperchloremia was associated with poor graft recovery on POD 2 in the whole study population and in PS-matched patients (Table 6). After PS adjustment, hyperchloremia remained an independent factor related to poor graft recovery.

Table 6. Association of hyperchloremia with poor early graft function (eGFR < 60 ml/min/1.73 m^2) on postoperative day 2 in living donor kidney transplantation.

	Multivariable Logistic Regression Analysis			
	β	Odds ratio	95% CI	*p*
In the whole patients (n = 301)				
Hyperchloremia adjusted for PS	0.592	1.808	1.053–3.104	0.032
In the PS-matched patients (n = 200)				
Hyperchloremia adjusted for PS	0.721	2.057	1.146–3.694	0.016

Abbreviation: CI, confidence interval; PS, propensity score.

3.6. Postoperative Clinical Outcomes in PS-Matched Patients

In the hyperchloremia group, five (5.0%) patients required RRT due to poor graft function, five (5.0%) patients suffered graft rejection, and two (2.0%) patients died. In the non-hyperchloremia group, two (2.0%) patients required RRT, one (1.0%) patient suffered graft rejection, and one (1.0%) patient died. These postoperative outcomes did not differ significantly between groups.

4. Discussion

The main finding of our study was that hyperchloremia was associated with poor early recovery of graft function after LDKT in an analysis adjusted for clinical factors related to kidney graft function by PS matching. Patients without hyperchloremia showed appropriate graft function recovery during POD 2, as indicated by the increase in proportion of patients with eGFR > 60 mL/min/1.73 m^2 and decrease in the proportion of patients with eGFR < 30 mL/min/1.73 m^2. The proportion of patients with adequate graft function (i.e., eGFR > 60 mL/min/1.73 m^2) on POD 2 was larger in the non-hyperchloremia group than in the hyperchloremia group.

Many studies have examined the impact of hyperchloremia on AKI in critically ill patients, but debate persists regarding the relation between hyperchloremia and the occurrence of AKI [5,6,23,30,31]. A study of severely septic patients in the ICU showed that hyperchloremia was common in these patients due to aggressive fluid resuscitation, but that neither hyperchloremia nor an increase in the serum chloride level was associated with an increased risk of AKI development within the first three days of ICU admission [23]. In patients undergoing craniotomy for intracranial hemorrhage, hyperchloremia due to infusion of 0.9% NaCl solution was related to a decrease in the water shift across the blood–brain barrier, leading to metabolic acidosis, but did not directly cause AKI [30,32]. However, in another study of patients undergoing craniotomy for primary brain tumor resection, the occurrence of hyperchloremia within 3 PODs appeared to aggravate early kidney function [33]. In a study of patients with subarachnoid hemorrhage in the neurocritical care unit, those who developed AKI had a higher average serum chloride level than did those without AKI, despite similar chloride loading [5]. Suetrong et al. [6] suggested that the maximum serum chloride level (i.e., ≥ 110 mmol/L) and an increase ≥ 5 mmol/L within 48 hours after ICU admission due to severe sepsis or septic shock were the predominant factors associated with the development of AKI. Another study conducted by Marouli et al. [12] suggested that a high intraoperative chloride load (i.e., > 500 mEq) played a significant role in the development of AKI within 48 hours after major abdominal surgery. In a prospective ICU study, a lesser intravenous chloride supply was associated with significant reduction in the worst stages of AKI and the requirement for RRT. In fluid management, the infusion of a chloride-restrictive fluid (i.e., Plasma-Lyte 148), rather than a chloride-liberal fluid (i.e., 0.9% normal saline), may effectively attenuate the increase in serum creatinine level from baseline to peak during the ICU stay [34].

Patients with chronic kidney dysfunction and those undergoing RRT have been routinely excluded from many studies of AKI because the initial kidney status is one of the most critical factors contributing to the development of AKI after surgery or ICU admission [35]. In contrast, our study included patients with end-stage renal disease, most of whom were receiving dialysis, with kidney grafts rendered vulnerable by ischemic injury [1]. The impact of hyperchloremia on graft function recovery in the early period has not been investigated fully in such LDKT settings. As various preoperative and intraoperative risk factors may be related to postoperative graft function, these clinical risk factors were matched between patients with and without hyperchloremia to reduce selection bias using a PS-based method [29,36]. Therefore, the results of the present study suggest that hyperchloremia is an independent risk factor for inappropriate graft recovery after LDKT. The intraoperative infusion of a large amount of 0.9% normal saline may be related to an increase in the chloride load and consequent effects on kidney grafts because 0.9% saline contains 50% more chloride than serum (154 vs. 100 mEq/L) [37]. Postoperatively, however, the sodium and potassium levels did not differ between our study groups, suggesting that they are not related to an increased risk of AKI development, consistent with previous findings [5,6]. In animal experiments [38,39], a potential explanation for chloride-load kidney injury was suggested to be the dysregulation of tubuloglomerular feedback caused by chloride reaching the macula densa, which caused renal afferent arteriole vasoconstriction related to decreased renal cortical tissue perfusion and the development of tissue ischemia. A second explanation was proposed to involve renal interstitial edema related to fluid overload resulting in intracapsular hypertension or vasomotor nephropathy. Although the specific pathophysiology of the relationship between hyperchloremia and graft dysfunction in patients undergoing LDKT remains unclear, exposure of the kidney graft to high serum chloride levels may have a negative effect on functional recovery and prolong the recovery period.

This study had some limitations. First, although confounding factors were adjusted between patients with and without hyperchloremia by PS matching, hidden biases attributable to unknown factors could not be completely excluded. Second, we were not able to determine the amounts of chloride infused from the patients' records, so the analysis was based on the serum chloride concentrations. Third, our observations did not elucidate the pathophysiology underlying the relationship between hyperchloremia and kidney graft function recovery. Fourth, because of the possibility of graft failure requiring RRT, such as arteriovenous fistula [40], we did not routinely perform arterial procedures, such as ABGA. We were unable to determine the effects of metabolic acidosis on early graft recovery. Finally, the power to identify associations of hyperchloremia with the requirement for RRT, rejection, and mortality was limited because the sample was small.

5. Conclusions

Exposure to hyperchloremia may have a negative effect on the early recovery of kidney grafts injured by ischemia in LDKT. The infusion of large amounts of chloride-rich fluid seems to be a major factor contributing to increased serum chloride levels, and this chloride load may play a role in prolonging kidney graft recovery in the early postoperative period. Previous studies have shown that chloride loads cause renal vasoconstriction and interstitial edema, thereby decreasing renal blood flow and perfusion, and consequently reducing the GFR and urine output [41,42]. However, the potential pathophysiological relationships in the KT-specific setting have not been clarified. Therefore, further studies are required to determine the association between the chloride load and transplanted kidney graft functional recovery.

Author Contributions: Conceptualization, M.S.C.; methodology, M.S.C.; software, M.S.C.; validation, M.S.C.; formal analysis, J.G., S.-C.P., S.-S.Y., J.P., J.-W.S., H.M.L., Y.-S.K., Y.E.M., S.H.H., and M.S.C.; investigation, J.G., S.P., S.-S.Y., J.P., J.-W.S., H.M.L., Y.-S.K., Y.E.M., S.H.H., and M.S.C.; resources, J.G., J.K., and M.S.C.; data curation, J.G. and J.K.; writing—original draft preparation, J.G. and M.S.C.; writing—review and editing, M.S.C.; visualization, M.S.C.; supervision, M.S.C.

Conflicts of Interest: No author has any conflict of interest regarding the publication of this article.

Abbreviations

AKI	acute kidney injury
KT	kidney transplantation
LDKT	living donor kidney transplantation
ICU	intensive care unit
RRT	renal replacement therapy
CVP	central venous pressure
POD	postoperative day
eGFR	estimated glomerular filtration rate
MDRD	Modification of Diet in Renal Disease
BMI	body mass index
PS	propensity score

References

1. Cooper, J.E.; Wiseman, A.C. Acute kidney injury in kidney transplantation. *Curr. Opin. Nephrol. Hypertens.* **2013**, *22*, 698–703. [CrossRef] [PubMed]
2. Lee, S.Y.; Chung, B.H.; Piao, S.G.; Kang, S.H.; Hyoung, B.J.; Jeon, Y.J.; Hwang, H.S.; Yoon, H.E.; Choi, B.S.; Kim, J.I.; et al. Clinical significance of slow recovery of graft function in living donor kidney transplantation. *Transplantation.* **2010**, *90*, 38–43. [CrossRef] [PubMed]
3. Tyson, M.; Castle, E.; Andrews, P.; Heilman, R.; Mekeel, K.; Moss, A.; Mulligan, D.; Reddy, K. Early graft function after laparoscopically procured living donor kidney transplantation. *J. Urol.* **2010**, *184*, 1434–1439. [CrossRef] [PubMed]
4. Berend, K.; van Hulsteijn, L.H.; Gans, R.O. Chloride: the queen of electrolytes? *Eur. J. Intern. Med.* **2012**, *23*, 203–211. [CrossRef] [PubMed]

5. Sadan, O.; Singbartl, K.; Kandiah, P.A.; Martin, K.S.; Samuels, O.B. Hyperchloremia Is Associated With Acute Kidney Injury in Patients With Subarachnoid Hemorrhage. *Crit. Care Med.* **2017**, *45*, 1382–1388. [CrossRef] [PubMed]

6. Suetrong, B.; Pisitsak, C.; Boyd, J.H.; Russell, J.A.; Walley, K.R. Hyperchloremia and moderate increase in serum chloride are associated with acute kidney injury in severe sepsis and septic shock patients. *Crit. Care (Lond., Engl.)* **2016**, *20*, 315. [CrossRef] [PubMed]

7. Toyonaga, Y.; Kikura, M. Hyperchloremic acidosis is associated with acute kidney injury after abdominal surgery. *Nephrology (Carlton, Vic.)* **2017**, *22*, 720–727. [CrossRef] [PubMed]

8. Oh, T.K.; Song, I.A.; Jeon, Y.T.; Jo, Y.H. Fluctuations in Serum Chloride and Acute Kidney Injury among Critically Ill Patients: A Retrospective Association Study. *J. Clin. Med.* **2019**, *8*, 447. [CrossRef] [PubMed]

9. McCluskey, S.A.; Karkouti, K.; Wijeysundera, D.; Minkovich, L.; Tait, G.; Beattie, W.S. Hyperchloremia after noncardiac surgery is independently associated with increased morbidity and mortality: a propensity-matched cohort study. *Anesth. Analg.* **2013**, *117*, 412–421. [CrossRef]

10. Raghunathan, K.; Shaw, A.; Nathanson, B.; Sturmer, T.; Brookhart, A.; Stefan, M.S.; Setoguchi, S.; Beadles, C.; Lindenauer, P.K. Association between the choice of IV crystalloid and in-hospital mortality among critically ill adults with sepsis. *Crit. Care Med.* **2014**, *42*, 1585–1591. [CrossRef]

11. Shaw, A.D.; Raghunathan, K.; Peyerl, F.W.; Munson, S.H.; Paluszkiewicz, S.M.; Schermer, C.R. Association between intravenous chloride load during resuscitation and in-hospital mortality among patients with SIRS. *Intensive Care Med.* **2014**, *40*, 1897–1905. [CrossRef] [PubMed]

12. Marouli, D.; Stylianou, K. Preoperative Albuminuria and Intraoperative Chloride Load: Predictors of Acute Kidney Injury Following Major Abdominal Surgery. *J. Clin. Med.* **2018**, *7*, 431. [CrossRef] [PubMed]

13. Hamdani, G.; Zhang, B.; Liu, C.; Goebel, J.; Zhang, Y.; Nehus, E. Outcomes of Pediatric Kidney Transplantation in Recipients of a Previous Non-Renal Solid Organ Transplant. *Am. J. Transplant.* **2017**, *17*, 1928–1934. [CrossRef] [PubMed]

14. Scurt, F.G.; Ewert, L.; Mertens, P.R.; Haller, H.; Schmidt, B.M.W.; Chatzikyrkou, C. Clinical outcomes after ABO-incompatible renal transplantation: a systematic review and meta-analysis. *Lancet (Lond., Engl.)* **2019**, *393*, 2059–2072. [CrossRef]

15. Stites, E.; Wiseman, A.C. Multiorgan transplantation. *Transplant. Rev. (Orlando, Fla.)* **2016**, *30*, 253–260. [CrossRef] [PubMed]

16. Yeo, S.M.; Kim, Y.; Kang, S.S.; Park, W.Y.; Jin, K.; Park, S.B.; Park, U.J.; Kim, H.T.; Cho, W.H.; Han, S. Long-term Clinical Outcomes of Kidney Re-transplantation. *Transplant. Proc.* **2017**, *49*, 997–1000. [CrossRef]

17. Zhang, H.; Wei, Y.; Liu, L.; Li, J.; Deng, R.; Xiong, Y.; Yuan, X.; He, X.; Fu, Q.; Wang, C. Different Risk Factors for Graft Survival Between Living-Related and Deceased Donor Kidney Transplantation. *Transplant. Proc.* **2018**, *50*, 2416–2420. [CrossRef] [PubMed]

18. Lich Jr, R.; Howerton, L.W.; Davis, L.A. Childhood urosepsis. *J. Ky. Med. Assoc.* **1961**, *59*, 1177–1179.

19. Taguchi, Y.; Klauber, G.T.; MacKinnon, K.J. Implantation of transplant ureters: a technique. *J. Urol.* **1971**, *105*, 194–195. [CrossRef]

20. Lugo-Baruqui, J.A.; Ayyathurai, R.; Sriram, A.; Pragatheeshwar, K.D. Use of Mannitol for Ischemia Reperfusion Injury in Kidney Transplant and Partial Nephrectomies-Review of Literature. *Curr. Urol. Rep.* **2019**, *20*, 6. [CrossRef]

21. Voldby, A.W.; Brandstrup, B. Fluid therapy in the perioperative setting-a clinical review. *J. Intensive Care* **2016**, *4*, 27. [CrossRef] [PubMed]

22. Othman, M.M.; Ismael, A.Z.; Hammouda, G.E. The impact of timing of maximal crystalloid hydration on early graft function during kidney transplantation. *Anesth. Analg.* **2010**, *110*, 1440–1446. [CrossRef]

23. Yessayan, L.; Neyra, J.A.; Canepa-Escaro, F.; Vasquez-Rios, G.; Heung, M.; Yee, J. Effect of hyperchloremia on acute kidney injury in critically ill septic patients: a retrospective cohort study. *BMC Nephrol.* **2017**, *18*, 346. [CrossRef]

24. Levey, A.S.; Coresh, J.; Greene, T.; Stevens, L.A.; Zhang, Y.L.; Hendriksen, S.; Kusek, J.W.; van Lente, F. Using standardized serum creatinine values in the modification of diet in renal disease study equation for estimating glomerular filtration rate. *Ann. Intern. Med.* **2006**, *145*, 247–254. [CrossRef] [PubMed]

25. Levey, A.S.; Coresh, J.; Balk, E.; Kausz, A.T.; Levin, A.; Steffes, M.W.; Hogg, R.J.; Perrone, R.D.; Lau, J.; Eknoyan, G. National Kidney Foundation practice guidelines for chronic kidney disease: evaluation, classification, and stratification. *Ann. Intern. Med.* **2003**, *139*, 137–147. [CrossRef] [PubMed]

26.	Foster, M.C.; Hwang, S.J.; Massaro, J.M.; Jacques, P.F.; Fox, C.S.; Chu, A.Y. Lifestyle factors and indices of kidney function in the Framingham Heart Study. *Am. J. Nephrol.* **2015**, *41*, 267–274. [CrossRef] [PubMed]

27.	Solez, K.; Axelsen, R.A.; Benediktsson, H.; Burdick, J.F.; Cohen, A.H.; Colvin, R.B.; Croker, B.P.; Droz, D.; Dunnill, M.S.; Halloran, P.F.; et al. International standardization of criteria for the histologic diagnosis of renal allograft rejection: the Banff working classification of kidney transplant pathology. *Kidney Int.* **1993**, *44*, 411–422. [CrossRef]

28.	Stuart, E.A. Matching methods for causal inference: A review and a look forward. *Stat. Sci.* **2010**, *25*, 1–21. [CrossRef]

29.	Yang, J.Y.; Webster-Clark, M.; Lund, J.L.; Sandler, R.S.; Dellon, E.S.; Sturmer, T. Propensity score methods to control for confounding in observational cohort studies: a statistical primer and application to endoscopy research. *Gastrointest. Endosc.* **2019**. [CrossRef]

30.	Oh, T.K.; Jeon, Y.T.; Sohn, H.; Chung, S.H.; Do, S.H. Association of Perioperative Hyperchloremia and Hyperchloremic Metabolic Acidosis with Acute Kidney Injury After Craniotomy for Intracranial Hemorrhage. *World Neurosurg.* **2019**. [CrossRef]

31.	Oh, T.K.; Song, I.A.; Kim, S.J.; Lim, S.Y.; Do, S.H.; Hwang, J.W.; Kim, J.; Jeon, Y.T. Hyperchloremia and postoperative acute kidney injury: A retrospective analysis of data from the surgical intensive care unit. *Crit. Care (Lond., Engl.)* **2018**, *22*, 277. [CrossRef] [PubMed]

32.	Shackford, S.R.; Zhuang, J.; Schmoker, J. Intravenous fluid tonicity: effect on intracranial pressure, cerebral blood flow, and cerebral oxygen delivery in focal brain injury. *J. Neurosurg.* **1992**, *76*, 91–98. [CrossRef] [PubMed]

33.	Oh, T.K.; Kim, C.Y.; Jeon, Y.T.; Hwang, J.W.; Do, S.H. Perioperative hyperchloremia and its association with postoperative acute kidney injury after craniotomy for primary brain tumor resection: A Retrospective, Observational Study. *J. Neurosurg. Anesthesiol.* **2018**. [CrossRef] [PubMed]

34.	Yunos, N.M.; Bellomo, R.; Hegarty, C.; Story, D.; Ho, L.; Bailey, M. Association between a chloride-liberal vs chloride-restrictive intravenous fluid administration strategy and kidney injury in critically ill adults. *Jama* **2012**, *308*, 1566–1572. [CrossRef] [PubMed]

35.	Chawla, L.S.; Eggers, P.W.; Star, R.A.; Kimmel, P.L. Acute kidney injury and chronic kidney disease as interconnected syndromes. *N. Engl. J. Med.* **2014**, *371*, 58–66. [CrossRef] [PubMed]

36.	Redfield, R.R.; Scalea, J.R.; Zens, T.J.; Muth, B.; Kaufman, D.B.; Djamali, A.; Astor, B.C.; Mohamed, M. Predictors and outcomes of delayed graft function after living-donor kidney transplantation. *Transpl. Int.* **2016**, *29*, 81–87. [CrossRef] [PubMed]

37.	Myburgh, J.A.; Mythen, M.G. Resuscitation fluids. *N. Engl. J. Med.* **2013**, *369*, 2462–2463. [CrossRef]

38.	Stone, H.H.; Fulenwider, J.T. Renal decapsulation in the prevention of post-ischemic oliguria. *Ann. Surg.* **1977**, *186*, 343–355. [CrossRef] [PubMed]

39.	Wilcox, C.S. Regulation of renal blood flow by plasma chloride. *J. Clin. Investig.* **1983**, *71*, 726–735. [CrossRef] [PubMed]

40.	De Jonge, H.; Bammens, B.; Lemahieu, W.; Maes, B.D.; Vanrenterghem, Y. Comparison of peritoneal dialysis and haemodialysis after renal transplant failure. *Nephrol. Dial. Transplant.* **2006**, *21*, 1669–1674. [CrossRef]

41.	Bell, P.D.; Komlosi, P.; Zhang, Z.R. ATP as a mediator of macula densa cell signalling. *Purinergic Signal.* **2009**, *5*, 461–471. [CrossRef] [PubMed]

42.	Ren, Y.; Garvin, J.L.; Liu, R.; Carretero, O.A. Role of macula densa adenosine triphosphate (ATP) in tubuloglomerular feedback. *Kidney Int.* **2004**, *66*, 1479–1485. [CrossRef] [PubMed]

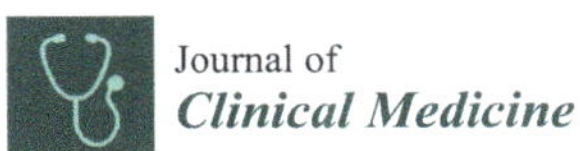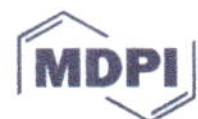

Journal of
Clinical Medicine

Article

Phenotypic and Genotypic Characterization of *Escherichia coli* Causing Urinary Tract Infections in Kidney-Transplanted Patients

Jonas Abo Basha [1], Matthias Kiel [2], Dennis Görlich [3], Katharina Schütte-Nütgen [1], Anika Witten [4], Hermann Pavenstädt [1], Barbara C. Kahl [5], Ulrich Dobrindt [2,†,*] and Stefan Reuter [1,†,*]

[1]   Department of Medicine D, Division of General Internal Medicine, Nephrology and Rheumatology, University Hospital Münster, 48149 Münster, Germany
[2]   Institute of Hygiene, University of Münster, 48149 Münster, Germany
[3]   Institute of Biostatistics and Clinical Research, University of Münster, 48149 Münster, Germany
[4]   Institute for Human Genetics, University of Münster, 48149 Münster, Germany
[5]   Institute of Medical Microbiology, University Hospital Münster, 48149 Münster, Germany
*   Correspondence: dobrindt@uni-muenster.de (U.D.); sreuter@uni-muenster.de (S.R)
†   These authors contributed equally to this work.

Received: 3 June 2019; Accepted: 5 July 2019; Published: 7 July 2019

Abstract: Urinary tract infection (UTI), frequently caused by uropathogenic Escherichia coli (UPEC), is the most common infection after kidney transplantation (KTx). Untreated, it can lead to urosepsis and impairment of the graft function. We questioned whether the UPEC isolated from KTx patients differed from the UPEC of non-KTx patients. Therefore, we determined the genome sequences of 182 UPEC isolates from KTx and control patients in a large German university clinic and pheno- and genotypically compared these two isolated groups. Resistance to the β-lactams, trimethoprim or trimethoprim/sulfamethoxazole was significantly higher among UPEC from KTx than from control patients, whereas both the isolated groups were highly susceptible to fosfomycin. Accordingly, the gene content conferring resistance to β-lactams or trimethoprim, but also to aminoglycosides, was significantly higher in KTx than in control UPEC isolates. *E. coli* isolates from KTx patients more frequently presented with uncommon UPEC phylogroups expressing higher numbers of plasmid replicons, but interestingly, less UPEC virulence-associated genes than the control group. We conclude that there is no defining subset of virulence traits for UPEC from KTx patients. The clinical history and immunocompromised status of KTx patients enables *E. coli* strains with low uropathogenic potential, but with increased antibiotic resistance to cause UTIs.

Keywords: Uropathogenic E. coli; UPEC; phylogeny; genomics; antibiotic resistance; virulence traits; kidney transplantation

---

1. Introduction

Kidney transplantation (KTx) is the best treatment for patients with end-stage renal disease (ESRD). Despite routine screening, treatment and prophylaxis, the prevalence of urinary tract infections (UTIs) in KTx patients is high; more than every third patient is affected [1]. While lower UTI/cystitis usually does not limit graft prognosis, pyelonephritis and urosepsis limit the same, not only in the acute setting, but also in the long run, impairing graft function and prognosis [2,3]. Older age, duration of catheterization, acute rejection periods and deceased donor KTx are known risk factors for UTI after KTx [1]. In addition, female patients are at a higher risk for UTIs. Recently, we concluded that a male donor kidney is a new risk factor [4]. Further potential that predisposes host factors are, e.g., excessive immunosuppression, diabetes mellitus, and the instrumentation of the urinary tract [5].

Uropathogenic *Escherichia coli* (UPEC) are the most common clinical isolates in UTI patients after KTx [6]. UPEC encode virulence factors including adhesins, toxins, capsules, and factors involved in biofilm formation [7]. Resistances to certain antibiotics are common, as patients are frequently treated by antimicrobial compounds, for, e.g., the prophylaxis of *Pneumocystis* pneumonia, UTIs, or in perioperative/periprocedural settings.

As clinical variables and features of patients and UTIs are significantly different from non-transplanted patients, we hypothesized that UPEC isolates from both groups are also different. Therefore, we sought to characterize phylogeny, virulence traits, and antibiotic susceptibility of UPEC from KTx patients and non-transplanted patients to ultimately assist transplant physicians in the management of UTI in KTx patients.

2. Experimental Section

Detailed methods are provided in the Supplemental Information.

2.1. Study Population

We prospectively collected and analyzed 182 UPEC isolates from 167 patients who were diagnosed with an UPEC-associated UTI between July and December 2016 at the Department of Nephrology or the emergency room at the University Clinic of Muenster. We included 62 KTx patients (71 isolates) and 105 non-transplanted controls (111 isolates). Urine samples were taken in case of clinically relevant UTI symptoms or pyuria and included if $\geq 10^5$ colony forming units (CFU)/mL urine were detected. Additional blood or respiratory tract samples were collected if required. More than one isolate per patient was included if genotypically different strains were identified from samples.

2.2. Patients' Characteristics

Patients' and donors' characteristics were collected from the patients' files. All non-KTx patients treated at the Department of Nephrology or the emergency room during the study period served as controls. The study was permitted by the local ethics committee (Ethikkommission der Ärztekammer Westfalen-Lippe und der Medizinischen Fakultät der Westfälischen Wilhelms-Universität, No. 2014-381-f-N).

2.3. Bacterial Strains and Culture Conditions

We analyzed *E. coli* samples from urine ($n = 164$), blood ($n = 8$), and respiratory tract ($n = 10$).

2.4. Phenotypic Tests

Hemolytic capacity, bacteriocin production, expression of type 1 fimbriae and biofilm formation were analyzed.

2.5. Genome Sequencing

Genome sequencing was carried out as described in the Supplemental Information.

2.6. Draft Genome Comparison and Typing

Multi-Locus Sequence Typing (MLST) was conducted on all UPEC isolates and UPEC virulence-associated genes were detected.

2.7. Statistical Analysis

The data were statistically analyzed using the IBM SPSS statistics 24 for Windows (IBM Corporation, Somers, NY, USA). All baseline variables were described using standard univariate analysis, while bivariate analysis such as the Fisher's exact test and the t-test were performed for comparing the two groups' results with each other. The *p*-values were interpreted as exploratory, not confirmatory. If the *p*-values were ≤0.05, the result was considered as statistically significant.

3. Results

3.1. Patients' Characteristics

The mean age at the time of infection was comparable between the KTx recipients (79% females) and the control group (70.5% females) (56.7 ± 15.1 vs. 53.45 ± 21.82, respectively). The KTx recipients had a higher BMI (26.19 ± 4.58 kg/m^2 vs. 24.62 ± 4.41, *p* = 0.0251) and showed a higher frequency of hypertension than control patients (80.6% vs. 35.3%), while the frequency of diabetes did not differ between the groups (Table 1). Causes of ESRD are given in Supplemental Table S1. The recipients' glomerular filtration rate at the time of UTI was 58.4 ± 32.48 mL/min in KTx patients and 70.21 ± 35.67 mL/min in the control group. To note, the kidney function in KTx patients is based on one working kidney (the transplant) only. More than every fourth recipient and more than every fifth control patient experienced acute renal injury at the time of infection. Lower UTI was observed in ~80% of KTx and controls. 24.5% of KTx and 39.3% controls had been hospitalized for UTI (Table 1). Interestingly, within three months before the UTI diagnosis, KTx patients differed significantly from control patients by being more often hospitalized, having a ureteral stent or urinary catheter, and by antibiotic treatment with cephalosporines, TMP/SMX and fosfomycin mainly for treatments of UTIs and for prophylaxis, e.g., for UTIs and/or Pneumocystis jirovecii infection (Table 1).

Table 1. Clinical data.

Clinical data at UTI diagnosis			
	KTx Recipients	**Controls**	***p***
Sex (female/male)	49 (79%)/13 (21%)	74 (70.5%)/31 (29.5%)	0.1512
Age (mean/median/σ in yr)	56.67/58.75/15.09	53.45/ 55/21.82	0.2902
BMI (mean/median/σ)	26.19/26.03/4.58	24.62/24.21/4.41	**0.0251**
Hypertension (%)	80.6%	35.3%	**0**
Diabetes mellitus (%)	21%	14.7%	0.3922
Immunosuppression (%)	100%	9.7%	**0**
Previous tumor diagnosis (%)	0%	10.7%	**0.0072**
Time from last KTx to UTI (mean/median/σ in yr)	5.4/3.2/6.2	-	-
Ureteral stent or urinary catheter (%)	16.1%	5.8%	0.0539
Lower UTI (%)	80.3%	80.4%	1
Upper UTI (%)	19.7%	19.6%	1
eGFR (mean/median/σ in mL/min)	58.4/54.45/32.48	70.21/66.5/35.67	**0.0406**
Acute kidney injury (%)	28.3%	23.1%	0.5658
Hospitalization	24.5%	39.3%	0.0527
Clinical data of a three-month period before the UTI diagnosis			
Hospitalization	40.3%	20%	**0.0068**
Surgery	21%	10.5%	0.0709
Ureteral stent or urinary catheter	29%	12.4%	**0.0125**
Antibiotic therapy			
Beta-lactam	6.5%	1.9%	0.1961
Cephalosporine	25.8%	4.8%	**0.0002**

Table 1. *Cont.*

Clinical data at UTI diagnosis			
	KTx Recipients	**Controls**	*p*
Fluoroquinolone	9.7%	2.9%	0.0787
Trimethoprim/ Sulfonamide	30.6%	2.9%	0
Fosfomycin	11.3%	2.9%	0.0401
Carbapenem	0%	1%	1
Reason for antibiotic treatment			
Prophylaxis	29%	4.8%	0
UTI	25.8%	7.6%	0.0024
Other infection	12.9%	7.6%	0.2855

σ = standard variation, BMI= body mass index, eGFR = estimated glomerular filtration rate, KTx = kidney transplantation, *p*-values were obtained using t-test.

3.2. Epidemiological Classification of Urine Isolates from KTx and Control Patients

The 182 *E. coli* urine isolates were allocated to phylogenetic lineages and to sequence types (STs) as published by Clermont et al. [8] (Figure 1). 60.5% of all KTx isolates were allocated to phylogroups B2 and A, to which the majority of UPEC primarily belong (Table 2).

Table 2. Distribution of phylogroups in relation to KTx and control UPEC isolates.

Phylogroup	Total	KTx		Controls		*p*
	No. of Isolates	**No. of Isolates**	**%**	**No. of Isolates**	**%**	
A	25	16	22.5	9	8.1	**0.0061**
B1	24	10	14.1	14	12.6	0.4706
B2	88	27	38	61	55	**0.0394**
C	8	1	1.4	7	6.3	0.1117
D	23	9	12.7	14	12.6	0.5805
E	2	2	2.8	0	0	0.1509
F	10	5	7	5	4.5	0.3389
Clade V	2	1	1.4	1	0.9	0.6293

No. = number, KTx = strains of kidney transplanted patients, *p*-values were obtained using Fisher's exact test.

78 different STs were identified. The top ranked STs, representing 93 isolates (51.1% of all isolates), are shown in Supplementary Table S2. Isolates from the KTx and control groups could not be distinguished based on STs. ST10 and ST69 were the most prevalent STs in KTx isolates. ST73 and ST131 were most frequently detected in the control group (Supplementary Table S2). Isolates of KTx patients with a BMI > 25 kg/m^2 showed a higher number of ST10 and ST131, and a fewer number of ST23 compared to control patients' isolates. Age did not affect the ST distribution. The prevalence of ST127 and ST73 isolates was markedly higher in the control group supporting our finding that the phylogroup B2 strains are overrepresented in this group.

The O serogroups were highly variable in the urine isolates. Table 3 shows the most frequently predicted O serogroups in 98 isolates (53.8% of all isolates). The O antigen could be typed for 161 isolates leading to the identification of 46 different O antigen types (Table 3). O8 and O89 (9.9% each) were most prevalent in KTx isolates, whereas O6 (15.2%) and O8 (9.8%) were the most prevalent O serotypes in the control group. Typical UPEC O serotypes, i.e., O6, were less prevalent among the KTx isolates. In contrast, KTx isolates more frequently belonged to the O89 serotype than strains of the control group.

Table 3. Distribution of O serotypes in relation to KTx and control UPEC isolates.

Serogroups	Total	KTx		Controls		p
	No. of Isolates	No. of Isolates	%	No. of Isolates	%	
O2	14	5	7	9	7.1	0.5159
O4	8	3	4.2	5	5	0.6187
O6	20	3	4.2	17	15.2	**0.0148**
O8	18	7	9.9	11	9.8	0.6013
O15	10	6	8.5	4	3.6	0.1435
O16	5	2	2.8	3	2.7	0.6485
O25	11	4	5.6	7	6.3	0.5608
O83	5	1	1.4	4	3.6	0.3515
O89	10	7	9.9	3	2.7	**0.0432**
not typeable	21	10	14.1	11	10	nd
other serotypes	60	23	32.4	31	33.9	nd

No. = Number, KTx = strains of kidney transplanted patients, nd = not determined, *p*-values were obtained using Fisher's exact test.

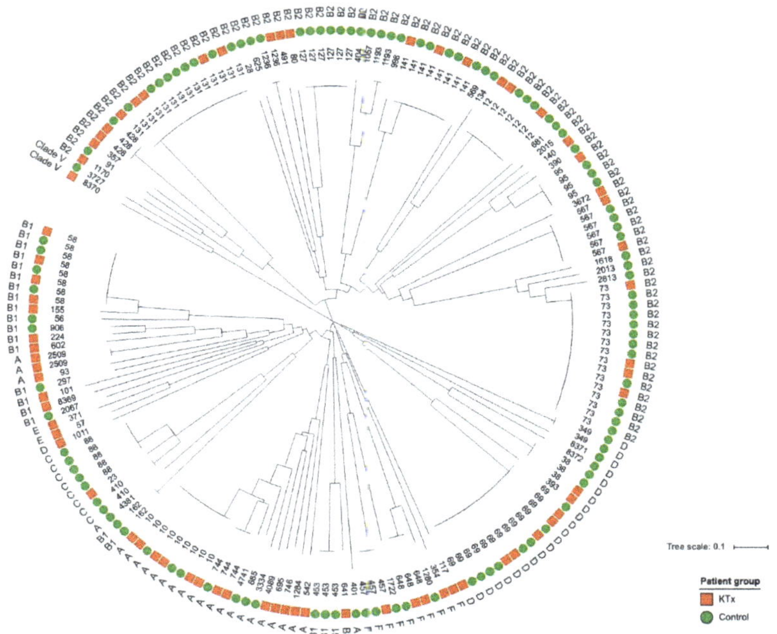

Figure 1. Phylogenetic diversity of the UPEC isolated from KTx and control patients. The neighboring joining tree is based on the MLST of seven housekeeping genes performed with Ridom SeqSphere+ (https://www.ridom.de/seqsphere/) and was created with iTOL (https://itol.embl.de/). The sequence type (ST), the corresponding phylogroup and the isolate group is indicated for each UPEC isolate. The allocation to the two isolate groups (KTx or control) is indicated by different colors. Phylogenetic diversity of UPEC isolated from KTx and control patients. The neighboring joining tree is based on the MLST of seven housekeeping genes and was created with the Ridom SeqSphere+ (https://www.ridom.de/seqsphere/). The sequence type (ST), the corresponding phylogroup and the isolate group (KTx patient yes or no) is indicated for each UPEC isolate. The allocation to different phylogroups is indicated by different colors.

3.3. Prevalence of UPEC Virulence-ASSOCIATED genes

The binary matrix with colored gradation of presence/absence ratios of the virulence factors (VFs) and their functional categories are shown in Figure 2. Of the 1154 VFs tested, 889 were found in at least one isolate. In general, both isolate groups exhibited a similar VF pattern. The overall VF content was slightly higher in the control than in the KTx patient isolates (Figure 2). 113 VFs showed a tendency to be overrepresented either in isolates of the KTx or the control group. Only three VFs (FimB, FocB, SfaB), representing type 1- or S/F1C fimbriae, were significantly associated with control group isolates when a Bonferroni correction was applied (Supplementary Table S3; Supplementary Figure S2). VFs with a tendency of overrepresentation in KTx patient isolates included bacteriocins, adhesins (e.g., Ybg, Yfc, Yhc), ABC transporter (ets), group 4 capsule (GfcABCDE-Etp), type 3 secretion system components, and three autotransporters. VFs enriched in the isolates of control UTI patients comprised VFs which were described for UPEC and phylogroup B2 isolates, including S-/F1C fimbriae, other chaperone-usher family adhesins, group II capsule, the polyketide colibactin and the CjrABC-SenB gene products. The VF binary matrix was used to examine the grouping of isolates according to the VF presence/absence matrix, phylogeny and the isolate group by the principle coordinates analysis. We could not observe a correlation between the source of isolation (KTx vs. control group) and the VF content or phylogroup. Nevertheless, phylogroup B2 strains clustered separately from isolates from other phylogroups.

3.4. Antibiotic Susceptibility

A significant number of resistance genes (RGs) was detected in the isolates except for fosfomycin (0.5% of all isolates) and fluoroquinolones (5% of all isolates). UPEC isolates of KTx patients presented more RGs than control UPEC strains (Table 4, Supplementary Table S4). Higher prevalence of the same in KTx patient isolates were observed for trimethoprim, β-lactam, and aminoglycoside resistance determinants. Some resistance genes with high prevalence in the KTx group were less frequently observed in control strains, such as *bla*TEM-1B, *sul2*, *strA* and *strB* (Supplementary Table S4). Clinical susceptibility tests showed that UPEC strains of the KTx and control groups differed significantly in their resistance phenotypes (Table 5).

Table 4. Distribution of resistance genes (RGs) present in relation to KTx and control UPEC isolates.

Antibiotic		>1 RGs present		No RGs present		p
		No. of Isolates	%	No. of Isolates	%	
Beta-Lactam	KTx	42	59.2	29	40.8	0.0033
	Controls	41	36.9	70	63.1	
Trimethoprim	KTx	34	47.9	37	52.1	0.0061
	Controls	31	27.9	80	72.1	
Sulfonamides	KTx	35	49.3	36	50.7	0.0763
	Controls	40	36.0	71	64.0	
Fosfomycin	KTx	0	0.0	71	100	1
	Controls	1	0.9	110	99.1	
Fluoroquinolones	KTx	3	4.2	68	95.8	1
	Controls	6	5.4	105	94.6	
Aminoglycosides	KTx	42	59.2	29	40.8	0.0101
	Controls	44	39.6	67	60.4	

No. = number, KTx = strains of kidney transplanted patients, RG = resistance gene, nd = not determined, *p*-values were obtained using Fisher's exact test.

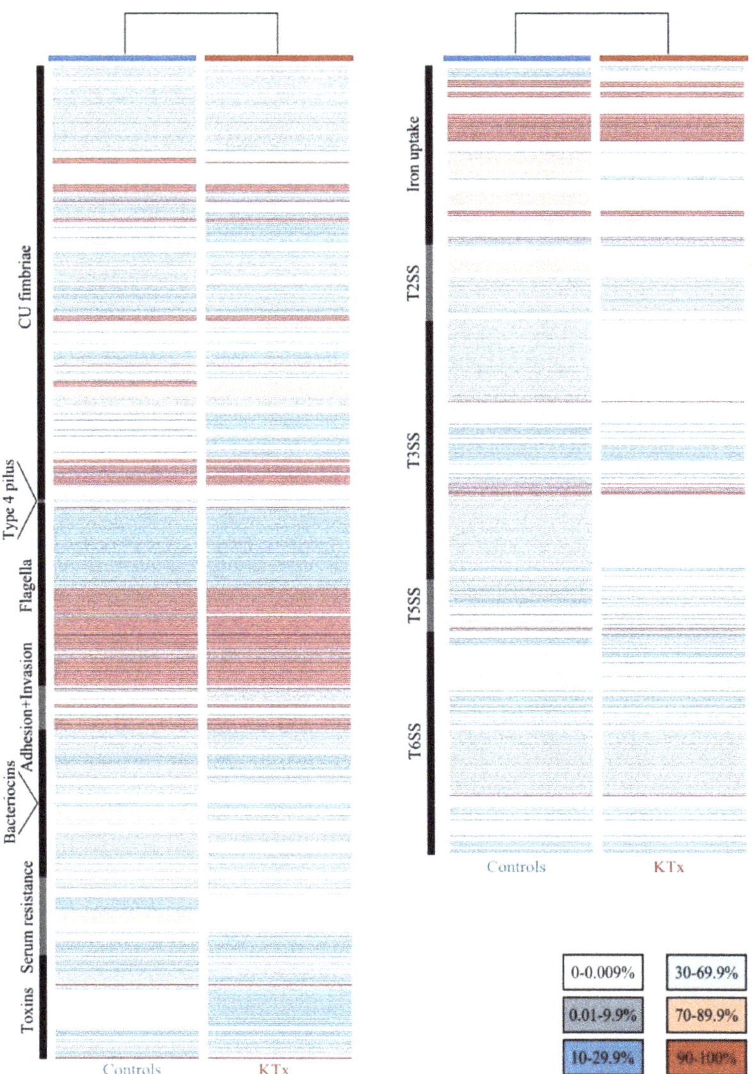

Figure 2. Heatmap displaying the distribution of virulence factors present in KTx and control UPEC isolates. Each row represents one virulence factor. The prevalence of each virulence factor (VF) in KTx and control strains is coded by a color gradient. Vertical black and grey bars indicate the functional VF group: CU-fimbriae = chaperone-usher fimbriae, T2SS = type 2 secretion system, T3SS = type 3 secretion system, T5SS = type 5 secretion system, T6SS = type 2 secretion system. The color code indicates the prevalence of the corresponding VF (calculated as percentage) in the KTx and control group, respectively.

Table 5. Susceptibility patterns of KTx and control UPEC isolates.

Antibiotic		Susceptible		Intermediate		Resistant		*p*
		No. of Isolates	%	No. of Isolates	%	No. of Isolates	%	
Beta- Lactam (AMP+AMX)	KTx	27	38	0	0	44	62	0.0015
	Controls	69	62.2	0	0	42	37.8	
Beta- Lactam + inhibitor (SAM)	KTx	50	70.4	0	0	21	29.6	0.1734
	Controls	88	79.3	0	0	23	20.7	
Beta- Lactam (CFX)	KTx	58	81.7	0	0	13	18.3	0.2147
	Controls	98	88.3	0	0	13	11.7	
Trimethoprim	KTx	33	50	0	0	33	50	0.0029
	Controls	70	72.9	0	0	26	27.1	
TMP/SMX	KTx	37	52.1	0	0	34	47.9	0.0132
	Controls	78	70.3	0	0	33	29.7	
Fosfomycin	KTx	66	98.5	0	0	1	1.5	1
	Controls	96	98	0	0	2	2	
Fluoroqinolones (CIP+LVX)	KTx	55	77.5	1	1.4	15	21.1	0.6588
	Controls	92	82.9	1	0.9	18	16.2	
Aminoglycosides (GEN)	KTx	66	93	0	0	5	7	0.4637
	Controls	106	95.5	0	0	5	4.5	

No. = number, KTx = strains of kidney transplanted patients, AMP = ampicillin, AMX = amoxicillin, SAM= ampicillin/sulbactam, CFX = Cefuroxime, TMP = trimethoprim, SMX = sulfamethoxazole, CIP = ciprofloxacin, LVX = levofloxacin, GEN = gentamicin, *p*-values were obtained using Fisher's exact test.

3.5. Plasmid Types

Virulence and resistance determinants are frequently located on plasmids. We identified 25 different plasmid replicon types in 149 isolates. UPEC isolates of the control group were more often plasmid-free than isolates from the KTx group. IncFIB, IncFII, Col156 and Inc1 were the most frequently identified replicon types among all strains. IncFIB, IncFII, IncFIC, IncI1 and IncQ1 replicons were more prevalent in the KTx than in the control group. The Col156 replicon was more frequently found in control isolates. The seven most prevalent plasmid types are summarized in Table 6.

Table 6. Distribution of the most frequent plasmid replicon types in relation to KTx and control UPEC isolates.

Plasmid Type	Total No. of Isolates	KTx		Controls		*p*
		No. of Isolates	%	No. of Isolates	%	
IncFIA	24	10	14.1	14	12.6	0.4706
IncFIB	114	49	69	65	58.6	0.1025
IncFIC	27	16	22.5	11	9.9	**0.0178**
IncFII	100	40	56.3	60	54.1	0.4411
IncI1	33	17	23.9	16	14.4	0.0773
IncQ1	20	13	18.3	7	6.3	**0.0120**
Col156	35	9	12.7	26	23.4	0.0526
Other replicons	68	30	42.3	38	34.2	0.1751
None	33	7	9.9	26	23.4	**0.0150**

No. = number, KTx = strains of kidney transplanted patients, *p*-values were obtained using Fisher's exact test.

3.6. Phenotypic Assays

Almost all the analyzed UPEC isolates (97.8%) carried the type 1 fimbrial adhesin gene *fimH*. 156 strains (85.7%), and functionally expressed type 1 fimbriae (KTx: 84.5% vs. controls: 86.5%). α-Hemolysin was produced in 18.1% of isolates without any significant differences between both groups. UPEC from KTx patients (63.4%) more often expressed often bacteriocins killing *E. coli* DH5α than control UPEC (49.5%) (Figure 3). Cellulose and curli expression are important for biofilm formation of *E. coli* (Figure 4, Supplementary Tables S5 and S6). The corresponding rdar/ras morphotype expression was more prevalent at lower growth temperatures and decreased with increasing temperature. Rdar/ras morphotype expression was more frequently observed in the UPEC of KTx patients. Increased expression of the "saw" morphotype correlated with increasing incubation temperature and occurred more often in the control group. The rare mucoid morphotype appeared more often in the KTx isolates.

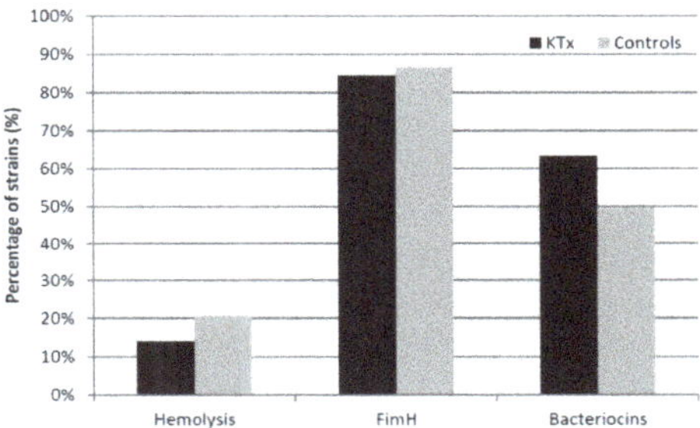

Figure 3. Phenotypic characteristics of the KTx and control UPEC isolates. The percentage of strains phenotypically tested positive for the expression of α-hemolysin, type 1 fimbriae and bacteriocins killing *E.coli* DH5α has been compared between the KTx and control groups.

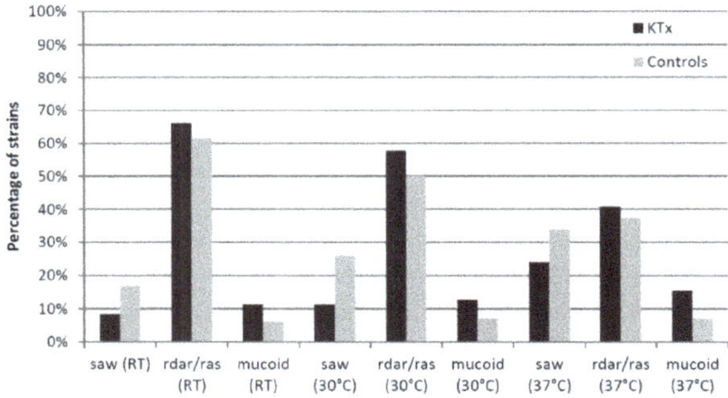

Figure 4. Expression of biofilm morphotypes in KTx and control UPEC isolates. The percentage of strains expressing different biofilm morphotypes at different growth temperatures is compared between the KTx and control groups.

4. Discussion

UTI results from complex pathogen–host interactions and is affected by host risk factors, bacterial traits and the host immune response [9]. Risk factors for uncomplicated and complicated UTI in adults have been defined before [10]. Genetic factors involved in host susceptibility to acute pyelonephritis have been described including polymorphisms that reduce expression of the interferon regulatory factor 3 (IRF3) or CXCR1 coding for the IL-8 receptor [11].

Our main objectives were to evaluate if the KTx-related factors, such as antibiotic therapy, immunosuppression or host characteristics, impact on UPEC, the major pathogen causing UTI after

KTx [1]. We herein present the genotypic and phenotypic characteristics of the UPEC isolated from KTx patients first.

Prior use of antibiotics promotes the risk of UTI due to (multi-)resistant uropathogens as frequent antibiotic prescription leads to a selection of more resistant bacteria, which is also highlighted by our data which shows increased antibiotic resistances in the KTx group isolates (Tables 4 and 5). Antibiotic susceptibility rates are significantly lower in hospital- than in community-acquired UTIs [12]. Immunocompromised patients often display co-morbidities and are more often hospitalized than immunocompetent patients. Accordingly, the former are more likely to develop UTI caused by multi-drug resistant pathogens [13]. Accordingly, comparing the KTx patients with controls three months prior to the UTI diagnosis, there were significant differences in clinical parameters such as hospitalization rate or application of devices (ureteral stents, urinary catheter); all of which seem to facilitate UTIs in KTx patients. In the transplant setting, invasive procedures such as the instrumentation of the urinary tract as well as antimicrobial prophylaxis against opportunistic microorganisms and treatment of infections are common and are more frequently performed than in controls (Table 1). These interventions affect the microbiome composition, fostering urinary dysbiosis in KTx patients [14]. *E. coli* was found seven times more often in KTx recipients than in controls. Rani and colleagues concluded that UTIs follow the disruption of the local microbial homeostasis and arise from bacteria being part of the colonizing microbiome [14]. Patients suffering from recurrent UTI or with frequent occurrence of symptomatic episodes are at a higher risk of being infected with resistant uropathogenic strains [15–18]. Interestingly, we more frequently observed treated UTIs in KTx patients within a three-month period before the sample acquisition. Thus, factors promoting the selection of virulent UPEC should be minimized and therapeutic or probiotic modification of the colonizing microbiome may mitigate frequency and/or severity of UTIs. Against this background, depletion of intestinal reservoirs of UPEC [19] or fecal microbiota transplantation [20] are promising approaches to tackling such infections.

In particular, treatment of asymptomatic bacteriuria led to a significant exposure to antibiotics in KTx patients. Recent studies suggest against the treatment this condition, which seems to be a step in the right direction [21].

In Germany, the resistance rate of UPEC in uncomplicated UTI was 25.9% for TMP/SMX, 34.9% for ampicillin, 3.7% for ciprofloxacin, and 0.8% for fosfomycin [22]. International data shows higher resistance rates for all antibiotic classes in UPEC from KTx recipients [6,23,24]. Similarly, we found relevant resistance rates among our KTx patients as they have received more frequently antibiotic treatments, e.g., with TMP/SMX, and the UPEC carried more trimethoprim, sulfonamide, and β-lactam resistance genes. In particular, the carriage of blaTEM-1B, strA and strB genes was significantly higher than in control strains (Table 4, Supplementary Table S4). Accordingly, the high resistance rates to antibiotics are clinically important (Table 5). Especially for TMP/SMX, one should balance the high resistance rate against the benefit of the *P. jirovecii* prophylaxis [25]. In line with international findings, we only identified a few fosfomycin resistance determinants leading to reasonable susceptibility rates of UPEC [26]. In this regard, our data are relevant for the clinical decision-making.

Several reports focused on "common" O serogroups linked with UTIs [27], but data regarding O serogroups of *E. coli* causing UTIs in KTx patients is limited. In an analysis of 40 urine isolates from KTx patients, *E. coli* ST131 (O25:H4) was identified to be the most prevalent clone [28]. We detected most of the previously reported "common" UPEC O serogroups, including O25 in KTx isolates with the highest prevalence of serogroups O8 and O89 [28]. In general, distinct O serogroups could not be correlated with KTx isolates (Table 3). In contrast to Rice et al., who proposed a unique pattern of UPEC O serogroups in their US patient cohort with acute kidney injury (AKI) at the time of UTI, we did not find such an association [28]. Our AKI rate was lower and there was a similarity between KTx and controls. The fact that the renal function of KTx patients is based on one working kidney (the transplant) only might confound this analysis because two kidneys might better compensate for affections, especially when one kidney is infected (pyelonephritis). Also, the definition of AKI varied between studies. Interestingly, the hospitalization rate was lower in KTx patients than in controls, although the types of UTI were comparable between the groups.

The majority of *E. coli* strains with an increased potential to cause UTIs belong to phylogroups B2 and D, whereas isolates of other phylogenetic lineages display a reduced extraintestinal virulence potential. Phylogroups A and B1 often comprise commensals or diarrheagenic pathogens [29]. In our study, the B2 strains were overrepresented among UPEC isolates of the control group, while phylogroup A strains occurred more frequently in KTx patients. Similarly, Tashk et al. observed that *E. coli* urine isolates from KTx patients more frequently belonged to phylogroups which are uncommon for UPEC, such as phylogroups A, B1, and F, while typical UPEC phylogroups (B2 and D) were overrepresented among the fecal strains of these patients [30].

Recent analyses of UPEC phylogeny describe ST14, ST69, ST73, ST95 and ST131 as the most prevalent clones causing UTI [31]. ST131 is a pandemic clone responsible for a high incidence of extraintestinal infections worldwide [32]. Among our isolates, ST131 was one of the three most prevalent STs. In congruence with the results obtained for the phylogroup distribution, seven out of the ten most prevalent STs in our cohort represent phylogenetic lineages B2 and D (Supplementary Table S1), whereas ST127 significantly correlated with UPEC isolates of controls, and no ST was significantly associated with KTx UPEC.

Only a few selected UPEC virulence traits have been studied in the isolates of KTx patients ($n = 36$) and of non-transplanted patients ($n = 27$) without differences between groups [33]. This result was confirmed in our genome-wide approach. Although 113 virulence-associated gene products showed the tendency to be overrepresented in either the KTx or the control group, only three VFs (FimB, SfaB, FocB) proved to be significantly associated with one group, i.e., the control group. S/F1C fimbriae, as well as the other VFs, are important virulence-associated factors of *E. coli* strains of the phylogroups B2 and D [34]. Additionally, the presence of the B2 phylogroup-enriched cjrABC-senB gene products correlates with increased urovirulence [35,36]. Our PCoA underlines that the prevalence of VFs does not strictly correlate with the isolate groups, but rather with their phylogenetic background (Supplementary Figure S3). As the phylogenetic background plays a critical role for the overall genome content, the VF distribution correlates with phylogeny [37,38]. Typical phylogroup B2 VFs were more frequently found in controls; while in the KTx group, other VFs, including phylogroup A-associated Yhc fimbriae, were overrepresented.

Our analysis of plasmid replicons present in both isolate groups partly corresponds with recent studies [39]. Plasmids are common in UPEC with IncFIB, with IncFII being the most common replicon types. This is in congruence with our data. We identified a large number of colicin plasmids. Col-type plasmids frequently harbor resistance, as well as UPEC virulence-associated genes. Interestingly, isolates from control groups carried almost twice as many colicin plasmids as isolates from KTx patients.

Phenotypic characteristics like α-hemolysin, bacteriocin, and type 1 fimbriae expression or biofilm formation have not been studied in UPEC from KTx patients so far. In this isolate group, the bacteriocin expression was significantly higher than in the UPEC of controls. The rdar/ras morphotype was the most prevalent biofilm-related property in both isolate groups, always slightly higher when expressed in KTx patients' isolates. The slightly increased ability of the KTx isolates to express the rdar biofilm morphotype is an aspect that needs further investigations.

In summary, we show significant differences regarding the phylogenetic background of the UPEC isolates from KTx patients compared to non-transplanted patients. As the prevalence of individual VFs correlates with the phylogroup allocation, the observed differences in the VF distribution among the two isolate groups can be explained. Regarding their phylogenetic background, plasmid content and overall VF distribution, *E. coli* isolates from UTI in non-KTx patients who often share these traits with the typical UPEC described for uncomplicated UTI cases. In contrast, isolates from KTx patients included typical UPEC clones and carried less UPEC virulence-associated genes at a lesser frequency. These strains rather exhibited a weak uropathogenic potential. Our findings suggest that in immunocompromised KTx patients, even *E. coli* strains lacking typical UPEC VFs can cause UTIs, whereas the establishment of UTI in non-transplanted patients requires an increased uropathogenic potential. Clinically important are our findings that UPEC from KTx patients show a higher resistance to several groups of commonly used antibiotics, phenotypically and genotypically. Our study adds important aspects to the concept that UTI establishment results from multiple independent factors including the pathogenic potential of the invading pathogens, its interaction with the host and the host's clinical history and susceptibility.

Supplementary Materials: The following are available online at http://www.mdpi.com/2077-0383/8/7/988/s1. Figure S1: Representative biofilm morphotypes expressed by UPEC isolates on Congo Red agar plates, Figure S2: Manhattan Plot of Fisher's exact test p-values for the prevalence of individual virulence factors (VF) in an isolate group (KTx or control). The red line separates VFs with p-values < 0.05 from VFs without significant association with an isolate group. The green line separates VFs with significant association (p < 0.05) after the Bonferroni correction, Figure S3: Principal Coordinates Analysis (PCoA) to examine the grouping of UPEC isolates according to the presence/absence of virulence-associated genes, their phylogenetic group and their isolate group (KTx vs. control group). The axes are scaled with eigenvalue scaling using the square root of the eigenvalue and indicate the percentage of variation explained in the PCoA. KTx strains are marked with (+) and control strains are marked with (•). The phylogroup of each strain is color coded (phylogroup A = blue, phylogroup B1 = light green, phylogroup B2 = dark green, phylogroup C = brown, phylogroup D = pink, phylogroup E = red, phylogroup F = orange, clade V = black), Table S1: Additional KTx recipient and donor data, Table S2: Distribution of sequence types (STs) in relation to KTx and control UPEC isolates, Table S3: List of VFs significantly associated (Fisher's exact test) with either KTx or control UPEC isolates, Table S4: Resistance genes (RGs) with the largest differences between KTx and control isolates, Table S1: Distribution of the rdar/ras, saw and mucoid morphotypes expressed by KTx and control UPEC isolates, Table S6: Calcofluor binding KTx and control UPEC isolates.

Author Contributions: S.R., B.K. and U.D. conceived and designed the study. B.K. acquired the samples. J.A.B. conducted the experiments. A.W. analyzed the data, S.R., K.S.-N. and H.P. provided clinical data. J.A.B., M.K., B.K., D.G., S.R. and U.D. analyzed and interpreted the data. J.A.B., S.R. and U.D. wrote the main manuscript text. All authors reviewed the manuscript.

Funding: J.A.B. was supported by the Medical Faculty of the University of Münster (Doctoral program "Medizinerkolleg MedK"). H.P., M.K., and U.D. have received funding from the German Research Foundation (grant number SFB1009, TP B05 and B10). Support from the Münster Graduate School of Evolution (MGSE) to M.K. is gratefully acknowledged. We also acknowledge support by the Open Access Publication Fund of the University of Münster.

Conflicts of Interest: The authors declare no conflict of interest.

References

1. Wu, X.; Dong, Y.; Liu, Y.; Li, Y.; Sun, Y.; Wang, J.; Wang, S. The prevalence and predictive factors of urinary tract infection in patients undergoing renal transplantation: A meta-analysis. *Am. J. Infect. Control.* **2016**, *44*, 1261–1268. [CrossRef] [PubMed]

2. Al-Hasan, M.N.; Razonable, R.R.; Kremers, W.K.; Baddour, L.M. Impact of Gram-negative bloodstream infection on long-term allograft survival after kidney transplantation. *Transplantation* **2011**, *91*, 1206–1210. [CrossRef] [PubMed]

3. Bodro, M.; Sanclemente, G.; Lipperheide, I.; Allali, M.; Marco, F.; Bosch, J.; Cofan, F.; Ricart, M.J.; Esforzado, N.; Oppenheimer, F.; et al. Impact of urinary tract infections on short-term kidney graft outcome. *Clin. Microbiol. Infect.* **2015**, *21*, 1104.e1–1104.e8. [CrossRef] [PubMed]

4. Tholking, G.; Schuette-Nuetgen, K.; Vogl, T.; Dobrindt, U.; Kahl, B.C.; Brand, M.; Pavenstadt, H.; Suwelack, B.; Koch, R.; Reuter, S. Male kidney allograft recipients at risk for urinary tract infection? *PLoS ONE* **2017**, *12*, e0188262. [CrossRef] [PubMed]

5. de Souza, R.M.; Olsburgh, J. Urinary tract infection in the renal transplant patient. *Nat. Clin. Pract. Nephrol.* **2008**, *4*, 252–264. [CrossRef] [PubMed]

6. Vidal, E.; Torre-Cisneros, J.; Blanes, M.; Montejo, M.; Cervera, C.; Aguado, J.M.; Len, O.; Carratala, J.; Cordero, E.; Bou, G.; et al. Spanish Network for Research in Infectious Diseases (REIPI) Bacterial urinary tract infection after solid organ transplantation in the RESITRA cohort. *Transpl. Infect. Dis.* **2012**, *14*, 595–603. [CrossRef] [PubMed]

7. Luthje, P.; Brauner, A. Virulence factors of uropathogenic E. coli and their interaction with the host. *Adv. Microb. Physiol.* **2014**, *65*, 337–372. [CrossRef]

8. Clermont, O.; Christenson, J.K.; Denamur, E.; Gordon, D.M. The Clermont Escherichia coli phylo-typing method revisited: Improvement of specificity and detection of new phylo-groups. *Environ. Microbiol. Rep.* **2013**, *5*, 58–65. [CrossRef]

9. O'Brien, V.P.; Dorsey, D.A.; Hannan, T.J.; Hultgren, S.J. Host restriction of Escherichia coli recurrent urinary tract infection occurs in a bacterial strain-specific manner. *PLoS Pathog.* **2018**, *14*, e1007457. [CrossRef]

10. Guidelines on Urological Infections. Available online: https://uroweb.org/wp-content/uploads/19-Urological-infections_LR2.pdf (accessed on 30 June 2019).

11. Ragnarsdottir, B.; Lutay, N.; Gronberg-Hernandez, J.; Koves, B.; Svanborg, C. Genetics of innate immunity and UTI susceptibility. *Nat. Rev. Urol.* **2011**, *8*, 449–468. [CrossRef]

12. Sanchez, G.V.; Babiker, A.; Master, R.N.; Luu, T.; Mathur, A.; Bordon, J. Antibiotic Resistance among Urinary Isolates from Female Outpatients in the United States in 2003 and 2012. *Antimicrob. Agents Chemother.* **2016**, *60*, 2680–2683. [CrossRef] [PubMed]

13. Khawcharoenporn, T.; Vasoo, S.; Singh, K. Urinary Tract Infections due to Multidrug-Resistant Enterobacteriaceae: Prevalence and Risk Factors in a Chicago Emergency Department. *Emerg. Med. Int.* **2013**, *2013*, 258517. [CrossRef] [PubMed]

14. Rani, A.; Ranjan, R.; McGee, H.S.; Andropolis, K.E.; Panchal, D.V.; Hajjiri, Z.; Brennan, D.C.; Finn, P.W.; Perkins, D.L. Urinary microbiome of kidney transplant patients reveals dysbiosis with potential for antibiotic resistance. *Transl. Res.* **2017**, *181*, 59–70. [CrossRef] [PubMed]

15. Wright, S.W.; Wrenn, K.D.; Haynes, M.L. Trimethoprim-sulfamethoxazole resistance among urinary coliform isolates. *J. Gen. Intern. Med.* **1999**, *14*, 606–609. [CrossRef]

16. Killgore, K.M.; March, K.L.; Guglielmo, B.J. Risk factors for community-acquired ciprofloxacin-resistant Escherichia coli urinary tract infection. *Ann. Pharmacother.* **2004**, *38*, 1148–1152. [CrossRef] [PubMed]

17. Cohen-Nahum, K.; Saidel-Odes, L.; Riesenberg, K.; Schlaeffer, F.; Borer, A. Urinary tract infections caused by multi-drug resistant Proteus mirabilis: Risk factors and clinical outcomes. *Infection* **2010**, *38*, 41–46. [CrossRef] [PubMed]

18. Smithson, A.; Chico, C.; Ramos, J.; Netto, C.; Sanchez, M.; Ruiz, J.; Porron, R.; Bastida, M.T. Prevalence and risk factors for quinolone resistance among Escherichia coli strains isolated from males with community febrile urinary tract infection. *Eur. J. Clin. Microbiol. Infect. Dis.* **2012**, *31*, 423–430. [CrossRef] [PubMed]

19. Spaulding, C.N.; Klein, R.D.; Ruer, S.; Kau, A.L.; Schreiber, H.L.; Cusumano, Z.T.; Dodson, K.W.; Pinkner, J.S.; Fremont, D.H.; Janetka, J.W.; et al. Selective depletion of uropathogenic E. coli from the gut by a FimH antagonist. *Nature* **2017**, *546*, 528–532. [CrossRef]

20. Biehl, L.M.; Cruz Aguilar, R.; Farowski, F.; Hahn, W.; Nowag, A.; Wisplinghoff, H.; Vehreschild, M.J.G.T. Fecal microbiota transplantation in a kidney transplant recipient with recurrent urinary tract infection. *Infection* **2018**, *46*, 871–874. [CrossRef]

21. Origuen, J.; Lopez-Medrano, F.; Fernandez-Ruiz, M.; Polanco, N.; Gutierrez, E.; Gonzalez, E.; Merida, E.; Ruiz-Merlo, T.; Morales-Cartagena, A.; Perez-Jacoiste Asin, M.A.; et al. Should Asymptomatic Bacteriuria Be Systematically Treated in Kidney Transplant Recipients? Results From a Randomized Controlled Trial. *Am. J. Transplant.* **2016**, *16*, 2943–2953. [CrossRef]

22. Schito, G.C.; Naber, K.G.; Botto, H.; Palou, J.; Mazzei, T.; Gualco, L.; Marchese, A. The ARESC study: An international survey on the antimicrobial resistance of pathogens involved in uncomplicated urinary tract infections. *Int. J. Antimicrob. Agents* **2009**, *34*, 407–413. [CrossRef] [PubMed]

23. Azap, O.; Togan, T.; Yesilkaya, A.; Arslan, H.; Haberal, M. Antimicrobial susceptibilities of uropathogen Escherichia coli in renal transplant recipients: Dramatic increase in ciprofloxacin resistance. *Transplant. Proc.* **2013**, *45*, 956–957. [CrossRef] [PubMed]

24. Korayem, G.B.; Zangeneh, T.T.; Matthias, K.R. Urinary Tract Infections Recurrence and Development of Urinary-Specific Antibiogram for Kidney Transplant Recipients. *J. Glob. Antimicrob. Resist.* **2018**, *12*, 119–123. [CrossRef] [PubMed]

25. Singh, R.; Bemelman, F.J.; Hodiamont, C.J.; Idu, M.M.; Ten Berge, I.J.; Geerlings, S.E. The impact of trimethoprim-sulfamethoxazole as Pneumocystis jiroveci pneumonia prophylaxis on the occurrence of asymptomatic bacteriuria and urinary tract infections among renal allograft recipients: A retrospective before-after study. *BMC Infect. Dis.* **2016**, *16*, 90. [CrossRef] [PubMed]

26. Kerstenetzky, L.; Jorgenson, M.R.; Descourouez, J.L.; Leverson, G.; Rose, W.E.; Redfield, R.R.; Smith, J.A. Fosfomycin tromethamine for the Treatment of Cystitis in Abdominal Solid Organ Transplant Recipients With Renal Dysfunction. *Ann. Pharmacother.* **2017**, *51*, 751–756. [CrossRef] [PubMed]

27. Poolman, J.T.; Wacker, M. Extraintestinal Pathogenic Escherichia coli, a Common Human Pathogen: Challenges for Vaccine Development and Progress in the Field. *J. Infect. Dis.* **2016**, *213*, 6–13. [CrossRef]

28. Rice, J.C.; Peng, T.; Kuo, Y.F.; Pendyala, S.; Simmons, L.; Boughton, J.; Ishihara, K.; Nowicki, S.; Nowicki, B.J. Renal allograft injury is associated with urinary tract infection caused by Escherichia coli bearing adherence factors. *Am. J. Transplant.* **2006**, *6*, 2375–2383. [CrossRef]

29. Tourret, J.; Denamur, E. Population Phylogenomics of Extraintestinal Pathogenic Escherichia coli. *Microbiol. Spectr.* **2016**, *4*. [CrossRef]

30. Tashk, P.; Lecronier, M.; Clermont, O.; Renvoise, A.; Aubry, A.; Barrou, B.; Hertig, A.; Lescat, M.; Tenaillon, O.; Denamur, E.; et al. Molecular epidemiology and kinetics of early Escherichia coli urinary tract infections in kidney transplant recipients. *Nephrol. Ther.* **2017**, *13*, 236–244. [CrossRef]

31. Yun, K.W.; Kim, D.S.; Kim, W.; Lim, I.S. Molecular typing of uropathogenic Escherichia coli isolated from Korean children with urinary tract infection. *Korean J. Pediatr.* **2015**, *58*, 20–27. [CrossRef]

32. Nicolas-Chanoine, M.H.; Blanco, J.; Leflon-Guibout, V.; Demarty, R.; Alonso, M.P.; Canica, M.M.; Park, Y.J.; Lavigne, J.P.; Pitout, J.; Johnson, J.R. Intercontinental emergence of Escherichia coli clone O25:H4-ST131 producing CTX-M-15. *J. Antimicrob. Chemother.* **2008**, *61*, 273–281. [CrossRef] [PubMed]

33. Mercon, M.; Regua-Mangia, A.H.; Teixeira, L.M.; Irino, K.; Tuboi, S.H.; Goncalves, R.T.; Santoro-Lopes, G. Urinary tract infections in renal transplant recipients: Virulence traits of uropathogenic Escherichia coli. *Transplant. Proc.* **2010**, *42*, 483–485. [CrossRef] [PubMed]

34. Boyd, E.F.; Hartl, D.L. Chromosomal regions specific to pathogenic isolates of Escherichia coli have a phylogenetically clustered distribution. *J. Bacteriol.* **1998**, *180*, 1159–1165. [PubMed]

35. Cusumano, C.K.; Hung, C.S.; Chen, S.L.; Hultgren, S.J. Virulence plasmid harbored by uropathogenic Escherichia coli functions in acute stages of pathogenesis. *Infect. Immun.* **2010**, *78*, 1457–1467. [CrossRef]

36. Mao, B.H.; Chang, Y.F.; Scaria, J.; Chang, C.C.; Chou, L.W.; Tien, N.; Wu, J.J.; Tseng, C.C.; Wang, M.C.; Chang, C.C.; et al. Identification of Escherichia coli genes associated with urinary tract infections. *J. Clin. Microbiol.* **2012**, *50*, 449–456. [CrossRef] [PubMed]

37. Leimbach, A.; Hacker, J.; Dobrindt, U. E. coli as an all-rounder: The thin line between commensalism and pathogenicity. *Curr. Top. Microbiol. Immunol.* **2013**, *358*, 3–32. [CrossRef]

38. Touchon, M.; Hoede, C.; Tenaillon, O.; Barbe, V.; Baeriswyl, S.; Bidet, P.; Bingen, E.; Bonacorsi, S.; Bouchier, C.; Bouvet, O.; et al. Organised genome dynamics in the Escherichia coli species results in highly diverse adaptive paths. *PLoS Genet.* **2009**, *5*, e1000344. [CrossRef]

39. Bengtsson, S.; Naseer, U.; Sundsfjord, A.; Kahlmeter, G.; Sundqvist, M. Sequence types and plasmid carriage of uropathogenic Escherichia coli devoid of phenotypically detectable resistance. *J. Antimicrob. Chemother.* **2012**, *67*, 69–73. [CrossRef]

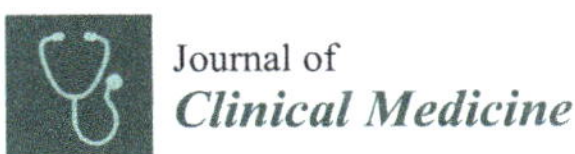

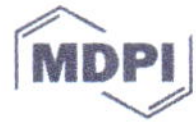

Article

Comparison of Glucose Tolerance between Kidney Transplant Recipients and Healthy Controls

Hisao Shimada [1], Junji Uchida [1,*], Shunji Nishide [1], Kazuya Kabei [1], Akihiro Kosoku [1], Keiko Maeda [2], Tomoaki Iwai [1], Toshihide Naganuma [1], Yoshiaki Takemoto [1] and Tatsuya Nakatani [1]

[1]   Department of Urology, Osaka City University Graduate School of Medicine, Osaka 545-8585, Japan
[2]   Department of Nursing, Osaka City University Hospital, Osaka 545-8585, Japan
*   Correspondence: uchida@msic.med.osaka-cu.ac.jp; Tel.: +81-6-6645-3857

Received: 24 May 2019; Accepted: 24 June 2019; Published: 27 June 2019

Abstract: Post-transplant hyperglycemia and new-onset diabetes mellitus after transplantation (NODAT) are common and important metabolic complications. Decreased insulin secretion and increased insulin resistance are important to the pathophysiologic mechanism behind NODAT. However, the progression of glucose intolerance diagnosed late after kidney transplantation remains clearly unknown. Enrolled in this study were 94 kidney transplant recipients and 134 kidney transplant donors, as the healthy controls, who were treated at our institution. The 75 g-oral glucose tolerance test (OGTT) was performed in the recipients, and the healthy controls received an OGTT before donor nephrectomy. We assessed the prevalence of glucose intolerance including impaired fasting glucose and/or impaired glucose tolerance, as well as insulin secretion and insulin resistance using the homeostasis model assessment, and compared the results between the two groups. Multivariate analysis after adjustment for age, gender, body mass index, estimated glomerular filtration rate, and systolic blood pressure showed that the prevalence of glucose intolerance, insulin resistance, insulin secretion, and 2 h plasma glucose levels were significantly higher in the kidney transplant recipients compared to the healthy controls. Elevation of insulin secretion in kidney transplant recipients may be compensatory for increase of insulin resistance. Impaired compensatory pancreas β cell function may lead to glucose intolerance and NODAT in the future.

Keywords: kidney transplantation; glucose intolerance; insulin secretion; insulin resistance; oral glucose tolerance test; healthy subject

---

1. Introduction

Post-transplant hyperglycemia and new-onset diabetes mellitus after transplantation (NODAT) are common and significant metabolic complications in kidney transplant recipients (KTRs) which can lead to increased mortality and cardiovascular morbidity [1–3]. Similar to type 2 diabetes mellitus (DM), decreased insulin secretion and increased insulin resistance are important to the pathophysiologic mechanism behind NODAT [4]. Previous reports have shown that impaired insulin secretion is a more dominant mechanism for the development of NODAT compared to type 2 DM [5]. However, the exact mechanism of glucose intolerance diagnosed late after kidney transplantation remains unknown [6], although immunosuppressive agents such as calcineurin inhibitors, steroids, and mammalian target of rapamycin inhibitors are thought to cause glucose intolerance following kidney transplantation [1–3]. The increased prevalence of cardiovascular events in transplant recipients is an issue that remains to be solved. Abnormal glucose homeostasis is considered to be one of the established risk factors for the development of cardiovascular events following kidney transplantation [7], but there have been few reports comparing glucose tolerance between KTRs and healthy subjects.

The oral glucose tolerance test (OGTT) has many advantages over fasting plasma glucose for diagnosing glucose intolerance, as it not only accurately identifies persons with DM but also identifies those with impaired fasting glucose (IFG) and impaired glucose tolerance (IGT). Abnormal glucose tolerance determined by the OGTT is a risk factor for the future development of type 2 DM in general populations [8,9], and the OGTT has also been established as a sensitive tool to detect NODAT and glucose intolerance in KTRs [10,11]. The homeostasis model assessment (HOMA) model is a well-known method used for the quantitative verification of insulin resistance and insulin secretion. In this model, fasting glucose levels and fasting insulin levels are mainly defined by feedback of glucose release from the liver and insulin secretion from pancreatic β cells [12]. The aim of this study was to compare glucose tolerance between KTRs and healthy subjects using the OGTT, and we assessed the prevalence of glucose intolerance including IFG and/or IGT as well as insulin secretion and insulin resistance using the HOMA. The correct homeostasis model assessment evaluation using a computer program was reported to be another verification of insulin sensitivity and pancreatic β cell function [13]. However, we used the homeostasis model assessment of insulin resistance (HOMA-R) and homeostasis model assessment of β cell function (HOMA-β) in this study, because we had previously reported on glucose intolerance in kidney transplant recipients using these methods [11].

2. Patients and Methods

2.1. Study Design and Participants

This study was a single-center, cross-sectional, observational investigation conducted at Osaka City University Graduate School of Medicine. Ninety-four out of 101 KTRs who underwent a transplant at our institution and consented to participate in this study were enrolled (KTR group) (Figure S1). To compare glucose tolerance between KTRs and healthy subjects, 134 kidney transplant donors who underwent a nephrectomy at our institution between 2006 and 2017 were enrolled in this study as the healthy controls (HC group). A 75 g-OGTT was performed in the KTR group from October 2010 to April 2012, and the HC group received a 75 g-OGTT before donor nephrectomy. For the KTR group, the inclusion criteria were as follows: (1) stable calcineurin inhibitor (CNI) levels for the last 6 months, (2) no prior evidence of DM, (3) at least a year after transplantation, (4) serum creatinine below 2.0 mg/dL, and (5) stable renal function for the last 6 months. The following recipients were excluded from this study: (1) patients with acute infection, liver dysfunction, abnormal thyroid tests, history of gastrectomy, or chronic pancreatitis and (2) patients who had histories of hepatitis B virus and/or hepatitis C virus infection irrespective of being treated or untreated. This study was approved by the Ethics Committee of Osaka City University Graduate School of Medicine (No. 4120). We provided patients with information explaining the proposed research plan (the purpose, required individual data, and duration of research) by means of an information website of our hospital and gave them the opportunity to opt out, and all the procedures were in accordance with the Helsinki Declaration of 2000 and the Declaration of Istanbul 2008.

2.2. Immunosuppressive Regimen

Standard immunosuppressive regimen for kidney transplantation consisted of basiliximab (BAS), methylprednisolone (MP), CNI (cyclosporine or tacrolimus), and antimetabolites (mycophenolate mofetil or mizoribine or azathioprine). CNI and antimetabolites were initiated 3 days before transplantation. BAS has been administered in all recipients since 2002 at a dose of 20 mg/day at the time of transplantation and 4 days after transplantation. MP was intravenously administered at a dose of 500 mg at the time of transplantation and orally administered at 40 mg/day 1 to 7 days after transplantation, the dose of which was decreased to 24, 12, 8, and 4 mg/day every week. For treatment of acute cellular rejection events, MP was intravenously administered at a dose of 500 mg/day for 3 days alone or in combination with deoxyspergualin (5 mg/kg/day: 5–7 days).

2.3. Data Collection

Patient characteristics (age, gender) and clinical data [estimated glomerular filtration rate (eGFR), fasting plasma glucose (FPG), fasting immunoreactive insulin, hemoglobin A1c, triglyceride, total cholesterol, high-density lipoprotein-cholesterol, low-density lipoprotein-cholesterol] were collected from electronic medical records in all subjects enrolled in this study. eGFR was estimated by the modified Modification of Diet in Renal Disease Equation using the Japanese coefficient [14]. Blood samples were obtained after overnight fasting. Body mass index (BMI) was calculated as body weight in kilograms divided by the square of body height in meters (kg/m^2). Blood pressure was reported as the average of five automated measurements taken at 3-min intervals. Clinical parameters of the KTR group such as type of CNIs, donor type, and post-transplant duration were collected. Dyslipidemia was defined by oral administration such as statin and polyunsaturated fatty acid, triglycerides over 150 mg/dL, or HDL cholesterol below 40 mg/dL, or LDL cholesterol over 140 mg/dL. Hypertension was defined by administration of antihypertensive drug, systolic blood pressure over 140 mmHg, or diastolic blood pressure over 90 mmHg. The administration of angiotensin converting enzyme inhibitor and/or angiotensin II receptor blocker, β-blocker, calcium channel blocker, loop diuretic, and thiazide diuretic were evaluated in all subjects.

2.4. Glucose Intolerance, Insulin Resistance, and β Cell Function

All patients underwent an OGTT in the morning after overnight fasting. Blood samples were drawn for determining plasma glucose and insulin before glucose loading and at 30 and 120 min after glucose loading. According to the World Health Organization [15], normal glucose tolerance (NGT) was defined as FPG and 2-h plasma glucose of <110 mg/dL and <140 mg/dL, IFG as 110–126 mg/dL and <140 mg/dL, IFG/IGT as 110–126 mg/dL and 140–200 mg/dL, and DM as ≥ 126 mg/dL and/or ≥200 mg/dL, respectively. Glucose intolerance consisted of IFG, IGT, IFG/IGT, and DM. Insulin resistance was estimated using the HOMA of insulin resistance (HOMA-R) according to the formula HOMA-R = fasting insulin (mU/L) × FPG (mg/dL)/405. For the assessment of pancreatic β cell function, we used the HOMA of β cell function (HOMA-β) according to the formula HOMA-β = 360 × fasting insulin (mU/L)/(FPG (mg/dL)-63), and the insulinogenic index = (insulin 30 min-fasting insulin (mU/L))/(plasma glucose 30 min-FPG (mg/dL)) [12].

2.5. Statistical Analysis

Categorical variables were expressed as count and percentage, and continuous variables were expressed as mean ± standard deviation, or median and interquartile range, or range. Differences between the groups were examined by Student's t-test or Mann-Whitney U-test. Categorical variables were compared using chi-squared analysis. Logistic regression analysis was used to test the influence of KTR group or HC group on the glucose intolerance (versus normal glucose tolerance). We also performed logistic regression analysis adjusted for multiple models (Model 1: Adjusted for age, gender, and BMI; Model 2: Adjusted for Model 1 and eGFR; Model 3: Adjusted for Model 2 and SBP). Linear regression analysis was used to test if the group (KTR group or HC group) was related to various dependent variables. We also performed linear regression analysis adjusted for multiple models (Model 1: Adjusted for age, gender, and BMI; Model 2: Adjusted for Model 1 and eGFR; Model 3: Adjusted for Model 2 and SBP). All statistical analyses were performed with SPSS version 22.0 for windows (IBM Japan, Tokyo, Japan). A *p*-value of less than 0.05 was considered statistically significant.

3. Results

3.1. Study Participants

The comparison of characteristics between the KTR and HC groups is presented in Table 1. The age in the KTR group was significantly younger than that in the HC group, while BMI in the HC group was significantly higher than that in the KTR group. Hemoglobin A1c levels in the KTR group were lower than those in the HC group. eGFR was lower in the KTR group compared to the HC group. The prevalence of hypertension in the KTR group was significantly higher than that in the HC group. The clinical parameters related to kidney transplantation in the KTR group are shown in Supplementary Table S1.

Table 1. Clinical characteristics of kidney transplant recipients and healthy controls.

Variables	KTR Group Median [IQR] or % $n = 94$	HC Group Median [IQR] or % $n = 134$	p
Age (years)	47 (37, 58)	57 (49, 65)	<0.001
Male gender (%)	48.9	39.6	0.176
Body mass index (kg/m^2)	20.36 (18.52, 22.52)	22.36 (20.74, 24.61)	<0.001
Serum creatinine (mg/dL)	1.21 (0.93, 1.43)	0.68 (0.59, 0.79)	<0.001
eGFR (mL/min/1.73 m^2)	47.02 (40.69, 55.65)	78.08 (69.93, 87.55)	<0.001
Hemoglobin (g/dL)	12.1 (11.1, 13.2)	13.8 (13.0, 14.8)	<0.001
Hematocrit (%)	36.35 (34.03, 39.08)	41.35 (39.23, 43.95)	<0.001
HbA1c (%)	5.4 (5.2, 5.8)	5.7 (5.5, 5.9)	<0.001
Triglycerides (mg/dL)	99 (74, 137)	94 (69, 138)	0.823
Total cholesterol (mg/dL)	197 (179, 217)	202 (181, 223)	0.231
HDL cholesterol (mg/dL)	66 (57, 74)	61 (50, 72)	0.077
LDL cholesterol (mg/dL)	111 (92, 128)	116 (101, 138)	0.036
Dyslipidemia (%)	38.3	43.3	0.494
Systolic blood pressure (mmHg)	120 (112, 126)	117 (106, 131)	0.478
Diastolic blood pressure (mmHg)	74 (68, 80)	71 (64, 78)	0.127
Hypertension (%)	76.6	15.7	<0.001
Administration of ARB (%)	53.2	12.7	<0.001
Administration of ACEi (%)	23.6	0.7	<0.001
Administration of β-blocker (%)	8.5	0	<0.001
Administration of calcium channel blocker (%)	44.7	8.2	<0.001
Administration of thiazide diuretics (%)	5.3	0.7	0.084
Administration of loop diuretics (%)	3.2	0	0.069
Post-transplant duration (years)	5.4 (2.8, 9.6)	-	-
Donor type (cadaver) (%)	16.0	-	-
CNI (Tacrolimus) (%)	39.4	-	-

KTR, kidney transplant recipients; HC, healthy controls; BMI, body mass index; eGFR, estimated glomerular filtration rate; HDL cholesterol, high-density lipoprotein cholesterol; LDL cholesterol, low-density lipoprotein cholesterol; ARB, angiotensin II receptor blocker; ACEi, angiotensin converting enzyme inhibitor; CNI, calcineurin inhibitors.

3.2. Insulin Secretion and Resistance in Subjects with NGT and Glucose Intolerance

In the KTR group, NGT was detected in 74 (78.7%) patients, while 20 (21.3%) had glucose intolerance including two with IFG, 10 with IGT, two with IFG/IGT, and six with DM. Meanwhile, in the HC group, NGT was detected in 107 (79.9%) patients, while 27 (20.1%) had glucose intolerance including four with IFG, 16 with IGT, three with IFG/IGT, and four with DM. There was no significant difference in the prevalence of glucose intolerance between the two groups. HOMA-R in the KTR group tended to be higher than that in the HC group ($p = 0.051$). HOMA-β in the KTR group was significantly higher than that in the HC group. There was also no significant change in the insulinogenic index between the two groups. There were no significant changes in FPG and 2 h plasma glucose levels between the two groups (Table 2).

Table 2. Glucose intolerance between kidney transplant recipients and healthy controls.

Variables	KTR Group Median [IQR] or % $n = 94$	HC Group Median [IQR] or % $n = 134$	p
Fasting plasma glucose (mg/dL)	95 (88, 99)	95 (90, 101)	0.471
2 h plasma glucose (mg/dL)	113 (96, 132)	114 (96, 129)	0.911
Fasting IRI (μU/mL)	6.5 (5.3, 8.7)	5.6 (4.0, 8.4)	0.027
Glucose intolerance (%)	19.4	20.1	1.000
HOMA-R (mIU/mmol L-2)	1.59 (1.15, 1.98)	1.37 (0.89, 2.00)	0.051
HOMA-β (mIU/mmol)	73.78 (53.65, 105.65)	64.02 (47.25, 92.59)	0.027
Insulinogenic Index (μU 10/mg)	0.80 (0.49, 1.22)	0.78 (0.39, 1.26)	0.804

KTR, kidney transplant recipients; HC, healthy controls; IRI, immunoreactive insulin; HOMA-R, homeostasis model assessment of insulin resistance; HOMA-β, homeostasis model assessment of β cell function. IQR, interquartile range.

3.3. Comparison of Prevalence of Glucose Intolerance by Multivariate Logistic Regression Analysis

Multivariate logistic regression analysis was performed to compare the prevalence of glucose intolerance between the two groups (Table 3). There was no significant association in the unadjusted Model and Model 1 (adjusted for age, gender, and BMI). In Model 2 (adjusted for Model 1 and eGFR), there was a statistically significant association between glucose intolerance and group (KTR group versus HC group) (OR = 3.544, 95% CI = 1.143–10.986, p = 0.028). In Model 3 (adjusted for Model 2 and SBP), there was a statistically significant association between glucose intolerance and group (KTR group versus HC group) (OR = 3.794, 95% CI = 1.200–11.996, p = 0.023).

Table 3. Multiple logistic regression analysis for prevalence of glucose intolerance (glucose intolerance versus normal glucose tolerance) between kidney transplant recipients and healthy controls.

	OR	95% CI	p
Unadjusted Model: KTR (vs. HC)	0.939	0.483, 1.825	0.852
Model 1: KTR (vs. HC) adjusted for age, gender, and BMI	1.374	0.645, 2.927	0.410
Model 2: KTR (vs. HC) adjusted for Model 1 and eGFR	3.544	1.143, 10.986	0.028
Model 3: KTR (vs. HC) adjusted for Model 2 and SBP	3.794	1.200, 11.996	0.023

KTR, kidney transplant recipients; HC, healthy controls; BMI, body mass index; eGFR, estimated glomerular filtration rate; SBP, systolic blood pressure; OR, odds ratio; 95% CI, 95% confidence interval.

3.4. Comparison of FPG and 2 h Plasma Glucose Levels by Multivariate Logistic Regression Analysis

The results of linear regression analysis of FPG and 2 h plasma glucose levels are shown in Table 4. In all models, there was no significant association between FPG and group (KTR group versus HC group). However, in Model 1, Model 2, and Model 3, there was a statistically significant association between 2 h plasma glucose levels and group (KTR group versus HC group) (Model 1: B = 10.713, S.E. = 4.861, p = 0.029; Model 2: B = 15.079, S.E. = 7.311, p = 0.040; Model 3: B = 15.091, S.E. = 7.329, p = 0.041).

Table 4. Correlation between fasting plasma glucose and 2 h plasma glucose with presence of kidney transplantation in adjusted linear regression analysis.

	FPG			2-hPG		
	B	S.E.	p	B	S.E.	p
Unadjusted Model: KTR (vs. HC)	−0.349	1.439	0.809	2.101	4.604	0.649
Model 1: KTR (vs. HC) adjusted for age, gender, and BMI	1.254	1.488	0.400	10.713	4.861	0.029
Model 2: KTR (vs. HC) adjusted for Model 1 and eGFR	4.062	2.226	0.069	15.079	7.311	0.040
Model 3: KTR (vs. HC) adjusted for Model 2 and SBP	4.068	2.229	0.069	15.091	7.329	0.041

FPG, fasting plasma glucose; 2-hPG, 2-h plasma glucose; KTR, kidney transplant recipients; HC, healthy controls; BMI, body mass index; eGFR, estimated glomerular filtration rate; SBP, systolic blood pressure; B, coefficient estimate; S.E., standard error.

3.5. Comparison of HOMA-R and HOMA-β by Multivariate Logistic Regression Analysis

Table 5 shows the results of linear regression analysis of HOMA-R and HOMA-β. In Model 1, Model 2, and Model 3, there was a statistically significant association between HOMA-R and group (KTR group versus HC group) (Model 1: B = 0.516, S.E. = 0.170, p = 0.003; Model 2: B = 0.615, S.E. = 0.256, p = 0.017; Model 3: B = 0.616, S.E. = 0.256, p = 0.017). In all models, there was a statistically significant association between HOMA-β and group (KTR group versus HC group) (unadjusted Model: B = 15.850, S.E. = 6.341; p = 0.013; Model 1: B = 24.581, S.E. = 6.417, p < 0.001; Model 2: B = 28.699, S.E. = 9.658, p = 0.003; Model 3: B = 28.715, S.E. = 9.689, p = 0.003).

Table 5. Correlation between HOMA-R and HOMA-β with presence of kidney transplantation in adjusted linear regression analysis.

	HOMA-R			HOMA-β		
	B	S.E.	p	B	S.E.	p
Unadjusted Model: KTR (vs. HC)	0.205	0.170	0.229	15.850	6.341	0.013
Model 1: KTR (vs. HC) adjusted for age, gender, and BMI	0.516	0.170	0.003	24.581	6.417	<0.001
Model 2: KTR (vs. HC) adjusted for Model 1 and eGFR	0.615	0.256	0.017	28.699	9.658	0.003
Model 3: KTR (vs. HC) adjusted for Model 2 and SBP	0.616	0.256	0.017	28.715	9.689	0.003

HOMA-R, homeostasis model assessment of insulin resistance; HOMA-β, homeostasis model assessment of β cell function; KTR, kidney transplant recipients; HC, healthy controls; BMI, body mass index; eGFR, estimated glomerular filtration rate; SBP, systolic blood pressure; B, coefficient estimate; S.E., standard error.

4. Discussion

In this study, multivariate regression analysis revealed that the prevalence of glucose intolerance in the KTR group was significantly higher than in the HC group. Moreover, insulin resistance in the KTR group was significantly higher than that in the HC group, and insulin secretion in the KTR group was also higher than that in the HC group. The elevation of insulin secretion may be compensatory for the increase of insulin resistance in the KTR group. To our knowledge, this is the first demonstration comparing glucose tolerance between KTRs and healthy subjects.

The pathophysiology of NODAT is similar to type 2 DM but with important differences. Previous reports have shown that the primary pathophysiological defect is more pancreatic β cell dysfunction in NODAT compared to type 2 DM [5]. However, the mechanism of glucose intolerance diagnosed late after kidney transplantation is not clear [6]. Because of the prolonged and elevated insulin resistance due to immunosuppressive agents such as steroids, CNIs, and mTOR inhibitors administered for a long time at a late post-transplant stage, long-term compensatory insulin secretion of pancreatic β cells may be required to prevent impaired glucose metabolism in KTRs. Additional risk factors of DM such as gaining weight after transplantation or aging may lead to the collapse of pancreatic β cells function in these patients. As a consequence, glucose intolerance and DM in KTRs may occur at a late post-transplant stage despite a concomitant decrease in steroid use and CNI blood levels.

It has been established that IGT and IFG are risk factors for developing type 2 DM in the future in general populations [6,7]. In our study, multivariate logistic regression analysis revealed that the prevalence of glucose intolerance based on the OGTT such as IFG, IGT, and DM in the KTR group was higher than that in the HC group. KTRs may therefore have a higher risk for new-onset DM compared to healthy subjects. One study reported that the occurrence of acute rejection and NODAT within the first post-transplantation year showed a similar impact on long-term transplant survival. Moreover, NODAT seems to be associated with death with a functioning graft [16]. As pre-stages of NODAT, IFG and IGT have been introduced as gluco-metabolic targets in an effort to reduce the risk of developing chronic transplant-associated morbidity and mortality by implementing proper management approaches during pre-and post-transplant stages [17]. Assessment of glucose intolerance based on the OGTT may also be more important for achieving excellent transplant outcomes in KTRs.

KTRs have an increased risk of premature death due to cardiovascular disease, malignancy, and infectious disease, as they are the predominant causes of mortality [18]. Immunosuppressive therapy may potentiate these risk factors. However, the increased long-term mortality after kidney transplantation cannot be fully explained by this. Hyperglycemia is reported to be a risk marker for cardiovascular disease and cancer among healthy subjects without DM [19,20]. In a previous study, 2-h post-load glucose concentrations indicated a risk of all cause and cardiovascular morbidity in a general population without known DM [21]. Multivariate regression analysis in our study identified that 2-h plasma glucose levels in the KTR group were higher than those in the HC group. Increased 2-h plasma glucose levels in KTRs may elevate the risk of all cause and cardiovascular morbidity, and KTRs may tend to have subclinical hyperglycemia.

This study has several important limitations. Because it was a cross-sectional, observational study, the risk for glucose intolerance was not completely clarified. Also, the risk factor data of NODAT, such as family history of DM and hypomagnesemia were not available [22,23]. However, this may be the first demonstration comparing glucose tolerance between KTRs and healthy subjects. Our study may be helpful for understanding the status of glucose tolerance in KTRs receiving immunosuppressive therapy. Prospective and cohort studies involving a much larger population are needed to identify the mechanism of glucose intolerance in KTRs.

5. Conclusions

In conclusion, insulin resistance as well as insulin secretion in the KTR group were significantly higher than those in the HC group. Moreover, the prevalence of glucose intolerance and 2-h plasma glucose levels in the KTR group were significantly higher than those in the HC group. The elevation of insulin secretion may be compensatory for the increase of insulin resistance in KTRs. In these recipients, the impaired compensatory pancreas β cell function may lead to NODAT and glucose intolerance late after kidney transplantation.

Supplementary Materials: The following are available online at http://www.mdpi.com/2077-0383/8/7/920/s1, Figure S1: Flow chart of patients' enrollment, Table S1: Clinical parameters of kidney transplant recipients.

Author Contributions: Conceptualization, J.U., Y.T. and K.K.; methodology, J.U., S.N. and T.N.; software, H.S.; validation, H.S., K.M. and J.U.; formal analysis, H.S.; investigation, H.S. and T.I.; resources, J.U.; data curation, H.S.; writing—original draft preparation, H.S. and A.K.; writing—review and editing, J.U.; visualization, H.S.; supervision, T.N.; project administration, J.U.

Conflicts of Interest: The authors declare no conflict of interest.

References

1. Kasiske, B.L.; Snyder, J.J.; Gilbertson, D.; Matas, A.J. Diabetes mellitus after kidney transplantation in the United States. *Am. J. Transplant.* **2003**, *3*, 178–185. [CrossRef] [PubMed]
2. Krentz, A.J.; Wheeler, D.C. New-onset diabetes after transplantation: A threat to graft and patient survival. *Lancet.* **2005**, *365*, 640–642. [CrossRef]
3. Cosio, F.G.; Kudva, Y.; van der Velde, M.; Larson, T.S.; Textor, S.C.; Griffin, M.D.; Stegall, M.D. New onset hyperglycemia and diabetes are associated with increased cardiovascular risk after kidney transplantation. *Kidney Int.* **2005**, *67*, 2415–2421. [CrossRef]
4. Ekstrand, A.V.; Eriksson, J.G.; Grönhagen-Riska, C.; Ahonen, P.J.; Groop, L.C. Insulin resistance and insulin deficiency in the pathogenesis of posttransplantation diabetes in man. *Transplantation* **1992**, *53*, 563–569. [CrossRef] [PubMed]
5. Nam, J.H.; Mun, J.I.; Kim, S.I.; Kang, S.W.; Choi, K.H.; Park, K.; Ahn, C.W.; Cha, B.S.; Song, Y.D.; Lim, S.K.; et al. beta-Cell dysfunction rather than insulin resistance is the main contributing factor for the development of postrenal transplantation diabetes mellitus. *Transplantation* **2001**, *71*, 1417–1423. [CrossRef] [PubMed]
6. Nagaraja, P.; Sharif, A.; Ravindran, V.; Baboolal, K. Long-term progression of abnormal glucose tolerance and its relationship with the metabolic syndrome after kidney transplantation. *Transplantation* **2014**, *97*, 576–581. [CrossRef]

7. Lee, H.C. Post-renal transplant diabetes mellitus in korean subjects: Superimposition of transplant-related immunosuppressant factors on genetic and type 2 diabetic risk factors. *Diabetes Metab. J.* **2012**, *36*, 199–206. [CrossRef] [PubMed]

8. Unwin, N.; Shaw, J.; Zimmet, P.; Alberti, K.G. Impaired glucose tolerance and impaired fasting glycaemia: The current status on definition and intervention. *Diabet. Med.* **2002**, *19*, 708–723.

9. Expert Committee on the Diagnosis and Classification of Diabetes Mellitus. Report of the expert committee on the diagnosis and classification of diabetes mellitus. *Diabetes Care* **2003**, *26*, S5–S20. [CrossRef]

10. Sharif, A.; Moore, R.H.; Baboolal, K. The use of oral glucose tolerance tests to risk stratify for new-onset diabetes after transplantation: An underdiagnosed phenomenon. *Transplantation* **2006**, *82*, 1667–1672. [CrossRef]

11. Uchida, J.; Iwai, T.; Kuwabara, N.; Machida, Y.; Iguchi, T.; Naganuma, T.; Kumada, N.; Kawashima, H.; Nakatani, T. Glucose intolerance in renal transplant recipients is associated with increased urinary albumin excretion. *Transpl. Immunol.* **2011**, *24*, 241–245. [CrossRef] [PubMed]

12. Matthews, D.R.; Hosker, J.P.; Rudenski, A.S.; Naylor, B.A.; Treacher, D.F.; Turner, R.C. Homeostasis model assessment: Insulin resistance and beta-cell function from fasting plasma glucose and insulin concentrations in man. *Diabetologia* **1985**, *28*, 412–419. [CrossRef] [PubMed]

13. Levy, J.C.; Matthews, D.R.; Hermans, M.P. Correct homeostasis model assessment (HOMA) evaluation uses the computer program. *Diabetes Care* **1998**, *21*, 2191–2192. [CrossRef] [PubMed]

14. Matsuo, S.; Imai, E.; Horio, M.; Yasuda, Y.; Tomita, K.; Nitta, K.; Yamagata, K.; Tomino, Y.; Yokoyama, H.; Hishida, A. Collaborators developing the Japanese equation for estimated GFR. Revised equations for estimated GFR from serum creatinine in Japan. *Am. J. Kidney Dis.* **2009**, *53*, 982–992. [CrossRef] [PubMed]

15. Gabir, M.M.; Hanson, R.L.; Dabelea, D.; Imperatore, G.; Roumain, J.; Bennett, P.H.; Knowler, W.C. The 1997 American Diabetes Association and 1999 World Health Organization criteria for hyperglycemia in the diagnosis and prediction of diabetes. *Diabetes Care* **2000**, *23*, 1108–1112. [CrossRef] [PubMed]

16. Cole, E.H.; Johnston, O.; Rose, C.L.; Gill, J.S. Impact of acute rejection and new-onset diabetes on long-term transplant graft and patient survival. *Clin. J. Am. Soc. Nephrol.* **2008**, *3*, 814–821. [CrossRef] [PubMed]

17. Bloom, R.D.; Crutchlow, M.F. New-onset diabetes mellitus in the kidney recipient: Diagnosis and management strategies. *Clin. J. Am. Soc. Nephrol.* **2008**, *3*, S38–S48. [CrossRef]

18. Briggs, J.D. Causes of death after renal transplantation. *Nephrol. Dial. Transplant.* **2001**, *16*, 1545–1549. [CrossRef]

19. Levitan, E.B.; Song, Y.; Ford, E.S.; Liu, S. Is nondiabetic hyperglycemia a risk factor for cardiovascular disease? A meta-analysis of prospective studies. *Arch. Intern. Med.* **2004**, *164*, 2147–2155. [CrossRef]

20. Stattin, P.; Björ, O.; Ferrari, P.; Lukanova, A.; Lenner, P.; Lindahl, B.; Hallmans, G.; Kaaks, R. Prospective study of hyperglycemia and cancer risk. *Diabetes Care* **2007**, *30*, 561–567. [CrossRef]

21. de Vegt, F.; Dekker, J.M.; Ruhé, H.G.; Stehouwer, C.D.; Nijpels, G.; Bouter, L.M.; Heine, R.J. Hyperglycaemia is associated with all-cause and cardiovascular mortality in the Hoorn population: The Hoorn Study. *Diabetologia* **1999**, *42*, 926–931. [CrossRef] [PubMed]

22. Pham, P.T.; Pham, P.M.; Pham, S.V.; Pham, P.A.; Pham, P.C. New onset diabetes after transplantation (NODAT): An overview. *Diabetes Metab. Syndr. Obes.* **2011**, *4*, 175–186. [CrossRef] [PubMed]

23. Shivaswamy, V.; Boerner, B.; Larsen, J. Post-Transplant Diabetes Mellitus: Causes, Treatment, and Impact on Outcomes. *Endocr. Rev.* **2016**, *37*, 37–61. [CrossRef] [PubMed]

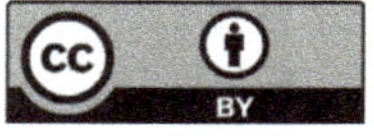

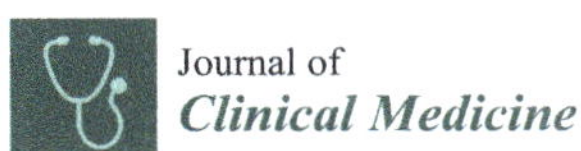

Journal of
Clinical Medicine

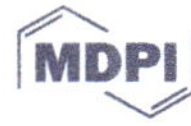

Article

The Effect of Donors' Demographic Characteristics in Renal Function Post-Living Kidney Donation. Analysis of a UK Single Centre Cohort

Maria Irene Bellini [1,*], Sotiris Charalampidis [1], Ioannis Stratigos [2], Frank J.M.F. Dor [1,3] and Vassilios Papalois [1,3]

[1] Renal and Transplant Directorate, Imperial College Healthcare NHS Trust, W120HS London, UK;
s.charalampidis@nhs.net (S.C.); Frank.dor@nhs.net (F.J.M.F.D.); vassilios.papalois@nhs.net (V.P.)
[2] Queen Mary University of London, E14NS London, UK; i.stratigos@se16.qmul.ac.uk
[3] Department of Surgery and Cancer, Imperial College London, SW72AZ London, UK
* Correspondence: Mariairene.bellini@nhs.net

Received: 23 May 2019; Accepted: 18 June 2019; Published: 20 June 2019

Abstract: Introduction: There is a great need to increase the organ donor pool, particularly for living donors. This study analyses the difference in post-living donation kidney function according to pre-donation characteristics of age, genetic relationship with the recipient, sex, ethnicity, and Body Mass Index (BMI). Methods: Retrospective single centre analysis of the trajectory of estimated Glomerular Filtration Rate (eGFR) post-living kidney donation, as a measure of kidney function. Mean eGFR of the different groups was compared at 6 months and during the 60 months follow up. Results: Mean age was 46 ± 13 years, 57% were female, and 60% Caucasian. Mean BMI was 27 ± 5 kg/m^2, with more than a quarter of the cohort having a BMI > 30 (26%), and the majority of the donors genetically related to their recipients (56%). The higher decline rate in eGFR was at 6 months after donation, with female sex, non-Caucasian ethnicity, and age lower than 60 years being independently associated with higher recovery in kidney function ($p < 0.05$). In the 60 months follow up, older age, genetic relationship with the recipient, and male sex led to higher percentual difference in eGFR post-donation. Conclusion: In this study, with a high proportion of high BMI living kidney donors, female sex, age lower than 60 years, and non-genetic relationship with recipient were persistently associated with higher increase in post-donation kidney function. Ethnicity and BMI, per se, should not be a barrier to increasing the living donor kidney pool.

Keywords: living donor; kidney transplantation; ethnicity; age; obesity; genetic relationship donor/recipient

---

1. Introduction

Living donor (LD) kidney transplantation provides the best long-term outcomes for patients with chronic kidney failure [1]. A careful selection to limit the potential risks related to living kidney donation is important, not only to safeguard these healthy individuals who should not be harmed as a result of their generous act, but also to keep expanding the organ donor pool [2]. The donor's demographic characteristics are currently a topic of interest to assess the potential risk of end stage renal disease (ESRD) among living donors.

It has been reported that high body mass index (BMI kg/m^2) has no higher perioperative risks for living kidney donors [3] but has a negative impact on post-donation kidney function [4]. However, there is no consensus regarding the BMI threshold for LD acceptance criteria; this is particularly important in populations where the average BMI is increasing [5,6].

Previous studies have also suggested that renal function reached at one year post-donation remains stable—at least over the next decade—but then declines with ageing [7,8]. Ibrahim et al. indicated that a younger age at the time of donation, a longer time since donation, and a higher eGFR at the time of donation were associated with a greater compensatory increase in the eGFR in the remaining kidney [9]. Conversely, Dols et al. reported that kidney donation by older donors is relatively safe over time since, in their experience, kidney function did not decline progressively [10,11]. A correlation with age and ethnicity has also been reported, with higher risk for ESRD for older Caucasians and younger Africans [12].

Regarding the donor's sex, there are reports that in males there is a more pronounced decline in the short-term renal function [13], but the absolute risk to develop ESRD is still very low: one per 2000, compared to one per 10000 in the general population (RR 8.83), according to a recent meta-analysis [14].

Living kidney donors with a first-degree genetic relationship to the recipient have an increased risk of developing ESRD [15], but a personalised estimation on the basis of donor characteristics still remains unavailable and controversial.

Risk estimation is critical for appropriate informed consent, so special consideration in potential living donors' relative risk triggered by certain demographics or conditions is massively important nowadays. This single centre study aims to establish the effect of the donor's sex, age, ethnicity, BMI, and genetic relationship to the recipient on the evolution of the eGFR as a marker of kidney function recovery after living kidney donation.

2. Methods

The study, performed in accordance with the Declaration of Helsinki principles, is a retrospective analysis on consecutive living kidney donors who had their operation in our centre during the period of 2000 and 2017, and with 60 months of follow up. After discharge, donors first came to our follow up clinic in 2 weeks' time, and then at six months and yearly (up to five years) post-donation for routine blood controls.

The data used were anonymised and extracted from an electronic database of medical records. The study fell under the category of research through the use of anonymised data of existing databases which, based on the Health Research Authority criteria [16], does not require proportional or full ethics review and approval.

Obesity was defined according to the World Health Organization (WHO) classification when BMI $\geq$ 30 kg/m^2, normal weight when BMI $\leq$ 25 kg/m^2, and overweight when 25 kg/m^2 < BMI < 30 kg/m^2. Donors were also stratified according to sex, ethnicity, and age below or above 60 years, which is the cut off between standard or extended criteria used in deceased donor organ donation [17]. Mean eGFR was compared using the CKD-EPI equations between groups, as this is recommended in view of the eligibility of potential living donors [18]. The decline in kidney function was analysed between different points of the 60 months follow up and donation. It was expressed as the percentual difference in eGFR (Δ eGFR), between mean eGFR at a given point of follow up and the eGFR at the time of donation.

Continuous variables were presented as mean $\pm$ standard deviation and compared using one-way ANOVA at 6, 12, 24, 36, 48, and 60 months follow up. Confidence interval was set to 95%, and *p* was considered significant at less than 0.05. A general linear model of repeated measures of ANOVA eGFR during the 60 months follow up was built to observe the percentual difference in eGFR recovery and assess the independent effect of donors' characteristics.

Statistical analysis was performed using SPSS (IBM SPSS Statistics for Windows, Version 20.0; IBM Corp, Armonk, NY, USA).

3. Results

A total of 889 consecutive living kidney donors were analysed (Table 1). Mean follow up was 44.1 $\pm$ 31.3 months. Full dataset at 6 months was available for 700 donors (79%), at 12 months for

635 (71%), at 24 months for 569 (64%), at 36 months for 489 (55%), at 48 months for 408 (46%), and at 60 months for 348 (39%) donors. The mean age at donation was 46 ± 13 years, with a mean BMI of 27 ± 5 kg/m^2. More than a quarter of the total LD cohort had a BMI > 30 (26%). Females were 57% and the prevalent ethnicity was Caucasian (60%). The majority of the donors were genetically related to the recipient (56%).

Table 1. Baseline demographic characteristics and eGFR reported in mL/min/1.73 m^2 at donation. In bold are highlighted statistically significant higher values. LRD: Living Related Donor; LURD: Living Unrelated Donor.

	eGFR Donation		
	Mean ± St. Dev.	***p* Value**	**Table *N* %**
Sex			
Female	**87 ± 22**	**<0.001**	57
Male	**95 ± 32**		43
Ethnicity			
Asian	**91 ± 19**	**<0.001**	25
African	**103 ± 23**		15
Caucasian	**87 ± 28**		60
Graft Type			
LRD	91 ± 26	0.94	56
LURD	90 ± 29		44
Age (years)	46 ± 13		100
< 60 years	**93 ± 24**	**<0.001**	85
> or = 60 years	**80 ± 39**		15
WHO classification BMI (kg/m^2)	27 ± 5		100
BMI < 25	92 ± 29	0.5	36
25 < or = BMI < or = 29	91 ± 30		38
BMI > or = 30	89 ± 20		26

Mean eGFR at donation was confirmed to be statistically significantly related to sex, age, and ethnicity ($p < 0.001$), but not to the BMI or the genetic relationship with the recipient (Table 1).

More specifically, females, donors aged > 60 years, and Caucasians had lower eGFR at donation. Mean eGFR was compared in the different groups during follow up, evaluating the evolution of kidney function recovery after donation. It was expressed as Δ eGFR, between mean eGFR at a given point of follow up and the eGFR at the time of donation. The lowest mean eGFR was after 6 months from donation ($p < 0.001$), with then a progressive decrease of Δ eGFR in the 60 months of follow up, mirroring a progressive recovery in kidney function after donation. Δ eGFR for the whole cohort at 6 months was 0.27 ± 16, Δ eGFR at 12 months 0.26 ± 15, Δ eGFR at 24 months 0.24 ± 15, Δ eGFR at 36 months 0.22 ± 16, Δ eGFR at 48 months 0.2 ± 17, and Δ eGFR at 60 months 0.18 ± 17 ($p < 0.001$). See Supplementary Table S1 for difference in Δ eGFR within different groups.

At 6 months of follow up, the nadir of the kidney function recovery, age older than 60 years, male sex, and Caucasian ethnicity were independent predictors for lower recovery in kidney function ($p < 0.05$). No effect was observed for different classes of BMI and genetic relationship with the recipient.

Figures 1–5 represent mean eGFR and the percentual difference from the donation eGFR during the 60 months follow up. The generalised repeated measures of ANOVA eGFR and Δ eGFR are stratified according to donor age, relationship with the recipient, sex, BMI, and ethnicity.

Mean eGFR post-donation was confirmed as persistently higher in the younger cohort ($p < 0.001$, Figure 1A). The percentual difference in eGFR during the 60 months follow up was also significantly different, with lower recovery from the original kidney function for donors aged > 60 years ($p = 0.037$, Figure 1B).

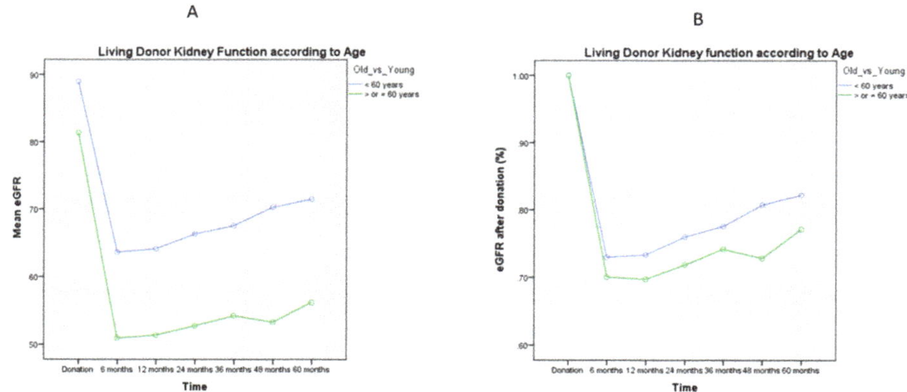

Figure 1. General Linear Model of Repeated Measures ANOVA of mean eGFR (Figure 1A) and mean Δ eGFR (Figure 1B) during the 60 months follow up. There is a decline in eGFR post-donation, with a statistical significant correlation with age > 60 years ($p < 0.001$). The percentual difference in eGFR is also statistically different, with lower recovery for age > 60 years ($p = 0.037$).

Figure 2A shows that although the genetic relationship with the recipient did not statistically affect mean eGFR during the follow up ($p = 0.168$), there was a difference in the kidney function recovery after donation (Figure 2B), in favor of living unrelated donors ($p = 0.007$).

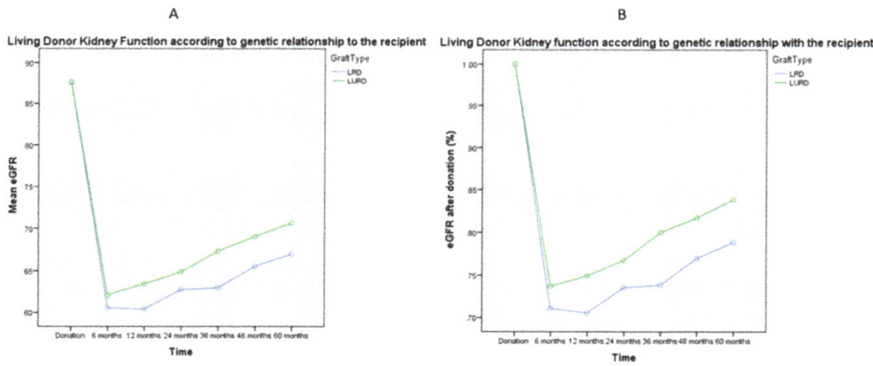

Figure 2. General Linear Model of Repeated Measures ANOVA of mean eGFR (Figure 2A) and mean Δ eGFR (Figure 2B) during the 60 months follow up. There is no difference in mean eGFR post-donation according to the genetic relationship with the recipient ($p = 0.168$), while the percentual recovery in eGFR is statistically different, being higher for live unrelated donor ($p = 0.007$). LRD: Living Related Donor; LURD: Living Unrelated Donor.

Males had higher mean eGFR at donation ($p > 0.001$), but there was no significant difference in mean eGFR after donation ($p = 0.3$, Figure 3A). The recovery of kidney function was persistently higher in females ($p < 0.001$, Figure 3B). This aspect could also be noted in Supplementary Table S1, where only at donation time male donors have a higher mean eGFR: 95 ± 32 mL/min/1.72 m^2 versus 87 ± 22 mL/min/1.72 m^2 for female donors ($p < 0.001$), and where the Δ eGFR is persistently higher for men during follow up ($p < 0.001$).

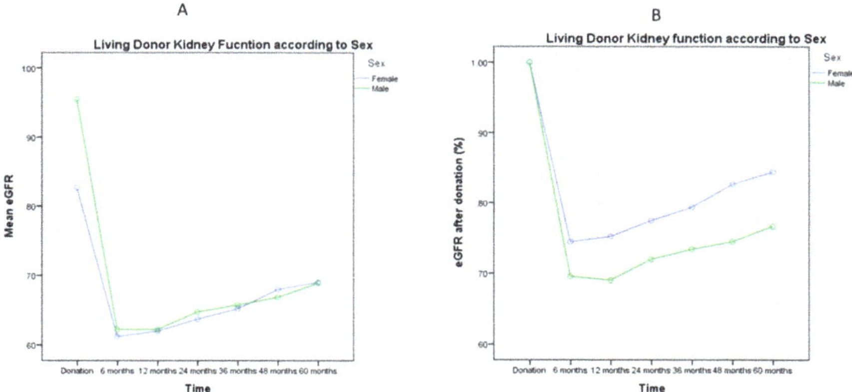

Figure 3. General Linear Model of Repeated Measures ANOVA of mean eGFR (Figure 3A) and mean Δ eGFR (Figure 3B) during the 60 months follow up. Mean eGFR at donation is lower in females ($p < 0.001$), but in the 60 months follow up mean eGFR is no longer significant ($p = 0.3$), because the mean percentual difference in eGFR is higher in males ($p < 0.001$).

Figure 4A,B represent kidney function according to different BMI classes; there was no significant difference pre- or post-donation, either in mean eGFR ($p = 0.53$) or in the percentual difference in kidney function recovery ($p = 0.79$) observed during the study period.

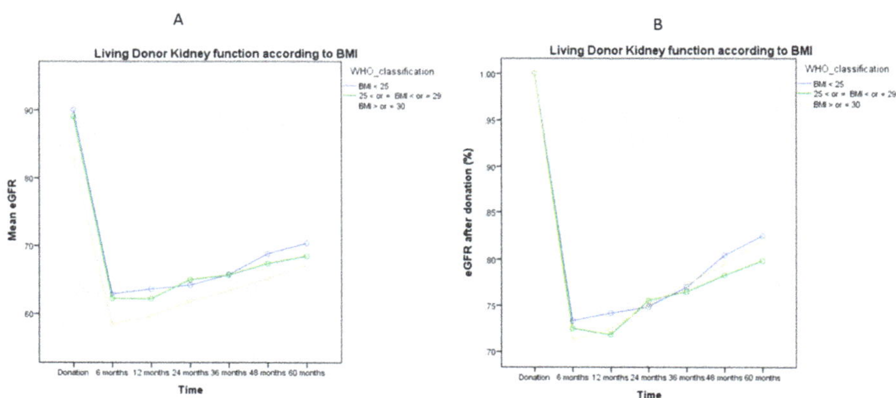

Figure 4. General Linear Model of Repeated Measures ANOVA of mean eGFR (Figure 4A) and mean Δ eGFR (Figure 4B) during the 60 months follow up. The mean eGFR post-donation does not differ according to BMI ($p = 0.53$), with no difference also in kidney function recovery after live donation ($p = 0.79$).

Finally, Caucasian ethnicity was related to a lower mean eGFR pre- and post-donation ($p < 0.001$, Table 1 and Figure 5A). There was also an ethnicity-related effect in the early kidney function recovery after donation at 6 months ($p = 0.005$) in favor of Africans and Asians, see also Supplementary Table S1. However, this ethnicity-related effect in kidney function recovery was not observed during the 60 months follow up, with no significant different mean Δ eGFR in the general linear model ($p = 0.38$, Figure 5B).

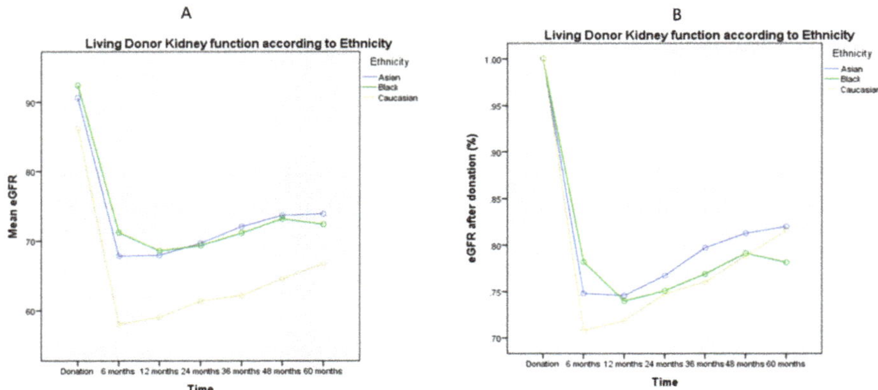

Figure 5. General Linear Model of Repeated Measures ANOVA of mean eGFR (Figure 5A) and mean Δ eGFR (Figure 5B) during the 60 months follow up. The mean eGFR post-donation confirmed to be lower for Caucasian ethnicity ($p < 0.001$), as well as the recovery in kidney function at 6 months ($p = 0.035$). There is not a statistically significance difference in the general linear model for the Δ eGFR at 60 months follow up ($p = 0.38$).

In a logistic regression with stepwise procedure, it was confirmed that only male sex and older age affected Δ eGFR in the long term.

4. Discussion

The present study investigated the kidney function recovery post-living donation in our centre at 6 months post-donation, and during 60 months follow up. Donors' demographic characteristics of age, genetic relationship to the recipient, sex, BMI, and ethnicity were analysed, aiming to assess long term risk, offer comprehensive information to potential donors, and further encourage living kidney donation [19].

Sixty percent of the living kidney donors in our study were Caucasian, the absolute majority for the cohort, but an inferior percentage compared to the rest of the UK, where 88% of the entire living donor pool are Caucasian [19]. The lack of an ethnicity-related effect to the recovery of kidney function could encourage potential living donors from African and Asian communities to proceed with donation; this is most important, considering the fact that these minority groups are more likely to deny consent for deceased organ donation, while at the same time they face prolonged waiting times due to difficulties in the matching process independently from the allocation policy [18,19]. In our centre, practicing in a multi-ethnic country like the UK, we focus on educational programmes directed to ethnic minorities to assure potential donors of the long-term safety of living kidney donation; the results of this study and similar findings in other cohorts [20,21] are informing the content of those programmes.

Similarly to other studies, we demonstrated that the lowest eGFR is within 6 months of follow up [20], and it is statistically significantly related to age older than 60 years [21] and male sex [15]. It is interesting to note that the mean eGFR is higher pre-donation for males, and after donation there is no difference during the 60 months follow up. This happens in relation to the higher Δ eGFR for the males versus females expressing their living donor kidney function recovery. The general longer life expectancy for women could also be a contributing factor [22].

Previous studies have demonstrated the overall safety of living kidney donation, even at older ages [10]. In our study, 15% of LDs were > 60 years old. Our data showed that the recovery of kidney function following living kidney donation was lower for the elderly, reflecting most probably the natural biological process [23]. However, the final mean eGFR for donors > 60 years old was

54 ± 11 mL/min/1.73 m^2, a very satisfactory outcome after 60 months of follow up (Figure 1A,B). Therefore, our centre policy is that living donation is not discouraged on the basis of age only.

Whether or not obesity plays a role in the deterioration of the kidney function following living kidney donation remains a hotly debated issue. Despite the recent report from Locke et al. of a 1.9-fold higher risk for ESRD when compared to normal BMI donors [4], the adjusted risk of ESRD associated with obesity is only 1.16 in living donors with obesity [24]. The 26% of living donors in our cohort had a BMI > 30, but there was no increased risk in terms of mean eGFRs and Δ eGFR or recovery in kidney function during the 60 months follow up (Figure 4A,B). As it is the case with age, our centre policy does not rely for LD risk on the basis of BMI only: Potential candidates are screened on the basis of a multi-disciplinary input and discussion with a multifactorial analysis, tailored on a case-by-case basis to consider the overall medical condition, rather than a single factor [25]. In our centre, we screen potential donors on the basis of a multi-disciplinary input and discussion. We investigate the past medical history, previous hospitalisation, and regular medications. Hypertension controlled with up to two medications is not a contraindication according to the British Transplant Society guidelines [26]; moreover, there is evidence that this does not affect long-term overall or cardiovascular mortality [27]. Proteinuria, diabetes, angina/heart disease, stroke, severe pulmonary disease, kidney stone (or other kidney disease), blood disorders, sickle cell disease, or active cancer are contraindications to donate. No BMI or age cut off are considered as standing only criteria to proceed with donation. All the potential donors undergo imaging of their kidneys and then decision to proceed is made if eGFR > 80 mL/min/1.73 m^2.

Finally, we found a statistically significant higher Δ eGFR after donation for genetically related donors (LRDs), as shown in Figure 2B. The concern that biologically-related living donors, especially first-degree relatives, may face increased risk of adverse renal outcomes after living kidney donation has been a topic of discussion in the transplant community for a long time [28,29]. Increased risks of renal failure in close biological relatives of ESRD patients have been observed in population-based and case-control studies among non-donors, regardless of whether recipient ESRD has a known hereditary cause [30,31]. In a study of Caucasian donors in Norway, the nine donors who developed ESRD were all biologically related to their recipients, and renal failure appeared mainly due to immunological diseases [21]. We believe that, although there is still controversy in the literature around whether LRDs are at increased risk compared to Living Unrelated Donors (LURDs) [32,33], the difference in mean eGFR after donation demonstrated in our study generates the responsibility for the transplant team to inform potential donors genetically related to the recipient about the potential increased risk of ESRD. A possible explanation for this finding, along with the latency of some genetic renal disorders running in the family, could be the presence of emotional factors [34] that push towards the decision to donate in a biologically related donor more than in an unrelated donor. It is also possible that the background risk of ESRD is dependent on several conditions, including family habits or life in a particular socio-economic area—and together, all of these may affect synergistically the eGFR trajectory more significantly than in unrelated donors.

The retrospective nature of this study has limited our analysis to those patients for whom we had complete data during the follow up period. The difficulty for a lifelong follow up in living kidney donors is possibly related to the fact that they are healthy individuals, therefore reluctant to come for tests after the first year post-donation. Another possible explanation could be the fact that as the years go by, donors move around the country and there is no continuity in their follow up.

5. Conclusions

The present study demonstrated that the higher decline rate in eGFR post-living kidney donation was at 6 months, with female sex, non-Caucasian ethnicity, and age lower than 60 years being independently associated with higher recovery in kidney function. At 60 months follow up, older age, genetic relationship with the recipient and male sex were related to a lesser recovery of eGFR, with male sex and older age confirmed at logistic regression analysis. BMI did not relate to kidney function pre or post living kidney donation.

Supplementary Materials: The following are available online at http://www.mdpi.com/2077-0383/8/6/883/s1, Table S1: Mean eGFR during follow up and percentual difference between mean eGFR during follow up and eGFR at donation (Δ eGFR).

Author Contributions: Conceptualisation, M.I.B. and V.P.s; Data curation, S.C. and I.S.; Formal analysis, M.I.B.; Investigation, M.I.B., S.C., F.J.M.F.D., and V.P.; Methodology, M.I.B., F.J.M.F.D., and V.P.; Project administration, M.I.B., S.C., I.S., and V.P.; Writing – original draft, M.I.B., F.J.M.F.D., and V.P.

Conflicts of Interest: The authors declare no conflict of interest.

Meeting Presentation: This work has been presented at the Association of Surgeons of Great Britain and Ireland meeting held in Telford, UK on the 7th–9th May 2019.

Abbreviations

BMI	Body Mass Index
CKD-EPI	Chronic Kidney Disease Epidemiology Collaboration
ECD	Extended Criteria Donor
eGFR	estimated Glomerular Filtration Rate
ESRD	End Stage Renal Disease
LD	Living Donor
LRD	Living Related Donor
LURD	Living Unrelated Donor
RR	Relative Risk
WHO	World Health Organization

References

1. Shapiro, R. End-stage renal disease in 2010: Innovative approaches to improve outcomes in transplantation. *Nat. Rev. Nephrol.* **2011**, *7*, 68–70. [CrossRef] [PubMed]
2. Ahmadi, A.R.; Lafranca, J.A.; Claessens, L.A.; Imamdi, R.M.; IJzermans, J.N.; Betjes, M.G.; Dor, F.J. Shifting paradigms in eligibility criteria for live kidney donation: A systematic review. *Kidney Int.* **2015**, *87*, 31–45. [CrossRef] [PubMed]
3. Lafranca, J.A.; Hagen, S.M.; Dols, L.F.; Arends, L.R.; Weimar, W.; IJzermans, J.N.; Dor, F.J. Systematic review and meta-analysis of the relation between body mass index and short-term donor outcome of laparoscopic donor nephrectomy. *Kidney Int.* **2013**, *83*, 931–939. [CrossRef] [PubMed]
4. Locke, J.E.; Reed, R.D.; Massie, A.; MacLennan, P.A.; Sawinski, D.; Kumar, V.; Segev, D.L. Obesity increases the risk of end-stage renal disease among living kidney donors. *Kidney Int.* **2017**, *91*, 699–703. [CrossRef] [PubMed]
5. Naik, A.S.; Cibrik, D.M.; Sakhuja, A.; Samaniego, M.; Lu, Y.; Shahinian, V.; Lentine, K.L. Temporal trends, center-level variation, and the impact of prevalent state obesity rates on acceptance of obese living kidney donors. *Am. J. Transplant.* **2018**, *18*, 642–649. [CrossRef] [PubMed]
6. Bellini, M.I.; Koutroutsos, K.; Galliford, J.; Herbert, P.E. One-Year Outcomes of a Cohort of Renal Transplant Patients Related to BMI in a Steroid-Sparing Regimen. *Transplant. Direct* **2017**, *3*, e330. [CrossRef] [PubMed]
7. Fehrman-Ekholm, I.; Norden, G.; Lennerling, A.; Rizell, M.; Mjornstedt, L.; Wramner, L.; Olausson, M. Incidence of end-stage renal disease among live kidney donors. *Transplantation* **2006**, *82*, 1646–1648. [CrossRef]
8. Janki, S.; Dols, L.F.; Timman, R.; Mulder, E.E.; Dooper, I.M.; van de Wetering, J.; IJzermans, J.N. Five-year follow-up after live donor nephrectomy—Cross-sectional and longitudinal analysis of a prospective cohort within the era of extended donor eligibility criteria. *Transpl. Int. Off. J. Eur. Soc. Organ Transplant.* **2017**, *30*, 266–276. [CrossRef]
9. Ibrahim, H.N.; Foley, R.; Tan, L.; Rogers, T.; Bailey, R.F.; Guo, H.; Matas, A.J. Long-term consequences of kidney donation. *New Engl. J. Med.* **2009**, *360*, 459–469. [CrossRef]
10. Dols, L.F.; Kok, N.F.; Roodnat, J.I.; Tran, T.C.; Terkivatan, T.; Zuidema, W.C.; IJzermans, J.N.M. Living kidney donors: Impact of age on long-term safety. *Am. J. Transplant. Off. J. Am. Soc. Transplant. Am. Soc. Transpl. Surg.* **2011**, *11*, 737–742. [CrossRef]

11. Dols, L.F.; Weimar, W.; Ijzermans, J.N. Long-term consequences of kidney donation. *New Engl. J. Med.* **2009**, *360*, 2371–2372. [PubMed]

12. Wainright, J.L.; Robinson, A.M.; Wilk, A.R.; Klassen, D.K.; Cherikh, W.S.; Stewart, D.E. Risk of ESRD in Prior Living Kidney Donors. *Am. J. Transplant.* **2018**, *18*, 1129–1139. [CrossRef] [PubMed]

13. Unger, L.W.; Feka, J.; Sabler, P.; Rasoul-Rockenschaub, S.; Gyori, G.; Hofmann, M.; Salat, A. High BMI and male sex as risk factor for increased short-term renal impairment in living kidney donors—Retrospective analysis of 289 consecutive cases. *Int. J. Surg. (Lond Engl.)* **2017**, *46*, 172–177. [CrossRef] [PubMed]

14. O'Keeffe, L.M.; Ramond, A.; Oliver-Williams, C.; Willeit, P.; Paige, E.; Trotter, P.; Evans, J.; Wadstrom, J.; Nicholson, M.; Collett, D.; Di Angelantonio, E. Mid- and Long-Term Health Risks in Living Kidney Donors: A Systematic Review and Meta-analysis. *Ann. Intern. Med.* **2018**, *20*, 276–284. [CrossRef] [PubMed]

15. Massie, A.B.; Muzaale, A.D.; Luo, X.; Chow, E.K.H.; Locke, J.E.; Nguyen, A.Q.; Segev, D.L. Quantifying Postdonation Risk of ESRD in Living Kidney Donors. *J. Am. Soc. Nephrol. JASN* **2017**, *28*, 2749–2755. [CrossRef] [PubMed]

16. Research Tissue Banks and Research Databases. Available online: https://www.hra.nhs.uk/planning-and-improving-research/policies-standards-legislation/research-tissue-banks-and-research-databases/ (accessed on 19 November 2018).

17. Metzger, R.A.; Delmonico, F.L.; Feng, S.; Port, F.K.; Wynn, J.J.; Merion, R.M. Expanded criteria donors for kidney transplantation. *Am. J. Transplant. Off. J. Am. Soc. Transplant. Am. Soc. Transpl. Surg.* **2003**, *3*, 114–125. [CrossRef]

18. Gaillard, F.; Courbebaisse, M.; Kamar, N.; Rostaing, L.; Jacquemont, L.; Hourmant, M.; Janbon, B. Impact of estimation versus direct measurement of predonation glomerular filtration rate on the eligibility of potential living kidney donors. *Kidney Int.* **2019**, *95*, 896–904. [CrossRef]

19. Transplant Activity Report. Available online: https://www.organdonation.nhs.uk/supporting-my-decision/statistics-about-organ-donation/transplant-activity-report/ (accessed on 15 March 2019).

20. Von Zur-Muhlen, B.; Berglund, D.; Yamamoto, S.; Wadstrom, J. Single-centre long-term follow-up of live kidney donors demonstrates preserved kidney function but the necessity of a structured lifelong follow-up. *Upsala J. Med. Sci.* **2014**, *119*, 236–241. [CrossRef]

21. Mjoen, G.; Hallan, S.; Hartmann, A.; Foss, A.; Midtvedt, K.; Oyen, O.; Line, P.D. Long-term risks for kidney donors. *Kidney Int.* **2014**, *86*, 162–167. [CrossRef]

22. Kiberd, B.A.; Tennankore, K.K. Lifetime risks of kidney donation: A medical decision analysis. *BMJ Open* **2017**, *7*, e016490. [CrossRef]

23. Stevens, L.A.; Coresh, J.; Greene, T.; Levey, A.S. Assessing kidney function—Measured and estimated glomerular filtration rate. *New Engl. J. Med.* **2006**, *354*, 2473–2483. [CrossRef] [PubMed]

24. Grams, M.E.; Sang, Y.; Levey, A.S.; Matsushita, K.; Ballew, S.; Chang, A.R.; Shalev, V. Kidney-Failure Risk Projection for the Living Kidney-Donor Candidate. *New Engl. J. Med.* **2016**, *374*, 411–421. [CrossRef] [PubMed]

25. Bellini, M.I.; Paoletti, F.; Herbert, P.E. Obesity and bariatric intervention in patients with chronic renal disease. *J. Int. Med. Res.* **2019**, 300060519843755. [CrossRef] [PubMed]

26. British Transplant Society. *Guidelines for Living Donor Kidney Transplantation*, 4th ed.; British Transplant Society: Macclesfield, UK, 2018.

27. Haugen, A.J.; Langberg, N.E.; Dahle, D.O.; Pihlstrøm, H.; Birkeland, K.I.; Reisaeter, A.; Midtvedt, K.; Hartmann, A.; Holdaas, H.; Mjøen, G. Long-term risk for kidney donors with hypertension at donation—A retrospective cohort study. *Transpl. Int.* **2019**. [CrossRef] [PubMed]

28. Matas, A.J. Transplantation: Increased ESRD and mortality risk for kidney donors? *Nat. Rev. Nephrol.* **2014**, *10*, 130–131. [CrossRef] [PubMed]

29. Muzaale, A.D.; Massie, A.B.; Anjum, S.; Liao, C.; Garg, A.X.; Lentine, K.L.; Segev, D.L. Recipient Outcomes Following Transplantation of Allografts from Live Kidney Donors Who Subsequently Developed End-Stage Renal Disease. *Am. J. Transplant. Off. J. Am. Soc. Transplant. Am. Soc. Transplant. Surg.* **2016**, *16*, 3532–3539. [CrossRef] [PubMed]

30. Lei, H.H.; Perneger, T.V.; Klag, M.J.; Whelton, P.K.; Coresh, J. Familial aggregation of renal disease in a population-based case-control study. *J. Am. Soc. Nephrol. Jasn.* **1998**, *9*, 1270–1276.

31. O'Dea, D.F.; Murphy, S.W.; Hefferton, D.; Parfrey, P.S. Higher risk for renal failure in first-degree relatives of white patients with end-stage renal disease: A population-based study. *Am. J. Kidney Dis. Off. J. Natl. Kidney Found.* **1998**, *32*, 794–801. [CrossRef]
32. Skrunes, R.; Svarstad, E.; Reisaeter, A.V.; Vikse, B.E. Familial clustering of ESRD in the Norwegian population. *Clin. J. Am. Soc. Nephrol. CJASN* **2014**, *9*, 1692–1700. [CrossRef]
33. Lentine, K.L.; Schnitzler, M.A.; Garg, A.X.; Xiao, H.; Axelrod, D.; Tuttle-Newhall, J.E.; Segev, D.L. Race, Relationship and Renal Diagnoses After Living Kidney Donation. *Transplantation* **2015**, *99*, 1723–1729. [CrossRef]
34. Jacobs, C.L.; Gross, C.R.; Messersmith, E.E.; Hong, B.A.; Gillespie, B.W.; Hill-Callahan, P.; Odim, J. Emotional and Financial Experiences of Kidney Donors over the Past 50 Years: The RELIVE Study. *Clin. J. Am. Soc. Nephrol. CJASN* **2015**, *10*, 2221–2231. [CrossRef] [PubMed]

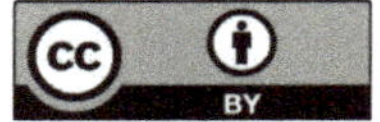

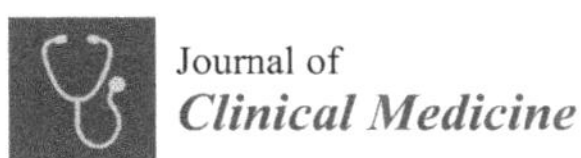

Journal of
Clinical Medicine

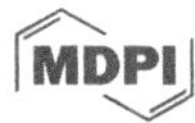

Article

Outcomes of Kidney Transplant Patients with Atypical Hemolytic Uremic Syndrome Treated with Eculizumab: A Systematic Review and Meta-Analysis

Maria L. Gonzalez Suarez [1,*], Charat Thongprayoon [2], Michael A. Mao [3], Napat Leeaphorn [4], Tarun Bathini [5] and Wisit Cheungpasitporn [1]

1   Division of Nephrology, Department of Medicine, University of Mississippi Medical Center, MS 39216, USA
2   Division of Nephrology and Hypertension, Mayo Clinic, Rochester, MN 55905, USA
3   Division of Nephrology and Hypertension, Mayo Clinic, Jacksonville, FL 32224, USA
4   Department of Nephrology, Department of Medicine, Saint Luke's Health System, Kansas City, MO 64111, USA
5   Department of Internal Medicine, University of Arizona, Tucson, AZ 85721, USA
*   Correspondence: malourdes.gonzalez@gmail.com or mgonzalezsuarez@umc.edu

Received: 19 May 2019; Accepted: 26 June 2019; Published: 27 June 2019

Abstract: Background: Kidney transplantation in patients with atypical hemolytic uremic syndrome (aHUS) is frequently complicated by recurrence, resulting in thrombotic microangiopathy in the renal allograft and graft loss. We aimed to assess the use of eculizumab in the prevention and treatment of aHUS recurrence after kidney transplantation. Methods: Databases (MEDLINE, EMBASE and Cochrane Database) were searched through February 2019. Studies that reported outcomes of adult kidney transplant recipients with aHUS treated with eculizumab were included. Estimated incidence rates from the individual studies were extracted and combined using random-effects, generic inverse variance method of DerSimonian and Laird. Protocol for this systematic review has been registered with PROSPERO (International Prospective Register of Systematic Reviews; no. CRD42018089438). Results: Eighteen studies (13 cohort studies and five case series) consisting of 380 adult kidney transplant patients with aHUS who received eculizumab for prevention and treatment of post-transplant aHUS recurrence were included in the analysis. Among patients who received prophylactic eculizumab, the pooled estimated incidence rates of recurrent thrombotic microangiopathy (TMA) after transplantation and allograft loss due to TMA were 6.3% (95%CI: 2.8–13.4%, $I^2 = 0\%$) and 5.5% (95%CI: 2.9–10.0%, $I^2 = 0\%$), respectively. Among those who received eculizumab for treatment of post-transplant aHUS recurrence, the pooled estimated rates of allograft loss due to TMA was 22.5% (95%CI: 13.6–34.8%, $I^2 = 6\%$). When the meta-analysis was restricted to only cohort studies with data on genetic mutations associated with aHUS, the pooled estimated incidence of allograft loss due to TMA was 22.6% (95%CI: 13.2–36.0%, $I^2 = 10\%$). We found no significant publication bias assessed by the funnel plots and Egger's regression asymmetry test ($p > 0.05$ for all analyses). Conclusions: This study summarizes the outcomes observed with use of eculizumab for prevention and treatment of aHUS recurrence in kidney transplantation. Our results suggest a possible role for anti-C5 antibody therapy in the prevention and management of recurrent aHUS.

Keywords: atypical hemolytic uremic syndrome; eculizumab; kidney transplantation; renal transplantation; meta-analysis

---

1. Introduction

Atypical hemolytic uremic syndrome (aHUS) is a microvascular occlusive disorder characterized by hemolytic anemia, thrombocytopenia and acute kidney injury that is not associated with Shiga toxin-producing Escherichia coli (STEC) or ADAMTS13 deficiency. Instead, it is typically associated with dysregulation of the alternative complement pathway [1,2]. Thrombotic microangiopathy (TMA) is the pathological lesion seen with aHUS, which represents a response to endothelial injury [3]. About 10% of hemolytic uremic syndrome (HUS) pediatric cases and the majority of cases in adults are due to atypical HUS [4].

Kidney transplantation in patients with aHUS has been linked to poor outcomes due to high recurrence rate and graft failure. Approximately 50% of patients with aHUS develop end stage renal disease (ESRD) with a high risk of recurrence after kidney transplantation [5]. Roughly 60–70% of aHUS patients have mutations in factors of the complement system or antibodies directed against complement factor H (*CFH*) [6]. In some cases, aHUS recurrence is noted early after transplantation, while other cases may be at lower risk of recurrence [7]. The risk of aHUS recurrence after transplant is higher in patients with gene mutations that encode circulating complement factors (*C3, CFH,* complement factor I (*CFI*)) when compared to patients with gene mutations that encode solid phase proteins such as CD46 [6,8,9]. Patients with no prior history of aHUS may also present with de novo aHUS after kidney transplantation.

Therapies described for management of aHUS in the post-transplant period include the use of plasma exchange (PLEX), rituximab (used for anti-Factor *H* autoantibodies; helps to maintain low levels of antibodies, preventing recurrence of aHUS after transplant) [10], simultaneous liver–kidney transplant for *CFH* mutations, and use of eculizumab (a humanized monoclonal antibody directed against complement protein C5 and thus inhibits terminal complement activation) [11–13]. Prior to the use of eculizumab, patients with gene mutations *CFH, CFH-CFHR1/3, CFI, C3,* and *CFB* had a 50% risk of progression to ESRD or death at onset of recurrent aHUS during the first year, and this risk increased to 75% after 3–5 years [14].

The KDIGO workgroup recommends the prophylactic use of eculizumab in kidney transplant patients at high risk of recurrence based on their genetic mutations [14]. Whether there is an advantage of preemptive use of eculizumab in all patients with a known pretransplant history of aHUS is currently unclear. In addition, eculizumab use is associated with an increased risk of infection due to terminal complement blockade such as meningococcal infections [15,16]. In this study, we aimed to assess the use of eculizumab in the prevention and treatment of aHUS recurrence after kidney transplantation.

2. Methods

2.1. Search Strategy and Literature Review

The protocol for the systematic review has been registered in PROSPERO (registration number: CRD42018089438; http://www.crd.york.ac.uk/PROSPERO). A systematic literature review of EMBASE (1988 to February 2019), MEDLINE (1946 to February 2019), and the Cochrane Database of Systematic Reviews (CDSR) (database inception to February 2019) was performed to assess the use of eculizumab in the prevention and treatment of aHUS recurrence after kidney transplantation. The systematic literature search was undertaken independently by two investigators (M.G.S. and C.T.) using a search approach that incorporated the terms of "kidney" OR "renal" AND "transplant" OR "transplantation" AND "eculizumab". The search strategy is provided in online Supplementary Data 1. No language restriction was applied. A manual literature search for conceivably pertinent studies using references of the included articles was also performed. This study was conducted by the PRISMA (Preferred Reporting Items for Systematic Reviews and Meta-Analysis) statement [17].

2.2. Selection Criteria

Eligible studies must be (1) clinical trials or observational studies (cohort, case-series, or cross-sectional studies) that reported use of eculizumab in the prevention and treatment of aHUS recurrence after kidney transplantation; (2) adult (age ≥ 18 years old) kidney transplant recipients; and (3) they must provide the data on outcomes of interest including rates of aHUS recurrence and allograft loss among patients who received prophylactic eculizumab and rates of allograft loss among patients who received eculizumab for treatment of post-transplant aHUS recurrence. The eculizumab treatment group included post-transplant patients with de novo or recurrent aHUS. We excluded case reports and studies with single cases treated with eculizumab. Retrieved studies were independently reviewed for eligibility by the two authors (M.L.G.S. and C.T.). Discrepancies were discussed and resolved by a third author (W.C.) and common consensus. Inclusion was not confined by the size of study. Newcastle-Ottawa quality assessment scale [18] was used to appraise the quality of observational studies and the Cochrane risk-of-bias tool correspondingly for clinical trials [19]. Detailed evaluation of each study is presented in online Supplementary Tables S1 and S2.

2.3. Data Abstraction

A structured information collecting form was used to obtain the following information from each study including title, name of the first author, publication year, country where the study was conducted, demographic data of kidney transplant patients, history of previous kidney transplantation, type of donor, genetic mutations associated with aHUS, eculizumab regimen, use of PLEX, and outcomes following kidney transplantation (rates of aHUS recurrence and allograft loss among patients who received prophylactic eculizumab and rates of allograft loss among patients who received eculizumab treatment for post-transplant aHUS recurrence).

2.4. Statistical Analysis

Analyses were conducted utilizing the Comprehensive Meta-Analysis 3.3 software (version 3; Biostat Inc., Englewood, NJ, USA). We estimated the pooled incidence rate of recurrent TMA, all-cause allograft loss, and allograft loss due to TMA by the generic inverse variance approach of DerSimonian and Laird, which designated the weight of each study based on its variance [20]. Due to the possibility of between-study variance, we used a random-effects model rather than a fixed-effect model. Sensitivity analysis was performed with restriction to only cohort studies with data on genetic mutations associated with aHUS. We used Cochran's Q test and I^2 statistic to assess the between-study heterogeneity. A value of I^2 of 0% to 25% represents insignificant heterogeneity, 26% to 50% low heterogeneity, 51% to 75% moderate heterogeneity and 76–100% high heterogeneity [21]. The presence of publication bias was assessed by both subjective inspections of funnel plot and the Egger test [22]. The raw data for this systematic review is publicly available through the Open Science Framework (URL: osf.io/2pz4k).

3. Results

A total of 1096 potentially eligible articles were identified using our search strategy. After the exclusion of 888 articles based on title and abstract for clearly not fulfilling inclusion criteria on the basis of type of article, study design, or population or outcome of interest, and exclusion of 172 articles due to being duplicates; 36 full-length articles were reviewed. Fifteen of these articles were subsequently excluded from full-length review because they were also duplicates [23–28], did not fulfill inclusion criteria [29–33], did not report the outcomes of interest, or data was unable to be abstracted [34–37]. An additional three articles were excluded because they were case reports or single cases treated with eculizumab [8,38,39]. Ultimately 18 studies (13 cohort studies and five case series) [5,9,15,40–54] consisting of 380 patients with a history of aHUS who received eculizumab for prevention and treatment of post-transplant recurrent aHUS were included into the final analysis. The literature review and selection process are shown in Figure 1. The characteristics of the included studies are presented in Tables 1 and 2.

Table 1. Use of eculizumab for treatment of atypical hemolytic uremic syndrome (aHUS) on patients after kidney transplantation.

Authors, Publication Year	Type of Study	Ktx Patients Treated with ecu, n	Median Age at Ktx, Months	Female, n	Patients with Prior Failed Ktx, n	Type of Donor	Ecu Initiation, Median Months	Duration of Therapy, Months	PLEX, %	Mean Follow up, Months	aHUS/TMA Recurrence after Ecu, n	Graft Loss, n	Acute Rejection, n
Legendre et al., 2017	Cohort from non-randomized clinical trial	26	41.5	16	8	-	2	25	61.5	18	3	0	-
Levi et al., 2017	Case series	2	24.9	1	1	DD,1	1.25	55	0	63.8	1 [a]	1	AMR, 1
Manani et al., 2017	Case series	2	42.5	1	0	LD, 1 DD, 1	0.5	1.5 [b]	100	4		2	AMR,1 CMR,1
Sheerin et al., 2016	Retrospective cohort	3	-	-	-	-	96 [c]	Ecu cont.	0	-	3	0	-
Mallett et al., 2015	Retrospective cohort	3	40	3	0	DD, 2 LR, 1	29 [d]	Ecu cont.	100	18.9	NM	2	AMR,1
Matar et al., 2014	Retrospective Cohort	3	38	2	2	LU,1 DD, 1 LR, 1	-	14.5 [e]	100	19.7	2	2	0
LeQuintrec et al., 2013	Retrospective multicenter cohort	3	38	-	3	-	3	-	100	24	0	0	0
Zuber et al., 2012	Retrospective multicenter cohort	11	34	-	9	-	-	16	90	15	4	2	AMR, 1
Kocak, et al., 2015	Retrospective cohort	4	30.5	3	0	LR,1	2	-	100	-	-	0	-
Modelli de Andrade et al., 2017	Prospective cohort	5	32	2	0	DD, 4 LD, 1	1.16	21	-	21	0	0	0
Cavero et al., 2017	Retrospective multicenter cohort	7	43	5	-	-	0.46	2	85.7	10.54	-	0	0
Zuber et al., 2017	Retrospective multicenter cohort	17	-	-	-	-	-	12	0	12	-	6	-
Siedlecki et al., 2019	Retrospective multicenter cohort	100	39.5	31	3	-	40	24	-	24	-	24	-
Aigner et al., 2018	Case series	4	28.5	4	0	-	-	-	100	72	0	0	-

(-) missing information from the original study. a. One patient had recurrence after discontinuation followed by graft loss. b. One patient continued with therapy at the time of Manani et al. 2017 publication. c. One patient was started at 24 h post-transplant. d. One patient was started early after kidney transplantation. e. One patient continued with therapy at the time of Matar et al. 2014 publication. Abbreviations: Ktx: Kidney transplantation; n: Number; Ecu: Eculizumab; cont.: Continued; DD: Deceased donor; LD: Living donor; LU: Living unrelated donor; LR: Living related donor; AMR: Antibody mediated rejection; CMR: Chronic antibody mediated rejection; PLEX: Plasma exchange; TMA: Thrombotic microangiopathy.

Table 2. Use of eculizumab for prevention of aHUS on patients after kidney transplantation.

Authors, Publication Year	Type of Study	Ktx Patients Received prophylaxis with Ecu, *n*	Median Age at Ktx, Months	Female, *n*	Patients with Prior Failed Ktx, *n*	Type of Donor	Ecu Initiation, Median Days (D)	Duration of Therapy, Months	PLEX, %	Mean Follow up, Months	aHUS/TMA Recurrence after Ecu, *n*	Graft Loss, *n*	Acute Rejection, *n*
Levi et al., 2017	Case series	10	41	5	4	DD, 7 LD, 3	D 0	Ecu cont. [a]	0	21	1 [b]	1	AMR, 2
Sheerin et al., 2015	Retrospective Cohort	8	-	-	-	-	-	-	-	-	0	0	-
Matar et al. 2014	Retrospective Cohort	4	39	3	3	LD, 1	D −1	6 [c]	0	20.5	0	0	0
Zuber et al., 2012	Retrospective multicenter cohort	9	25.6	-	-	DD, 3	D 5, 1 D 0, 2	Ecu cont.	66	14.5	0	1 [d]	AMR + ACR, 1
Modelli de Andrade et al., 2017	Prospective cohort	2	29	1	-	DD, 1	D 0	Ecu cont.	0	4	0	1 [e]	-
Zuber et al., 2017	Multicenter retrospective cohort	35	-	63	-	-	D 0	-	0	35	17	1	-
Bresin et al., 2013	Case series from 4 independent multinational cohorts	4	-	-	-	-	-	-	-	-	0	0	-
Kumar et al., 2016	Case series	9	-	8	-	LU, 7 DD, 2	-	-	-	31.2	0	0	0
Yelken et al. 2017	Retrospective single center cohort	7	-	-	-	-	-	-	-	28	0	0	
Favi et al., 2017	Retrospective single center cohort	12	-	-	-	-	-	-	-	26.5	0	1	3
	Comparison group with no Ecu	24	-	-	-	-	-	-	-	79	11	7	7
Siedlecki et al. 2019	Multicenter cohort	88	32.3	45	24	-	-	Ecu cont.	-	27	-	3	-

(-) missing information from the original study. a. One patient was discontinued at 28.7 m with no complement mutation identified. b. One patient had recurrence after discontinuation followed by graft loss. There were subclinical TMA lesions on kidney biopsy in 2 patients. c. One patient continued prophylaxis at the time of Matar et al. 2014 publication. d. Patient had immediate graft loss due to intestinal hemorrhage. e. Patient had intestinal hemorrhage at 4 m after kidney transplantation. Abbreviations: Ktx: Kidney transplantation; *n*: Number; Ecu: Eculizumab cont.: Continued; D: Day; DD: Deceased donor; LD: Living donor; LU: Living unrelated donor; AMR: Antibody mediated rejection; ACR: Acute cellular rejection.

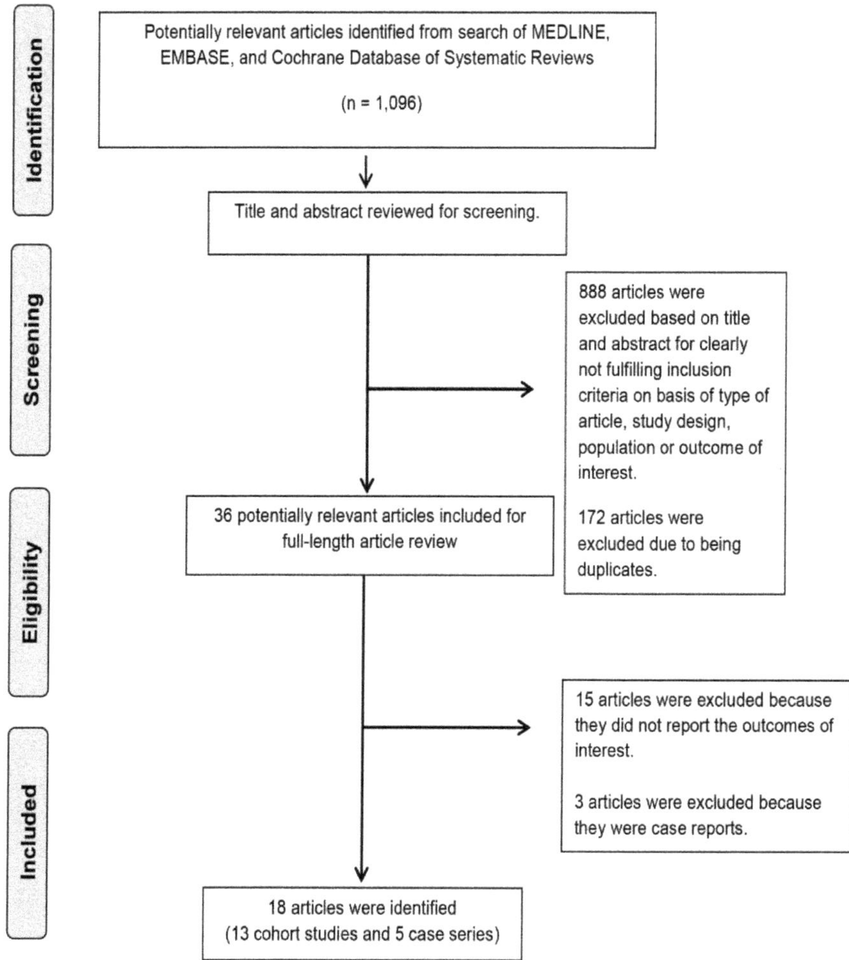

Figure 1. Preferred Reporting Items for Systematic Reviews and Meta-Analysis (PRISMA) flow diagram.

The baseline characteristics of kidney transplant patients and data on genetic mutations associated with aHUS are summarized in Table 3. There were 192 patients in the treatment group and 188 patients in the prophylaxis group, with a median age of 38 and 32.3 years, respectively. Females were predominant in both groups (59.4% vs. 84.4%, respectively). The most commonly reported genetic mutation in this our study population was CFH, followed by CFI and C3 in both groups.

Table 3. Baseline characteristics of kidney transplant patients included in the meta-analysis *.

Baseline Characteristics	Treatment Group	Prophylaxis Group
Patients received eculizumab *n*/total (%)	192	188
Age at time of transplant, years (range)	38 (18–69)	32.3 (18–51)
Female, *n*/total (%)	94/158 (59.4)	125/148 (84.4)
History of previous transplant, *n*/total (%)	26/165 (15.8)	31/102 (30.4)
Type of donor, *n* (%)		
Living	8 (4.2)	11 (5.9)
Deceased	9 (4.7)	13 (6.9)
Not mentioned	175 (91.1)	164 (87.2)
Gene mutation, *n* (%)		
CFH	45 (23.4)	39 (20.7)
CFI	11 (5.7)	9 (4.8)
CFH/CFI	4 (2.0)	1 (0.5)
C3	10 (5.2)	10 (5.3)
CFHR1	1 (0.5)	-
CFHR2	2 (1)	-
CFHR3	1 (0.5)	-
CFH/CFHR3	1 (0.5)	-
CFH/CFHR1	2 (1)	-
CFHR1/CHFR3	2 (1)	-
CFH/CFI/CFHR3	1 (0.5)	-
CFI/C3	1 (0.5)	-
CFB	1 (0.5)	1 (0.5)
Anti CFH antibodies	1 (0.5)	3 (1.6)
MCP	3 (1.5)	9 (4.8)
MCP/THBD	1 (0.5)	-
THBD	1 (0.5)	-
No mutation identified	22 (11.5)	5 (2.6)
Not mentioned/not specified	82 (42.7)	111 (59)
Initiation of Eculizumab	2 months (median)	One day prior to surgery, *n*(%) 1 (0.5) On day of surgery, *n*(%) 57 (30.3) On day 5 post-surgery, *n*(%) 1 (0.5) Timing not mentioned, *n*(%) 129 (68.6)
Median follow up, months (range)	18.9 (3.9–72)	26.7 (4–79)
Plasmapheresis, *n*/total (%)	68/165 (41.2)	22/95 (23.1)

* Percentages are calculated from total available data. *n* = number.

A history of aHUS prior to kidney transplantation was known in all patients included in this systematic review, except for de novo cases. The triggers for post-transplant aHUS were not reported in the majority of patients. The most commonly reported potential triggers were: Viral infections, urosepsis, *C. difficile* infection, tacrolimus use, and everolimus use. De novo aHUS was reported in 56 patients [15,42,47,49]. Tacrolimus was identified as a possible trigger in one of the de novo cases in which aHUS presented 16 years after transplant without any genetic mutations identified [49], while it was suspected in four other cases that had antibody-mediated rejection and their immunosuppression was switched from tacrolimus to sirolimus [42,49]. Urosepsis was reported as a trigger in one de novo case [47].

3.1. Use of Eculizumab in the Prevention of aHUS Recurrence after Kidney Transplantation

Data on the initiation of prophylactic eculizumab therapy are summarized in Table 3. Overall, among patients who received prophylactic eculizumab, the pooled estimated rates of aHUS recurrence and allograft loss due to TMA were 6.3% (95%CI: 2.8–13.4%, $I^2 = 0$%, Figure 2A) and 5.5% (95%CI: 2.9–10.0%, $I^2 = 0$%, Figure 2B), respectively.

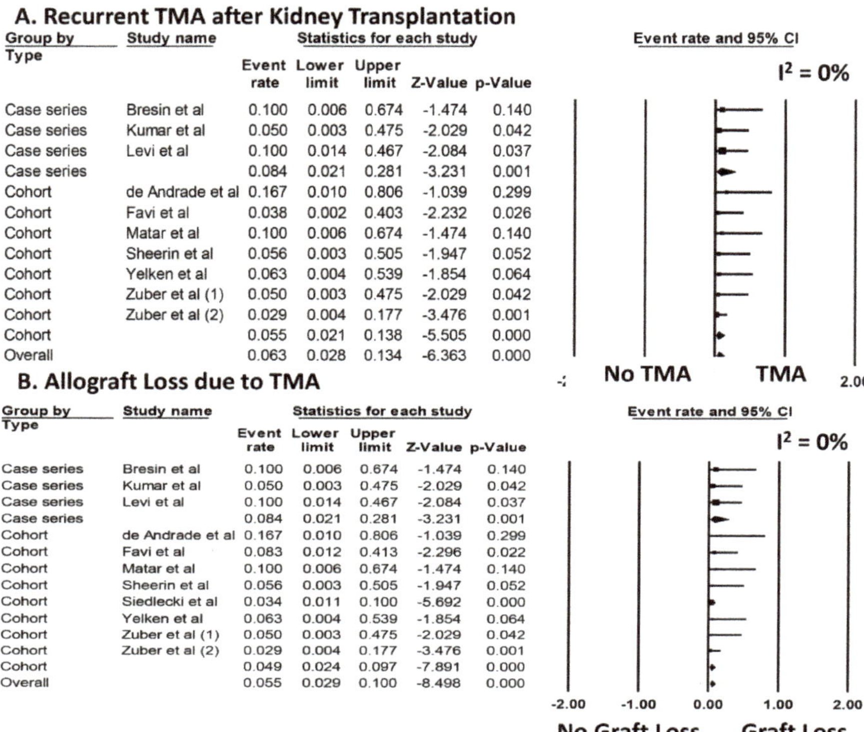

Figure 2. Incidence of (**A**) aHUS recurrence (recurrent TMA) and (**B**) allograft loss due to TMA after kidney transplantation with prophylactic eculizumab.

Sensitivity analysis excluding studies with potentially duplicated patients was performed, and showed the pooled estimated rates of aHUS recurrence and allograft loss due to TMA of 5.5% (95%CI: 1.9–14.6%, $I^2 = 0$%, Figure S1) and 5.3% (95%CI: 2.4–11.3%, $I^2 = 0$%, Figure S2), respectively. When analysis was limited only to studies with a mean follow-up time >12 month (mean follow up time range 21 to 35 months), we found pooled estimated rates of aHUS recurrence and allograft loss due to TMA of 4.6% (95%CI: 1.5–13.3%, $I^2 = 0$%) and 4.8% (95%CI: 2.1–10.7%, $I^2 = 0$%), respectively.

3.2. Use of Therapeutic Eculizumab for aHUS Recurrence after Kidney Transplantation

Data on the initiation of eculizumab treatment for post-transplant aHUS recurrence are summarized in Table 3. Among those who received eculizumab for treatment of post-transplant aHUS recurrence, the pooled estimated rates of allograft loss due to all causes was 24.4% (95%CI: 15.9–35.6%, $I^2 = 23$%, Figure 3A). The pooled estimated rates of allograft loss due to TMA was 22.5% (95%CI: 13.6–34.8%, $I^2 = 6$%, Figure 3B). Meta-regression analysis demonstrated no significant correlations between concomitant use of PLEX and rates of allograft loss due to all causes or due to TMA ($p = 0.61$ and 0.18, respectively).

A. Allograft Loss due to All Causes

Group by Type	Study name	Event rate	Lower limit	Upper limit	Z-Value	p-Value
Case series	Aigner et al	0.100	0.006	0.674	-1.474	0.140
Case series	Manani et al	0.833	0.194	0.990	1.039	0.299
Case series		0.421	0.017	0.968	-0.167	0.868
Cohort	Cavero et al	0.063	0.004	0.539	-1.854	0.064
Cohort	de Andrade et al	0.083	0.005	0.622	-1.623	0.105
Cohort	Kocak et al	0.100	0.006	0.674	-1.474	0.140
Cohort	Le Quintrec et al	0.125	0.007	0.734	-1.287	0.198
Cohort	Legendre et al	0.019	0.001	0.236	-2.781	0.005
Cohort	Levi et al	0.500	0.059	0.941	0.000	1.000
Cohort	Mallett et al	0.667	0.154	0.957	0.566	0.571
Cohort	Matar et al	0.667	0.154	0.957	0.566	0.571
Cohort	Sheerin et al	0.125	0.007	0.734	-1.287	0.198
Cohort	Siedlecki et al	0.240	0.166	0.333	-4.923	0.000
Cohort	Zuber et al (1)	0.182	0.046	0.507	-1.924	0.054
Cohort	Zuber et al (2)	0.353	0.168	0.596	-1.194	0.232
Cohort		0.241	0.156	0.353	-4.138	0.000
Overall		0.244	0.159	0.356	-4.119	0.000

$I^2 = 23\%$

Event rate and 95% CI — No Graft Loss / Graft Loss (-2.00, -1.00, 0.00, 1.00, 2.00)

B. Allograft Loss due to TMA

Group by Type	Study name	Event rate	Lower limit	Upper limit	Z-Value	p-Value
Case series	Aigner et al	0.100	0.006	0.674	-1.474	0.140
Case series	Manani et al	0.833	0.194	0.990	1.039	0.299
Case series		0.421	0.017	0.968	-0.167	0.868
Cohort	Cavero et al	0.063	0.004	0.539	-1.854	0.064
Cohort	de Andrade et al	0.083	0.005	0.622	-1.623	0.105
Cohort	Kocak et al	0.100	0.006	0.674	-1.474	0.140
Cohort	Le Quintrec et al	0.125	0.007	0.734	-1.287	0.198
Cohort	Legendre et al	0.019	0.001	0.236	-2.781	0.005
Cohort	Levi et al	0.500	0.059	0.941	0.000	1.000
Cohort	Mallett et al	0.333	0.043	0.846	-0.566	0.571
Cohort	Matar et al	0.333	0.043	0.846	-0.566	0.571
Cohort	Sheerin et al	0.125	0.007	0.734	-1.287	0.198
Cohort	Zuber et al (1)	0.182	0.046	0.507	-1.924	0.054
Cohort	Zuber et al (2)	0.353	0.168	0.596	-1.194	0.232
Cohort		0.221	0.132	0.344	-4.012	0.000
Overall		0.225	0.136	0.348	-3.985	0.000

$I^2 = 6\%$

Event rate and 95% CI — No Graft Loss / Graft Loss (-2.00, -1.00, 0.00, 1.00, 2.00)

Figure 3. Incidence of (**A**) allograft loss due to all causes and (**B**) allograft loss due to TMA after kidney transplantation with therapeutic eculizumab.

Sensitivity analysis excluding studies that potentially included duplicate patients was performed, and showed the pooled estimated rates of allograft loss due to all causes was 26.7% (95%CI: 13.0–46.9%, $I^2 = 33\%$, Figure S3) and the pooled estimated rates of allograft loss due to TMA was 20.0% (95%CI: 9.1–38.4%, $I^2 = 29\%$, Figure S4), respectively. Sensitivity analysis restricted only to cohort studies with data on genetic mutations associated with aHUS was performed. The pooled estimated incidence of allograft loss due to TMA in cohort studies with data on genetic mutations was 22.6% (95%CI: 13.2–36.0%, $I^2 = 10\%$ Figure 4).

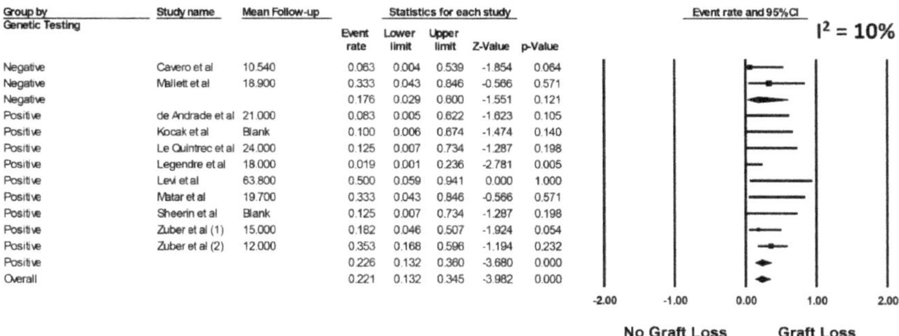

Group by Genetic Testing	Study name	Mean Follow-up	Event rate	Lower limit	Upper limit	Z-Value	p-Value
Negative	Cavero et al	10.540	0.063	0.004	0.539	-1.854	0.064
Negative	Mallett et al	18.900	0.333	0.043	0.846	-0.566	0.571
Negative			0.176	0.029	0.600	-1.551	0.121
Positive	de Andrade et al	21.000	0.083	0.005	0.622	-1.623	0.105
Positive	Kocak et al	Blank	0.100	0.006	0.674	-1.474	0.140
Positive	Le Quintrec et al	24.000	0.125	0.007	0.734	-1.287	0.198
Positive	Legendre et al	18.000	0.019	0.001	0.236	-2.781	0.005
Positive	Levi et al	63.800	0.500	0.059	0.941	0.000	1.000
Positive	Matar et al	19.700	0.333	0.043	0.846	-0.566	0.571
Positive	Sheerin et al	Blank	0.125	0.007	0.734	-1.287	0.198
Positive	Zuber et al (1)	15.000	0.182	0.046	0.507	-1.924	0.054
Positive	Zuber et al (2)	12.000	0.353	0.168	0.596	-1.194	0.232
Positive			0.226	0.132	0.360	-3.680	0.000
Overall			0.221	0.132	0.345	-3.982	0.000

Figure 4. Forrest plot evaluating for the incidence of allograft loss due to TMA in cohort studies with data on genetic mutations.

Subgroup analysis stratified by mean follow-up time was performed. We found the pooled estimated rates of allograft loss due to all causes was 25.5% (95%CI: 14.8–40.3%, $I^2 = 34\%$) at a mean follow-up time of 12 to 24 months and 26.0% (95%CI: 3.9–75.1%, I^2 = 13%) at a mean follow-up time of 60 to 72 months. The pooled estimated rates of allograft loss due to TMA were 22.6% (95%CI: 12.1–38.1%, I^2 = 8%) at a mean follow-up time of 12 to 24 months and 26.0% (95%CI: 3.9–75.1%, I^2 = 13%) at a mean follow-up time of 60 to 72 months.

3.3. Evaluation for Publication Bias

We found no significant publication bias as assessed by the funnel plots (Figure 5) and Egger's regression asymmetry test for the rates of aHUS recurrence and allograft loss due to TMA in patients treated with prophylactic eculizumab therapy (p = 0.48 and 0.28, respectively), nor for rates of allograft loss due to all causes and allograft loss due to TMA in patients treated with therapeutic eculizumab for aHUS recurrence after kidney transplantation (p = 0.78 and 0.20, respectively).

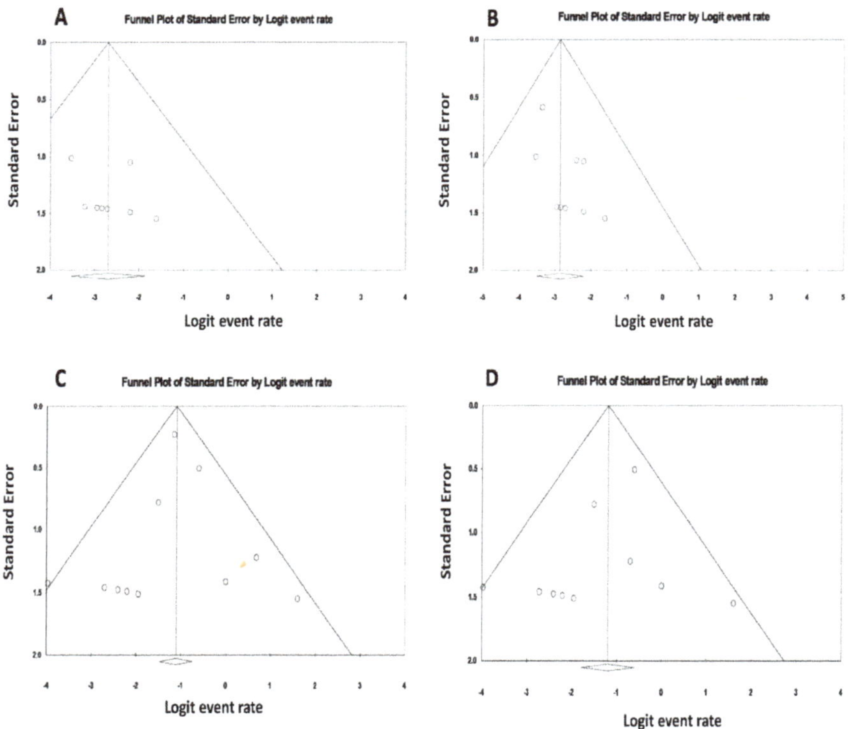

Figure 5. Funnel plots evaluating for publication bias for (**A**) the incidence of aHUS recurrence after kidney transplantation among patients who received prophylactic eculizumab; (**B**) the incidence of allograft loss due to TMA after kidney transplantation among patients who received prophylactic eculizumab; (**C**) the incidence of allograft loss due to all causes after kidney transplantation among patients with therapeutic eculizumab for aHUS recurrence; (**D**) the incidence of allograft loss due to TMA after kidney transplantation among patients with therapeutic eculizumab for aHUS recurrence.

4. Discussion

Atypical HUS recurrence after transplant is diagnosed with the presence of laboratory abnormalities such as renal failure, microangiopathic hemolytic anemia, thrombocytopenia and microvascular occlusion [1,48]. In many cases, aHUS recurrence is confirmed with a kidney biopsy–showing the usual findings of glomerular intracapillary thrombosis, congestion, endothelial swelling, and thickening of the capillary wall [4].

Our systematic review showed that mutations to genes encoding *CFH*, followed by mutations in *CFI* genes were the most commonly reported in patients with aHUS recurrence after transplant. This observation, however, is limited to the studies included in our analysis, which only included kidney transplant patients treated with eculizumab and did not include patients treated with alternative therapies. In our systematic review, mutations in *CFH* and *CFH/CFHR1* were more commonly associated with graft loss in patients who had received eculizumab therapy. The current literature describes the presence of complement factor genetic mutations in approximately 30% of patients who present with de novo HUS after kidney transplantation [6]. However, no mutations were identified in four patients who presented with de novo aHUS and had graft loss [47,49].

We found that in most pretransplant patients with a history of aHUS who had received eculizumab prophylaxis, this was started on the day of kidney transplant surgery (data abstracted from Mallet et al. [47] and Manani et al. [49] were not utilized for this subgroup analysis as only one case in each publication was prophylactically managed with eculizumab). Less than 6% of the patients who received eculizumab prophylaxis presented with aHUS recurrence, and recurrence was more likely to occur when eculizumab was discontinued. Yelken et al. reported their clinical experience in a retrospective cohort of seven patients with a prior history of aHUS who had received eculizumab prophylaxis and underwent kidney transplantation. None of them had presented with aHUS recurrence or graft loss during the follow-up period of 28 months [52]. More recently, a global registry for aHUS enrolled 1549 patients over a 5-year period. One hundred and eighty-eight patients underwent kidney transplantation. From those, 88 patients received eculizumab before or during transplant surgery. This group of patients presented significantly better graft function when compared to those patients who received eculizumab with aHUS recurrence or de novo aHUS in the post-transplant period [15].

The time for recurrence of aHUS after transplant in the eculizumab therapeutic group varied, with recurrence seen as early as 3 days and up to 6 years (median of 2 months). Our study shows that allograft outcomes of patients treated after early recurrence (3 days to 3 months post-transplant) [25,28,42,44,49] when compared to those patients treated for late recurrence (29–96 months post-transplant) [15,47,50] were similar. The effect of timing for therapeutic eculizumab is also unclear. Some studies have concluded that early therapy with eculizumab for aHUS recurrence has failed to show better allograft survival [9,47,48]. Future prospective randomized control trials would help elucidate whether early initiation of therapy has a beneficial effect for allograft survival.

In many cases, management for aHUS recurrence in kidney transplantation includes the use of PLEX. Previously, Le Quintrec et al. had reported a trend towards decreased aHUS recurrence in patients treated preemptively with PLEX [44]. Zuber et al.'s retrospective cohort had subsequently compared PLEX versus eculizumab in both therapeutic and prophylactic modalities. They found that eculizumab was superior when compared to PLEX in preventing and treating aHUS recurrence after kidney transplantation [51]. Other studies have shown no difference in graft survival independently of whether patients received PLEX or not [44,51]. More recently, Favi et al. reported a case-control study where patients with and without PLEX were compared with eculizumab prophylaxis alone. This is the only study that we encountered where a comparison group was used. Patients who did not receive eculizumab (whether they received prophylaxis with PLEX or not) were more likely to have higher graft loss recurrence and allograft rejection when compared to patients who had received eculizumab [54]. Our systematic review showed that 36.2% of individuals required eculizumab after PLEX therapy, while 23.1% received concomitant PLEX in the prophylaxis group. There is no data available regarding the use of PLEX in the rest of the cases. Those patients who received PLEX plus eculizumab had no significant difference in allograft survival and aHUS recurrence in comparison to those without PLEX, ($p = 0.65$). However, it remains difficult to conclude about the effects of concomitant PLEX and eculizumab use in aHUS post-transplant recurrence and associated graft loss due to the small number of patients analyzed, and these patients of interest may have had more severe risk markers that prompted dual therapy. PLEX is still considered an option in the management for aHUS recurrence [15].

Duration of eculizumab therapy has been controversial and so far is based on expert opinion, as there is no strong evidence to support lifelong therapy. We found that most patients who were prophylactically treated had continued eculizumab up to the time of their respective studies' publication. There is a report of one patient in whom no complement mutation was identified that stopped prophylactic eculizumab after 28.7 months. No aHUS recurrence was identified after 9 months of follow up [46]. The median duration of therapy was 18.9 months in the therapy patient group and 21 months in the prophylaxis patient group. While aHUS allograft recurrence after eculizumab cessation was reported in 5.2% of patients, it is difficult to conclude if other recurrent aHUS cases were missed due to the length of follow up after eculizumab therapy discontinuation.

Acute allograft rejection rates were similar in treatment and prophylactic groups. Despite receiving eculizumab treatment for aHUS post-transplant recurrence, graft loss was seen in 20.3% of the patients compared to 7.9% of patients who received eculizumab prophylaxis. While graft loss in the treatment group was likely associated with recurrence of aHUS, in the prophylaxis group, two cases of kidney allograft loss were associated with the presence of intestinal hemorrhage (one case immediately after transplant [45], the other case presented four months after transplant [47]). Whether there was a possible association of acute arterial allograft thrombosis with aHUS remains unclear.

We acknowledge the limitations inherent in this study. Firstly, this systematic review included only observational studies (cohorts and case series). Consequently, the majority of available studies also lacked a comparison (control) group. Only one of the included studies had a comparison group who did not receive eculizumab [54]. Recently, Duineveld C. et al. described 17 patients with aHUS who underwent living donor kidney transplantation without prophylactic eculizumab with median follow-up of 25 months after kidney transplantation [8]. Their institution's protocol emphasized lower target tacrolimus level and blood pressure control among these patients with aHUS. They found only one patient developed aHUS recurrence at 68 days after kidney transplantation, and was treated successfully with eculizumab. The investigators suggested that living donor kidney transplantation in aHUS without prophylactic eculizumab treatment appears feasible [8]. Secondly, inconsistencies in the reporting of certain variables such as type of donor, history of previous transplantation, genetic mutations, and immunosuppression regimen can make it difficult to draw firm associations between eculizumab prophylaxis or treatment on renal graft outcomes. Caution should be exercised in interpreting these data. Lastly, this study analysis was conducted on a highly selected study population. Only studies in which eculizumab was used were analyzed, and individuals who received an alternate treatment course or did not receive eculizumab were excluded from our analysis. Therefore, the frequency of mutations might not be representative. Although funnel plots and Egger's test of event rates demonstrated no statistical significance, a low risk of publication bias cannot be implied given the lack of comparison groups. Thus, future studies to assess the responsiveness to eculizumab based on certain aHUS genetic mutations (low risk vs. moderate risk vs. high risk of recurrence) [6] are needed.

In summary, our study describes the outcomes observed with use of eculizumab for prevention and treatment of aHUS recurrence in kidney transplantation. Our results suggest a possible advantageous role for anti-C5 antibody therapy in the prevention and management of recurrent aHUS. Future prospective studies and clinical trials are needed to evaluate for the efficacy of eculizumab, timing of initiation, and duration of prophylaxis and treatment therapy according to genetic mutations.

Supplementary Materials: The supplementary materials are available online at http://www.mdpi.com/2077-0383/8/7/919/s1.

Author Contributions: Conceptualization, M.L.G.S., C.T. and W.C.; Data curation, M.L.G.S., C.T. and W.C.; Formal analysis, W.C.; Investigation, M.L.G.S. and C.T.; Methodology, M.L.G.S. and W.C.; Project administration, N.L. and T.B.; Resources, M.A.M., N.L. and T.B.; Software, T.B. and W.C.; Supervision, M.A.M., N.L. and W.C.; Validation, M.L.G.S., C.T. and W.C.; Visualization, M.A.M. and W.C.; Writing, original draft, M.L.G.S.; Writing, review & editing, M.L.G.S., C.T., M.A.M. and W.C.

Acknowledgments: All authors had access to the data and played essential roles in writing of the manuscript.

Conflicts of Interest: The authors deny any conflicts of interest.

References

1. Barbour, T.; Johnson, S.; Cohney, S.; Hughes, P. Thrombotic microangiopathy and associated renal disorders. *Nephrol. Dial. Transplant.* **2012**, *27*, 2673–2685. [CrossRef] [PubMed]
2. Cataland, S.R.; Wu, H.M. How I treat: The clinical differentiation and initial treatment of adult patients with atypical hemolytic uremic syndrome. *Blood* **2014**, *123*, 2478–2484. [CrossRef] [PubMed]
3. Sridharan, M.; Go, R.S.; Willrich, M.A.V. Atypical hemolytic uremic syndrome: Review of clinical presentation, diagnosis and management. *J. Immunol. Methods* **2018**, *461*, 15–22. [CrossRef] [PubMed]
4. Noris, M.; Remuzzi, G. Atypical hemolytic-uremic syndrome. *N. Engl. J. Med.* **2009**, *361*, 1676–1687. [CrossRef] [PubMed]
5. Bresin, E.; Rurali, E.; Caprioli, J.; Sanchez-Corral, P.; Fremeaux-Bacchi, V.; Rodriguez de Cordoba, S.; Pinto, S.; Goodship, T.H.; Alberti, M.; Ribes, D.; et al. Combined complement gene mutations in atypical hemolytic uremic syndrome influence clinical phenotype. *J. Am. Soc. Nephrol.* **2013**, *24*, 475–486. [CrossRef] [PubMed]
6. Zuber, J.; Fakhouri, F.; Roumenina, L.T.; Loirat, C.; Fremeaux-Bacchi, V.; French Study Group for a HCG. Use of eculizumab for atypical haemolytic uraemic syndrome and C3 glomerulopathies. *Nat. Rev. Nephrol.* **2012**, *8*, 643–657. [CrossRef] [PubMed]
7. Bresin, E.; Daina, E.; Noris, M.; Castelletti, F.; Stefanov, R.; Hill, P.; Goodship, T.H.; Remuzzi, G.; International Registry of Recurrent and Familial HUS/TTP. Outcome of renal transplantation in patients with non-Shiga toxin-associated hemolytic uremic syndrome: Prognostic significance of genetic background. *Clin. J. Am. Soc. Nephrol.* **2006**, *1*, 88–99. [CrossRef] [PubMed]
8. Duineveld, C.; Verhave, J.C.; Berger, S.P.; Van De Kar, N.C.; Wetzels, J.F. Living Donor Kidney Transplantation in Atypical Hemolytic Uremic Syndrome: A Case Series. *Am. J. Kidney Dis.* **2017**, *70*, 770–777. [CrossRef]
9. Zuber, J.; Krid, S.; Bertoye, C.; Gueutin, V.; Lahoche, A.; Ardissino, G.; Chatelet, V.; Hourmant, M.; Niaudet, P.; Frémeaux-Bacchi, V.; et al. Eculizumab for Atypical Hemolytic Uremic Syndrome Recurrence in Renal Transplantation. *Am. J. Transplant.* **2012**, *12*, 3337–3354. [CrossRef]
10. Kwon, T.; Dragon-Durey, M.-A.; Macher, M.-A.; Baudouin, V.; Maisin, A.; Peuchmaur, M.; Fremeaux-Bacchi, V.; Loirat, C. Successful pre-transplant management of a patient with anti-factor H autoantibodies-associated haemolytic uraemic syndrome. *Nephrol. Dial. Transplant.* **2008**, *23*, 2088–2090. [CrossRef]
11. Mundra, V.R.R.; Mannon, R.B. Thrombotic Microangiopathy in a Transplant Recipient. *Clin. J. Am. Soc. Nephrol.* **2018**, *13*, 1251–1253. [CrossRef] [PubMed]
12. Fakhouri, F.; Fremeaux-Bacchi, V. Thrombotic microangiopathy: Eculizumab for atypical haemolytic uraemic syndrome: What next? *Nat. Rev. Nephrol.* **2013**, *9*, 495–496. [CrossRef] [PubMed]
13. Saland, J.M.; Ruggenenti, P.; Remuzzi, G. Liver-kidney transplantation to cure atypical hemolytic uremic syndrome. *JASN* **2009**, *20*, 940–949. [CrossRef] [PubMed]
14. Goodship, T.H.; Cook, H.T.; Fakhouri, F.; Fervenza, F.C.; Fremeaux-Bacchi, V.; Kavanagh, D.; Nester, C.M.; Noris, M.; Pickering, M.C.; Rodríguez de Córdoba, S.; et al. Atypical hemolytic uremic syndrome and C3 glomerulopathy: Conclusions from a "Kidney Disease: Improving Global Outcomes" (KDIGO) Controversies Conference. *Kidney Int.* **2017**, *91*, 539–551. [CrossRef] [PubMed]
15. Siedlecki, A.M.; Isbel, N.; Vande Walle, J.; James Eggleston, J.; Cohen, D.J. Eculizumab Use for Kidney Transplantation in Patients With a Diagnosis of Atypical Hemolytic Uremic Syndrome. *Kidney Int. Rep.* **2019**, *4*, 434–446. [CrossRef] [PubMed]
16. Milan Manani, S.; Virzi, G.M.; Ronco, C. Long-term Use of Eculizumab in Kidney Transplant Recipients. *Kidney Int. Rep.* **2019**, *4*, 370–371. [CrossRef] [PubMed]
17. Moher, D.; Liberati, A.; Tetzlaff, J.; Altman, D.G. Preferred reporting items for systematic reviews and meta-analyses: The PRISMA statement. *PLoS Med.* **2009**, *6*, e1000097. [CrossRef]
18. Stang, A. Critical evaluation of the Newcastle-Ottawa scale for the assessment of the quality of nonrandomized studies in meta-analyses. *Eur. J. Epidemiol.* **2010**, *25*, 603–605. [CrossRef]
19. Higgins, J.; Green, S.; Altman, D.; Sterne, J. Chapter 8: Assessing risk of bias in included studies. In *Cochrane Handbook for Systematic Reviews of Intervensions*; Version 510; 2011; Available online: https://handbook-5-1.cochrane.org/ (accessed on 15 February 2019).

20. DerSimonian, R.; Laird, N. Meta-analysis in clinical trials. *Control Clin. Trials.* **1986**, *7*, 177–188. [CrossRef]
21. Higgins, J.P.; Thompson, S.G.; Deeks, J.J.; Altman, D.G. Measuring inconsistency in meta-analyses. *BMJ* **2003**, *327*, 557–560. [CrossRef]
22. Easterbrook, P.J.; Berlin, J.A.; Gopalan, R.; Matthews, D.R. Publication bias in clinical research. *Lancet* **1991**, *337*, 867–872. [CrossRef]
23. Aigner, C.; Bohmig, G.; Eskandary, F.; Gaggl, M.; Kain, R.; Sunder-Plassmann, R.; Prohaszka, Z.; Schmidt, A.; Sunder-Plassmann, G. Preemptive Plasma Therapy and Eculizumab (ECU) Rescue for Atypical Hemolytic Uremic Syndrome (aHUS) Relapse Following Kidney Transplantation (KTX). *Am. J. Transplant.* **2018**, *18*, 793–794.
24. Alasfar, S.; Alachkar, N. Atypical hemolytic uremic syndrome post-kidney transplantation: Two case reports and review of the literature. *Front. Med.* **2014**, *1*, 52. [CrossRef] [PubMed]
25. Levi, C.; Fremeaux-Bacchi, V.; Rabant, M.; Scemla, A. Outcome after Eculizumab Therapy to Prevent Recurrence of Atypical Hemolytic Uremic Syndrome: Experience in Eleven Renal Transplant Recipients. *Transplant. Int.* **2015**, *28*, 230.
26. Zuber, J.; Le Quintrec, M.; Krid, S.; Gueuttin, V. Eculizumab for Preventing and Curing Post-Transplant Atypical Hemolytic Uremic Syndrome (aHUS) Recurrence. *Am. J. Transplant.* **2012**, *12*, A428. [CrossRef] [PubMed]
27. Legendre, C.; Greenbaum, L.; Sheerin, N.; Cohen, D.; Gaber, A.; Eitner, F.; Delmas, Y.; Furman, R.; Feldkamp, T.; Fouque, D.; et al. Eculizumab Efficacy in aHUS Pts with Progressing TMA, with or without Prior Renal Transplant. *Am. J. Transplant.* **2013**, *13*, 278.
28. Legendre, C.; Cohen, D.; Feldkamp, T.; Fouque, D.; Furman, R.; Gaber, A.O.; Greenbaum, L.; Goodship, T.; Haller, H.; Herthelius, M.; et al. Eculizumab in Atypical Haemolytic Uraemic Syndrome (aHUS) Patients with or without Prior Transplant. *Transplant. Int.* **2013**, *26*, 176.
29. Tanabe, K.; Okumi, M.; Unagami, K.; Kakuta, Y.; Inui, M.; Ishida, H. High Prevalence of Kidney Transplant-Associated Thrombotic Microangiopathy after ABO-Incompatible Kidney Transplantation: Risk Factors, Rapid Clinical Diagnosis, and Prompt Successful Treatment. *Am J Transplant.* **2018**, *18*, 517.
30. Tagle, R.; Rivera, G.; Walbaum, B.; Sepulveda, R. Atypical hemolytic uremic syndrome. Report of two cases treated with Eculizumab. *Rev. Med. Chile* **2018**, *146*, 254–259. [CrossRef]
31. Ikeda, T.; Okumi, M.; Unagami, K.; Kanzawa, T.; Sawada, A.; Kawanishi, K.; Omoto, K.; Ishida, H.; Tanabe, K. Two cases of kidney transplantation-associated thrombotic microangiopathy successfully treated with eculizumab. *Nephrology* **2016**, *21* (Suppl. 1), 35–40. [CrossRef]
32. Greenbaum, L.A.; Delmas, Y.; Fakhouri, F.; John, F.; Kincaid, C.L.; Minetti, E.E.; Mix, C.; Provôt, F.; Rondeau, E.; Sheerin, N.; et al. Eculizumab Prevents Thrombotic Microangiopathy: Long-Term Follow-up Study of Patients with Atypical Hemolytic Uremic Syndrome. *Blood* **2015**, *126*, 2252.
33. Le Quintrec, M.; Zuber, J.; Moulin, B.; Rondeau, E.; Delahousse, M.; Frémeaux-Bacchi, V. Genetic Factors Predict Graft Outcome in Adult Renal Transplant Recipients with Atypical Hemolytic Uremic Syndrome. *Am. J. Transplant.* **2012**, *12*, A427.
34. Zuber, J.; Caillard, S.; Frimat, M.; Kamar, N.; Gatault, P.; Petitprez, F.; Louis, M.; Chatelet, V.; Thierry, A.; Bertrand, D.; et al. Prophylactic use of eculizumab in patients at high risk of post-transplant aHUS recurrence improves graft outcomes. *Transplant. Int.* **2019**, (Suppl. 1), O33.
35. Zuber, J.; Jourde-Chiche, N.; Frimat, M.; Navarro, D.; Albano, L.; Arzouk, N.; Bamoulid, J.; Bertrand, D.; Boyer, O.; Caillard, S.; et al. Growing frequency of transplanted patients among the French cohort of atypical hemolytic uremic syndrome in the era of eculizumab. *Transplant. Int.* **2019**, (Suppl. 1), O84.
36. Chaturvedi, S.; Moliterno, A.R.; Merrill, S.A.; Braunstein, E.M.; Yuan, X.; Sperati, C.J.; Khneizer, G.; Brodsky, R.A. Chronic kidney disease, hypertension and cardiovascular sequelae during long term follow up of adults with atypical hemolytic uremic syndrome. *Blood* **2018**, *132*, 3754.
37. van den Brand, J.A.; Verhave, J.C.; Adang, E.M.; Wetzels, J.F. Cost-effectiveness of eculizumab treatment after kidney transplantation in patients with atypical haemolytic uraemic syndrome. *Nephrol. Dial. Transplant.* **2017**, *32*, i115–i122. [CrossRef] [PubMed]
38. Galindo, P.; Ramirez, M.; Perez Marfil, A.; Espigares, M.J.; Osoria, J.M.; Leiva, R.; Ruiz Fuentes, M.C.; De Gracia, C.; Osuna, A. Renal Transplant Immunosuppression in Patients With Hemolytic Uremic Syndrome: Four Case Reports. *Transplant. Proc.* **2018**, *50*, 572–574. [CrossRef]
39. Asif, A.; Nayer, A.; Haas, C. Atypical hemolytic uremic syndrome in the setting of complement-amplifying conditions: Case reports and a review of the evidence for treatment with eculizumab. *J. Nephrol.* **2017**, *30*, 347–362. [CrossRef]

40. Cavero, T.; Rabasco, C.; Lopez, A.; Roman, E.; Avila, A.; Sevillano, A.; Huerta, A.; Rojas-Rivera, J.; Fuentes, C.; Blasco, M.; et al. Eculizumab in secondary atypical haemolytic uraemic syndrome. *Nephrol. Dial. Transplant.* **2017**, *32*, 466–474. [CrossRef]

41. De Andrade, L.G.M.; Contti, M.M.; Nga, H.S.; Bravin, A.M.; Takase, H.M.; Viero, R.M.; Da Silva, T.N.; Chagas, K.D.N.; Palma, L.M.P. Long-term outcomes of the Atypical Hemolytic Uremic Syndrome after kidney transplantation treated with eculizumab as first choice. *PLoS ONE* **2017**, *12*, e0188155. [CrossRef]

42. Kocak, B.; Akyollu, B.; Karatas, C.; AkNc, S.; Arpali, E.; Yelken, B.; Görcin, S.; Demiralp, E.; Türkmen, A. Eculizumab for de novo HUS after kidney transplantation. *Transplant. Int.* **2015**, *28*, 247.

43. Kumar, A.; Stewart, Z.; Reed, A.; Orozco, D.; Smith, R.; Nester, C.; Thomas, C. Successful Prophylactic Use of Eculizumab in aHUS Kidney Transplant Patients: A report of 9 cases. *Am J Transplant.* **2016**, *16*, 742.

44. Le Quintrec, M.; Zuber, J.; Moulin, B.; Kamar, N.; Jablonski, M.; Lionet, A.; Chatelet, V.; Mousson, C.; Mourad, G.; Bridoux, F.; et al. Complement genes strongly predict recurrence and graft outcome in adult renal transplant recipients with atypical hemolytic and uremic syndrome. *Am J Transplant.* **2013**, *13*, 663–675. [CrossRef] [PubMed]

45. Legendre, C.M.; Campistol, J.M.; Feldkamp, T.; Remuzzi, G.; Kincaid, J.F.; Lommelé, Å.; Wang, J.; Weekers, L.E.; Sheerin, N.S. Outcomes of patients with atypical haemolytic uraemic syndrome with native and transplanted kidneys treated with eculizumab: A pooled post hoc analysis. *Transplant. Int.* **2017**, *30*, 1275–1283. [CrossRef] [PubMed]

46. Levi, C.; Frémeaux-Bacchi, V.; Zuber, J.; Rabant, M.; Devriese, M.; Snanoudj, R.; Scemla, A.; Amrouche, L.; Mejean, A.; Legendre, C.; et al. Midterm Outcomes of 12 Renal Transplant Recipients Treated With Eculizumab to Prevent Atypical Hemolytic Syndrome Recurrence. *Transplantation* **2017**, *101*, 2924–2930. [CrossRef] [PubMed]

47. Mallett, A.; Hughes, P.; Szer, J.; Tuckfield, A.; Van Eps, C.; Cambell, S.B.; Hawley, C.; Burke, J.; Kausman, J.; Hewitt, I.; et al. Atypical haemolytic uraemic syndrome treated with the complement inhibitor eculizumab: The experience of the Australian compassionate access cohort. *Intern. Med. J.* **2015**, *45*, 1054–1065. [CrossRef] [PubMed]

48. Matar, D.; Naqvi, F.; Racusen, L.C.; Carter-Monroe, N.; Montgomery, R.A.; Alachkar, N. Atypical hemolytic uremic syndrome recurrence after kidney transplantation. *Transplantation* **2014**, *98*, 1205–1212. [CrossRef] [PubMed]

49. Manani, S.M.; Virzì, G.M.; Giuliani, A.; Clementi, A.; Brocca, A.; Dissegna, D.; Martino, F.; Ronco, C. Hemolytic Uremic Syndrome and Kidney Transplantation: A Case Series and Review of the Literature. *Nephron* **2017**, *136*, 245–253. [CrossRef]

50. Sheerin, N.S.; Kavanagh, D.; Goodship, T.H.; Johnson, S. A national specialized service in England for atypical haemolytic uraemic syndrome-the first year's experience. *QJM* **2016**, *109*, 27–33. [CrossRef]

51. Zuber, J.; Kamar, N.; Frimat, M.; Le Quintrec, M.; Gatault, P.; Jourde-Chiche, N. Breakthrough in the Management of Atypical Hemolytic Uremic Syndrome after Kindey Transplantation: A Nationwide Study. *Transplant. Int.* **2017**, *30*, 99.

52. Yelken, B.; Gorcin, S.; Demir, E.; Karatas, C.; Arpali, E.; Akyollu, B.; Kocak, B.; Elbasi, O.; Eksioğlu, E.; Turkmen, A. The Promising Approach in Difficult Atypical Hemolytic Uremic Syndrome Series in Renal Transplantation. *Am. J. Transplant.* **2017**, *17*, 123.

53. Aigner, C.; Bohmig, G.; Eskandary, F.; Gaggl, M.; Kain, R.; Sunder-Plassmann, R.; Prohaszka, Z.; Schmidt, A.; Sunder-Plassmann, G. Preemptive plasma therapy and eculizumab rescue for atypical hemolytic uremic syndrome relapse following kidney transplantation. *Nephrol. Dial. Transplant.* **2018**, *33*, i592–i593. [CrossRef]

54. Favi, E.; Ardissino, G.; Cresseri, D.; Brocca, J.; Testa, S.; Tel, F.; Giussani, A.; Colico, C.; Beretta, C.; Ferraresso, M. Thirty-six consecutive kidney transplants in recipients with atypical hemolytic uremic syndrome: A single-centre experience. *Am. J. Transplant.* **2018**, *18*, 286.

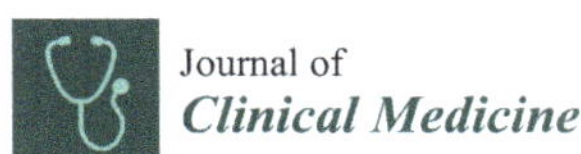 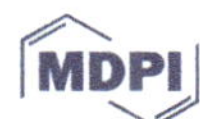

Journal of ***Clinical Medicine***

Review

Timing of Ureteric Stent Removal and Occurrence of Urological Complications after Kidney Transplantation: A Systematic Review and Meta-Analysis

Isis J. Visser [1], Jasper P. T. van der Staaij [1], Anand Muthusamy [1,2], Michelle Willicombe [1], Jeffrey A. Lafranca [1] and Frank J. M. F. Dor [1,2,*]

[1] Imperial College Renal and Transplant Centre, Imperial College NHS Healthcare Trust, Hammersmith Hospital, London W12 0HS, UK; isisjasmijn@hotmail.com (I.J.V.); jaspervanderstaay@hotmail.com (J.P.T.v.d.S.); anand.muthusamy@nhs.net (A.M.); michelle.willicombe@nhs.net (M.W.); j.a.lafranca@gmail.com (J.A.L.)

[2] Department of Surgery and Cancer, Imperial College, London W12 0HS, UK

*   Correspondence: frank.dor@nhs.net; Tel.: +44-0-2033135206

Received: 23 April 2019; Accepted: 13 May 2019; Published: 16 May 2019

Abstract: Implanting a ureteric stent during ureteroneocystostomy reduces the risk of leakage and ureteral stenosis after kidney transplantation (KTx), but it may also predispose to urinary tract infections (UTIs). The aim of this study is to determine the optimal timing for ureteric stent removal after KTx. Searches were performed in EMBASE, MEDLINE Ovid, Cochrane CENTRAL, Web of Science, and Google Scholar (until November 2017). For this systematic review, all aspects of the Cochrane Handbook for Interventional Systematic Reviews were followed and it was written based on the PRISMA-statement. Articles discussing JJ-stents (double-J stents) and their time of removal in relation to outcomes, UTIs, urinary leakage, ureteral stenosis or reintervention were included. One-thousand-and-forty-three articles were identified, of which fourteen articles (three randomised controlled trials, nine retrospective cohort studies, and two prospective cohort studies) were included (describing in total $n = 3612$ patients). Meta-analysis using random effect models showed a significant reduction of UTIs when stents were removed earlier than three weeks (OR 0.49, CI 95%, 0.33 to 0.75, $p = 0.0009$). Regarding incidence of urinary leakage, there was no significant difference between early (<3 weeks) and late stent removal (>3 weeks) (OR 0.60, CI 95%, 0.29 to 1.23, $p = 0.16$). Based on our results, earlier stent removal (<3 weeks) was associated with a decreased incidence of UTIs and did not show a higher incidence of urinary leakage compared to later removal (>3 weeks). We recommend that the routine removal of ureteric stents implanted during KTx should be performed around three weeks post-operatively.

Keywords: kidney transplantation; urological complications; ureteric stent; urinary tract infection; timing of removal

---

1. Introduction

Kidney transplantation (KTx) is considered the best option for end-stage renal disease (ESRD) management [1,2]. Kidney transplantation increases the life expectancy and quality of life of ESRD patients significantly compared to dialysis [3]. However, KTx is not without peri-operative complication risks; urinary tract infections (UTIs), urinary leakage, and ureteral stenosis are the most frequently seen urological complications. These complications are likely to compromise graft functions [4–7]. In order to minimize leakage and stenosis, in general, a stent is inserted in the ureter during implantation. Ureteric stents decrease the risk of these urological complications by five to ten-fold. [6,8,9] Most centres use a variation of a JJ-stent (double-J stent), with the typical pigtail end preventing stent migration by positioning one end in the pyelum. The other end remains in the bladder after the ureteroneocystostomy (UNC) is created. The stent can easily be removed by flexible cystoscopy later. Various randomised controlled trials demonstrate that JJ-stenting reduces urinary leakage and ureteral stenosis [5,10–12]. Meta-analyses by Wilson and Mangus [6,9] also confirmed these results. Although the use of a JJ-stent reduces the risk of urinary leakage and ureteral stenosis, it may also predispose to UTIs [12–16]. In the existing literature, there is no consensus about the preferred time of stent removal. The European Association of Urology states in its renal transplantation guideline that stent retention longer than 30 days is associated with an increased risk (6% versus 40%) of UTIs [12,17]. Therefore, the guideline advises stents to be removed earlier than six weeks post-transplant (which is protocol in most transplant centres) rather than later. Therefore, in the last two years, studies have started to investigate different timings of stent removal within one-month post-transplant [8,18–23]. Recently, Thompson et al. [24] published a review regarding this topic; however, the authors included fewer studies and did provide a robust conclusion about timing of stent removal as their focus was more on the difference between per-urethral and bladder indwelling stents.

The aim of this systematic review is to give a comprehensive overview of currently available literature and to investigate if meta-analysis can elucidate whether a more definite timing for stent removal can be determined.

2. Methods

All aspects of the Cochrane Handbook for Interventional Systematic Reviews were followed, and the study was written according to the Preferred Reporting Items for Systematic Reviews and Meta-Analyses (PRISMA) statement [25,26]. Details of the protocol for this systematic review were registered on PROSPERO (ID: CRD42018079867) and can be accessed online [27].

2.1. Literature Search Strategy

A literature search for all articles regarding JJ-stenting after KTx was performed in EMBASE, MEDLINE Ovid, CENTRAL (the Cochrane Library 2017, issue 11), Web of Science, and Google Scholar. The search was performed for articles published up to November 2017 relevant to outcomes of ureteric stent placement and timings of removal. The search strings for each respective database are attached in Appendix A. Reference lists of the identified relevant articles were manually scrutinized to ensure that no articles were missed.

2.2. Literature Screening

Study selection was performed independently by two authors (J.P.T.v.d.S. and I.J.V.). Study inclusion was carried out in two phases: after an initial title and abstract selection, full articles of the abstracts regarded as potentially eligible were retrieved and underwent complete review and assessment until a final inclusion was made. When a discrepancy in inclusion between the two authors occurred, articles were discussed with two senior authors (J.A.L., F.J.M.F.D.) in order to reach a consensus.

2.3. Data Extraction

Studies were assessed for timing of stent removal and the incidence of UTIs, urinary leakage, ureteral stenosis, and reintervention. Other parameters that were assessed were donor type, mean recipient age, the type of stent, technique of UNC, technique of stent removal, immunosuppressive therapy and antibiotic prophylaxis regimen. When the type of stent was not specified in a particular article, we reached out to the authors. If the authors did not respond, we noted the stent-type as "unspecified" but did not mark it as an exclusion criterium.

Studies were only included if they indicated time of stent removal and at least one of the following outcome parameters: UTI, urinary leakage, and/or ureteral stenosis. If a study stated an outcome as "major urological complication" (MUC) and we were not able to define whether this included stenosis or leakage, we analysed this outcome parameter separately as MUC.

To define UTI, we used the Guideline for Urological Infections of The European Association of Urology [28]. It states that a positive urine culture with a bacterial colony count of more than 10^5 colony-forming units per mL urine is defined as a UTI. However, if patients had lower counts of colony-forming units per mL urine but were reported to have symptoms of a UTI, we chose not to exclude them. When authors of the articles did not define a UTI, we assumed that the official definition was used.

We did not find an official guideline defining urinary leakage and ureteral stenosis. However, Dominguez et al. [10] stated the following definitions for urinary leakage and ureteral stenosis: leakage is defined as drainage or accumulation of perirenal fluid with characteristics of urine and ureteral stenosis is defined as impairment of adequate kidney drainage demonstrated at ultrasound (US) or intravenous pyelogram. When authors of the articles did not define urinary leakage and/or ureteral stenosis, we assumed the abovementioned definitions.

2.4. Critical Appraisal

The level of evidence of each selected paper was established using the GRADE tool [29]. The GRADE approach defines the quality of a body of evidence by consideration of within study risk of bias (methodological quality), directness of evidence, heterogeneity, precision of effect estimates, and risk of publication bias.

2.5. Statistical Analysis

Articles were assessed as to whether they were suitable for quantitative analysis. If articles compared two or more groups with different timings of stent removal and if those groups could be divided in an early and late timing of stent removal with a cut off at three weeks, they were included for meta-analysis.

Review Manager Software (RevMan 5.3; The Nordic Cochrane Centre, Copenhagen, Denmark) was used for meta-analysis [30]. Each study was weighted by sample size. Heterogeneity of time of stent removal effects between studies was tested using the Q (heterogeneity χ^2) and the I^2 statistics. A random effects model was used for calculating the summary estimates (odds ratio (OR)) and 95% confidence intervals (CIs) to account for possible heterogeneity. Overall, the effects were determined using a Z-test. In addition, sensitivity analyses were performed to examine whether removing a particular study would significantly change the results and were presented in funnel plots.

3. Results

Of the 1043 articles identified from the initial literature search, fourteen articles were within the scope of this systematic review; three randomised controlled trials (RCTs) [20,21,31], nine retrospective cohort studies [8,13,19,22,23,32–35] and two prospective studies [36,37]. A total of 3216 patients were included, of which 2406 patients (74.8%) underwent living donor KTx (two studies did not record if they used living or deceased donors [34,35]). Table 1 presents an overview of the included studies. In Figure 1, the PRISMA flowchart diagram for systematic reviews is presented. The quality assessment of the included studies is depicted in a Summary of Findings table in Figure 2.

We could not specify the type of stent in five studies. The authors of these five papers were contacted, but unfortunately, we received no response [19,34–37]. All studies reported the age of the recipients, except for the preliminary results in the three included abstracts [34–36]. Only four studies reported that they both included adults and children [19,21,23,37]. All articles described the incidence of UTIs, and nine articles also reported urinary leakage and/or ureteral stenosis [19–21,31–33,35–37]. Table 2 presents the incidence of the different outcome parameters for each study. Regarding the used UNC technique, seven out of the fourteen articles described the use of the Lich–Gregoir technique [13,20–23,31,32]. Seven articles did not specify which surgical technique was used [8,19,33–37]. Regarding stent removal, ten articles used a cystoscopy for removal [8,20–23,32–36]. In four studies, the stent was removed along with the urinary catheter seven days after transplantation [21,34–36]. Two studies removed the stent on the seventh day posttransplant by pulling on strings that were placed around the stent at the time of transplantation [8,20]. Four studies did not describe the technique of stent removal [13,31,37,38]. Ten studies reported the use of antibiotic prophylaxis to protect against UTI after KTx, of which seven studies also reported the duration of antibiotic prophylaxis regimen [13,20,21,23,31–33]. Six studies specified the use of co-trimoxazole as prophylaxis [13,21–23,31,32]. Four studies did not record the use of prophylactic antibiotics at all [8,36–38]. Seven studies reported which immunosuppressive regimen KTx recipients received [8,20,22,23,31–33]. An overview of all the characteristics of the included studies can be found in Table A1 in Appendix A. Four studies could not be included in the meta-analysis because the timing of stent removal was much earlier (e.g., earlier and later than four days) or much later (e.g., earlier and later than seven weeks) than the cut-off value of three weeks [18,39–41].

Table 1. Overview of the included studies.

Studies	Year	Sort Study	Timing of Stent Removal	Number of Patients	Urinary Tract Infection	Major Urological Complication	Urinary Leakage	Ureteral Stenosis
Yuksel et al. [23]	2017	Retrospective	5–7 days	153	x	x		
			8–14 days	165				
			15–21 days	283				
			>22 days	217				
Patel et al. [21]	2017	RCT	5 days	79	x	x	x	x
			6 weeks	126				
Sarier et al. [22]	2017	Retrospective	15–21 days	28	x			
			21–28 days	54				
			28–35 days	25				
Wingate et al. [8]	2017	Retrospective	<3 weeks	143	x			
			>3 weeks	161				
Liu et al. [20]	2016	RCT	7 days	52	x	x	x	x
			28 days	51				
Dadkhah et al. [37]	2016	Prospective	10 days	164	x	x	x	
			20 days	162				
			30 days	112				
Asgari et al. [38]	2016	Retrospective	10 days	30	x	x	x	
			20 days	31				
			30 days	30				
Gunawansa et al. [36]	2014(1)	Prospective randomised	6 days	203	x	x		x
			28 days	179				
Soldano et al. [35]	2014(2)	Retrospective	5 days	47	x	x	x	
			6 weeks	47				
Lee et al. [34]	2013(3)	Retrospective	5 days	26	x	x		
			6 weeks	26				
Huang et al. [33]	2012	Retrospective	3 weeks	179	x	x	x	x
			6 weeks	186				
Indu et al. [31]	2012	Prospective RCT	7 days	50	x	x	x	
			28 days	50				
Coskun et al. [13]	2011	Retrospective	13–14 days	10	x	x		
			>20 days	38				
Verma et al. [32]	2002	Retrospective	2 weeks	52	x	x	x	x
			4 weeks	57				

RCT: Randomised controlled trial. (1) Abstract of the 17th Congress of the European Society for Organ Transplantation; (2) Abstract of the the World Transplant Congress 2014; and (3) Abstract of the 16th Congress of the European Society for Organ Transplantation.

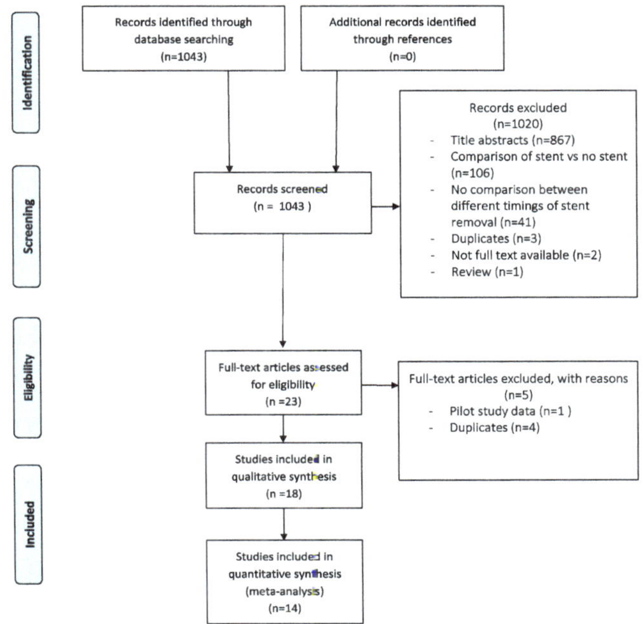

Figure 1. Preferred Reporting Items for Systematic Reviews and Meta-Analyses (PRISMA) flowchart.

Summary of findings:

Early vs late ureteric stent removal after kidney transplantation

Outcomes	Anticipated absolute effects* (95% CI)		Relative effect (95% CI)	№ of participants (studies)	Certainty of the evidence (GRADE)	Comments
	Risk with Late ureteric stent removal	Risk with Early ureteric stent removal				
Urinary Tract Infection	**Low**		OR 0.54 (0.33 to 0.87)	3216 (14 observational studies) [b]	⊕○○○ VERY LOW [c]	
	18 per 1.000 [a]	**10 per 1.000** (6 to 16)				
	High					
	447 per 1.000 [a]	**304 per 1.000** (211 to 413)				
Urinary Leakage	**Low**		OR 0.93 (0.29 to 2.94)	1353 (7 observational studies) [d]	⊕○○○ VERY LOW [c,e,f]	
	11 per 1.000	**10 per 1.000** (3 to 31)				
	High					
	64 per 1.000	**60 per 1.000** (19 to 167)				
Ureteral stenosis	Three studies reported zero incidences of ureteral stenosis. Patel et al. described one case in both the early and late stent removal group. Gunawansa et al described two cases with late stent removal.			587 (5 observational studies) [g]	⊕○○○ VERY LOW [c]	

*The risk in the intervention group (and its 95% confidence interval) is based on the assumed risk in the comparison group and the **relative effect** of the intervention (and its 95% CI).

CI: Confidence interval; **OR:** Odds ratio

GRADE Working Group grades of evidence
High certainty: We are very confident that the true effect lies close to that of the estimate of the effect
Moderate certainty: We are moderately confident in the effect estimate: The true effect is likely to be close to the estimate of the effect, but there is a possibility that it is substantially different
Low certainty: Our confidence in the effect estimate is limited: The true effect may be substantially different from the estimate of the effect
Very low certainty: We have very little confidence in the effect estimate: The true effect is likely to be substantially different from the estimate of effect

Explanations

a. The low and high risk values are the two extreme incidences of urinary tract infection in late stent removal from the studies included in this meta-analysis
b. 2 randomized controlled trials and 12 observational cohort studies
c. Not every study describe their type of antiobiotic profylaxe and immunosupression therapy, which is a possible comfounder. Furthermore studies never mention possible confounders .
d. 2 randomized controlled trials and 5 observational cohort studies
e. I²2 is very low (12%)

Figure 2. Quality assessment of the included studies.

Table 2. Overview of the measured outcome parameters.

Studies	Stent Removal	Number of Patients	Urinary Tract Infection (%)	Major Urological Complication	Ureteral Stenosis (%)	Urinary Leakage (%)	Surgical Reintervention (%)
Yuksel et al. [23]	5–7 days	153	0% *	11.0%			11.0%
	8–14 days	165	1.2% *	9.6%			9.6%
	15–21 days	283	1.1% *	1.7%			1.7%
	>22 days	217	3.2% *	1.3%			1.3%
Patel et al. [21]	5 days	79	7.6% *	3.7%	1.2%	2.5%	3.7%
	6 weeks	126	24.6% *	0.8%	0.8%	0%	0.8%
Sarier et al. [22]	15–21 days	28	7.1% *	x			
	21–28 days	54	5.6% *	x			
	28–35 days	25	12.0% *	x			
Wingate et al. [8]	<3 weeks	143	31.7% *	x			
	>3 weeks	161	51.6% *	x			
Liu et al. [20]	7 days	52	5.8% *	0%	0%	0%	0%
	28 days	51	29.4% *	0%	0%	0%	0%
Dadkhah et al. [37]	10 days	164	18.1%	1.0%		1.0%	
	20 days	162	5.7%	1.0%		1.0%	
	30 days	112	9.1%	2.8%		2.8%	
Asgari et al. [38]	10 days	30	20.0%	6.6%		6.6%	
	20 days	31	9.7%	6.4%		6.4%	
	30 days	30	26.7%	13.3%		13.3%	
Gunawansa et al. [36]	6 days	203	11.3%	0%	0%		
	28 days	179	10.6%	1.1%	1.1%		
Soldano et al. [35]	5 days	47	10.6% *	0%		0%	0%
	6 weeks	47	25.5% *	6.3%		6.3%	2.1%
Lee et al. [34]	5 days	26	53.0%	23.0%			
	6 weeks	26	30.0%	12.0%			
Huang et al. [33]	3 weeks	179	2.2% *	1.1%	0%	1.1%	1.1%
	6 weeks	186	8.1% *	1.1%	0%	1.1%	1.1%
Indu et al. [31]	7 days	50	14.0% *	2.0%		2.0%	0%
	28 days	50	38.0% *	0%		0%	0%
Coskun et al. [13]	13–14 days	10	10.0% *	0%			
	>20 days	38	45.0% *	0%			
Verma et al. [32]	2 weeks	52	25.0% *	5.8%	0%	5.8%	0%
	4 weeks	57	35.1% *	10.0%	0%	10.0%	0%

* Defined as urinary tract infection (UTI).

3.1. Urinary Tract Infection

Fourteen studies described the incidence of UTIs with different timings of stent removal and were included for meta-analysis (a total of 3216 patients). There was a significant difference between the groups in the risk of developing UTIs, favouring early stent removal (OR 0.49, CI 95%, 0.33 to 0.75 $p = 0.0009$) (Figure 3). Sensitivity analysis showed no change of significance. (Figure A1, Appendix A).

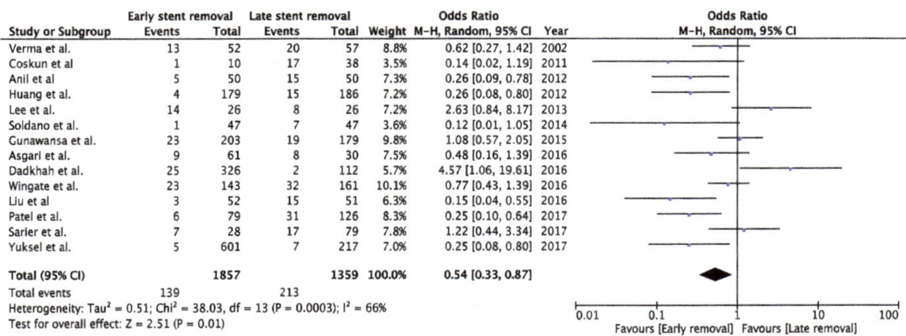

Figure 3. Forest plot of urinary tract infection for early (<3 weeks) versus late (>3 weeks) stent removal.

3.2. Urinary Leakage

Eight studies described the incidence of urinary leakage: three RCTs [20,21,31], one prospective study [37] and four retrospective studies [32,33,35,38]. One of these studies described zero events of urinary leakage; therefore, seven studies remained for meta-analysis, with a total of 1505 patients [21,31–33,35,37,38].

After pooling the data, there was no significant difference between groups in the risk of developing urinary leakage (OR 0.60, CI 95%, 0.29 to 1.23, $p = 0.16$) (Figure 4). Sensitivity analysis showed no change in significance (Figure A2, Appendix A).

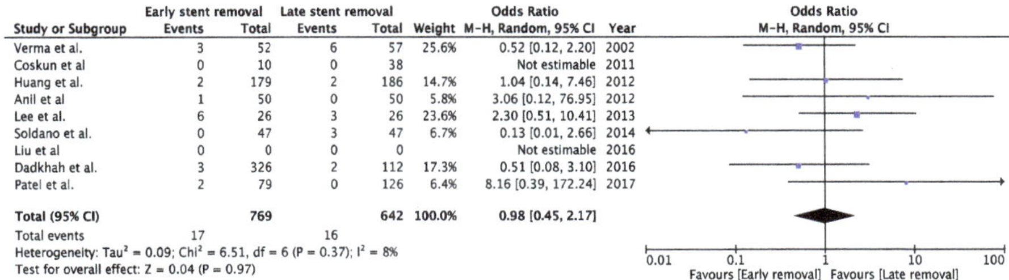

Figure 4. Forest plot urinary leakage for early (<3 weeks) versus late (>3 weeks) stent removal.

3.3. Ureteral Stenosis

Five studies described the incidence of ureteral stenosis [20,21,32,33,36]. Three out of these seven studies reported zero incidents of ureteral stenosis in both groups [20,32,33]. Patel et al. [21] described one case of ureteral stenosis in both the early and late group of stent removal (1.2% and 0.8%, respectively). Gunawansa et al. [36] reported two cases of ureteral stenosis in the late stent removal group (1.1%). No meta-analysis was performed given the low incidence of ureteral stenosis.

Dadkhah et al. [37] and Asgari et al. [19] recorded the incidence of hydronephrosis; however, they did not describe the cause of the hydronephrosis. Dadkhah et al. [37] reported eleven cases in the early stent removal group (3.4%) versus three (2.8%) in the late group of stent removal ($p = 0.122$). Asgari et al. [19] reported, respectively, seven (11.5%) and four (13.3%) cases in the early and late group of stent removal ($p = 0.71$).

Some studies only reported MUC without defining whether this was urinary leakage or ureteral stenosis [13,23,34]. We decided to perform an additional meta-analysis of MUC. We included data from those studies and combined ureteral stenosis and urinary leakage in a single MUC category. After pooling the data, there was no significant difference between groups in the risk of developing major urological complications (OR 1.01, CI 95%, 0.45 to 2.27, $p = 0.98$) (Figure A3, Appendix A). However, we think that ureteral stenosis and urinary leakage are fundamentally different because these complications have a different pathophysiology, so we should be careful with interpretation of these combined outcome parameters.

3.4. Reintervention

Yuksel et al. [23] described the incidence of surgical reintervention because of urological complications after renal transplantation at four different timings of stent removal. There was a clear difference between early (less than three weeks) and late (more than three weeks) stent removal (6.3% versus 1.3%). Patel et al. [21] reported three cases (3.7%) of major urological complications that required surgical revision in the early (five days) versus one case (0.8%) in the late (28 days) stent removal group. Indu et al. [31] reported one case (2.0%) of urinary leakage that required percutaneous nephrostomy in the early stent removal group. Huang et al. [33] reported two cases (1.1%) of urinary leakage that required surgical revision in both the early and late stent removal groups.

Verma et al. [32] reported zero surgical reintervention after major urological complications in both early and late stent removal group (two and four weeks, respectively).

Soldano et al. [35] and Liu et al. [20] investigated surgical reimplantation of the JJ-stent; Soldano et al. [35] reported one case (2.1%) of surgical reimplantation of the stent in the late stent removal group (six weeks), whereas Liu et al. did not report any reimplantation in both the early and late stent removal groups (one and four weeks, respectively).

4. Discussion

There is good evidence that stenting the UNC at the time of KTx is beneficial to reduce major urological complications. Intuitively, transplant professionals feel that ureteric stents should not be in situ for too long to reduce the incidence of infectious complications. However, the optimal timing of stent removal remains unclear. Previous studies show a wide range in the timing of stent removal after KTx (five days until 60 days) [42–45]. It is already known that the incidence of UTIs is higher when a stent is removed later than five weeks (24.6% to 44%) [13,21,22,34,35]. A UTI after KTx is associated with graft loss, higher morbidity rates, increased risk of rejection and increased hospitalisation rates [6,7,46–48]. For this reason, studies have been performed to investigate whether earlier stent removal (e.g., around three weeks) would reduce the incidence of UTIs [8,13,19,20,22,23,31,33,36,37]. We decided to perform a meta-analysis to further investigate if we could define a more optimal timing of stent removal.

Based on the results, we demonstrated that earlier (<three weeks) stent removal shows a significantly lower incidence of UTIs compared to later removal (>three weeks). Furthermore, earlier stent removal does not appear to lead to a higher incidence of urine leakage. Regarding ureteral stenosis and reintervention, no hard statements can be made, since we were not able to meta-analyse the results. However, overall, incidence or ureteral stenosis and reintervention is clearly very low in kidney transplant recipients (~1 and 3%).

4.1. Difficulty in Anastomosis

We realize that characteristics of the study population of both donors and recipients varies and that these are factors that can influence the difficulty of the ureteral anastomosis, and therefore, the outcome after KTx. Unfortunately, only a few studies describe the donor and recipient characteristics in detail; type of donor (living/deceased), type of deceased donor (donor after brainstem/circulatory death), pre-emptive status of the recipients and duration of dialysis are often not given.

Almost every study recorded whether they included a living and/or deceased donor. The majority of the included studies only involved living donor KTx [19,20,22,23,31,32,36,37]; Huang et al. [33] only included deceased donor kidneys. Three studies included both deceased and living donors [8,13,21]. Two studies did not record whether they included living and/or deceased donors [34,35].

Furthermore, Patel et al. [21] reported that of the deceased donors, the majority was a DBD—in the early stent group 81.2% and in the late stent group 64.4%. They recorded that in both the early and late stent removal group, 72% of the transplant patients were dialysis dependant before KTx. In the study by Huang et al. [33], all patients were receiving dialysis before KTx. In both groups, around 95% of the transplant patients underwent haemodialysis and 5% peritoneal dialysis. In the early and late stent removal groups, patients were respectively 25.7 and 24.8 months on dialysis prior to transplantation. Coskun et al. [13] only reported that duration of dialysis prior to transplantation varied between 1 and 168 months.

4.2. Urinary Tract Infection

The incidence of UTIs varied widely between included studies: 0 to 53% [8,13,19–23,31–37]. Most transplant centres used a similar triple-regimen immunosuppressive therapy, consisting of calcineurin inhibitors (tacrolimus or cyclosporine), mycophenolate mofetil and corticosteroids. For all details of the immunosuppressive therapy see Table A1 in appendix A. We noticed that some studies did not describe the immunosuppressive drugs nor the prophylactic antibiotics used. We assumed that in these cases, a calcineurin inhibitor-based triple-immunosuppressive regimen was used, and antibiotic prophylaxis was prescribed. Yuksel et al. [23] attribute the low incidence of UTIs to their strict regime of antibiotic prophylaxis. In addition, Sarier et al. [22] and Wilson et al. [6] stress the importance of prophylactic co-trimoxazole to protect against UTIs after transplantation. Furthermore, they state that previous in vivo and in vitro studies have demonstrated that the antibiotic types fluoroquinolones, aminoglycosides and beta-lactam antibiotics may be effective in prevention of the biofilm mechanism—a major problem in bacterial stent colonization [22].

Coskun et al. [13] state that UTIs should rather be treated with earlier stent removal opposed to the prescription of antibiotics. We agree with this statement and would advise transplant centres to remove the (potential) source of UTIs earlier rather than later as a best possible way to prevent UTIs.

Some studies investigated very early stent removal, around one week post-transplantation, and it showed promising results, specifically (and maybe only) regarding the incidence of UTIs [20,21,23,31,34,36].

Dadkhah et al. [37] showed a remarkably high incidence of UTIs in the early stent removal group (ten days), which was two times higher than for late stent removal (30 days). Surprisingly, they concluded that removal of the ureteral stent shortly after KTx has a statistically negligible impact on the rate of UTIs. We decided to include their controversial incidence of UTIs in our meta-analysis. However, one should keep in mind that this study had some paucity of data granularity, as the technique of UNC, length of follow up, immunosuppressive regimen, the use of antibiotic prophylaxis and technique of stent removal were not described.

4.3. Ureteral Leakage and Ureteral Stenosis

Included studies with wide varying timings of stent removal show that ureteral leakage and stenosis are complications with low incidences (0–3%). Three studies described a remarkably high incidence of urinary leakage [32,35,38]. Asgari et al. [38] reported 6.6% urinary leakage in the early stent removal group (ten days) and 13.3% in the late stent removal group (30 days). Soldano et al. [35] reported 6.3% urinary leakage in the late stent removal group (at six weeks). Verma et al. [35] reported 5.8% and 10% urinary leakage in the early (two weeks) and late (four weeks) stent removal groups. Because these remarkably high incidences were derived from (pilot) studies with small patient populations (each group containing respectively around 50 patients), we have to interpret these data very carefully.

Overall, the data implies that both leakage and stenosis can be successfully prevented with insertion of a stent but the duration of the stent being in situ does not have a great influence on the incidence of these urological complications [5,6,10–12]. Huang et al. [33] support this by concluding that stent removal at three weeks is as effective in preventing urological complications as removal at six weeks (with similar prophylactic antibiotics and immunosuppressive therapies). Furthermore, Patel et al. [21] demonstrate that very early stent removal (less than five days) results in a lower incidence of leakage and stenosis than in the un-stented population. Therefore, even when the stent is inserted for a brief period, it already shows benefit in preventing leakage and stenosis. The first two weeks after KTx are believed to have the highest incidence of urinary leakage and ureteral stenosis [8,13,23,32]. Yuksel et al. [23] conclude that stent removal earlier than fourteen days shows a significant increase of recurrent surgical UNC intervention. In addition, Coskun et al. [13] conclude that stent removal at two weeks results in acceptable mucosal healing of the anastomosis to prevent urological complications. In order to keep the incidence of urinary leakage and ureteral stenosis as low as possible, we recommend that stents should not be removed earlier than two weeks.

4.4. Additional Advantages

In addition to a lower incidence of UTIs, early stent removal has other advantages. Instead of a cystoscopy, stents can be removed less invasively together with the removal of the urinary catheter if tied to it at the time of transplantation. This procedure is considered far more comfortable for the patient [8,20]. Additionally, early stent removal provides the opportunity to remove the stent during the same admission, which leads to a reduction in costs and fewer forgotten stents [5,21,32,33].

4.5. Limitations

A meta-analysis can only be as good as the quality of the included studies. Unfortunately, most of the included studies are retrospective cohort studies. Only three RCTs were included [20,21,31]. We mention this limitation to alert the reader to carefully interpret the data. In the forest plot analysing urinary tract infections for early (<3 weeks) versus late (>3 weeks) stent removal (Figure 3), one can appreciate the relatively high heterogeneity (I^2 = 61%). The cause of this heterogeneity lies in the differences in study design; for example, not defining which type of stent has been used, technique of stent removal, technique of ureteroneocystostomy, use of prophylactic antibiotics or choice of immunosuppressive therapy. The latter two aspects are particularly important factors influencing UTI rates. Furthermore, urinary leakage and ureteral stenosis were not always defined, or no uniform definition was adhered to. This leads to assumptions, which may cause inadequate comparison. Studies often do not report at what time during follow-up, especially before or after stent removal, specific complications occurred.

Recently, Thompson et al. [24] also investigated the benefits of early stent removal. They concluded that early stent removal reduces the incidence of UTIs, while it was uncertain if there is a higher risk of MUC. Furthermore, the authors used incidence of MUC as a primary outcome and UTIs as a secondary outcome. In our study, UTIs and MUC were chosen as, respectively, primary and secondary outcome, because our main focus was to investigate whether early stent removal reduced the disadvantages of stenting (incidence of UTIs), without compromising the beneficial effects (preventing MUC).

Thompson et al. [24] classified early and late stent removal in a different manner; although they mention that early stent removal was defined as stent removal below fifteen days, they did not particularly use this definition in their analyses. The authors copied the "early" and "late" groups from included studies. As a consequence, there is no common cut-off value analysed in their study and meta-analysis.

Furthermore, the focus of their analysis was more on the specific type of stents used (bladder indwelling stent and per-urethral stents). In our opinion, we should first focus on the relation between duration of stenting and the incidence of UTIs rather than the influence of the type of stent.

5. Conclusions

The results of this systematic review clearly point favourably towards an earlier stent removal around three weeks opposed to the six weeks that is currently used in most transplant centres. Earlier stent removal (at or below three weeks) results in fewer UTIs without negatively affecting the anastomosis between ureter and bladder. We recommend at this stage that ureteric stents should not be removed earlier than two weeks. We would recommend initiating an RCT, randomising between very early stent removal at one week and stent removal at three weeks. Another option would be a three-armed RCT, adding an additional group of stent removal at six weeks.

Author Contributions: The study was conceptualized by F.J.M.F.D. and J.A.L., methodology was developed by I.J.V., J.P.T.v.d.S., J.A.L. and F.J.M.F.D. Formal analyses were done by I.J.V., J.P.T.v.d.S. and J.A.L. The original draft was written by I.J.V., J.P.T.v.d.S and J.A.L. The MS was further reviewed and edited by I.J.V., J.P.T.v.d.S., A.M., M.W., J.A.L. and F.J.M.F.D. The project was supervised by J.A.L. and F.J.M.F.D.

Acknowledgments: We thank Wichor Bramer for his expert assistance with the systematic literature search.

Conflicts of Interest: The authors declare no conflict of interest.

Appendix A

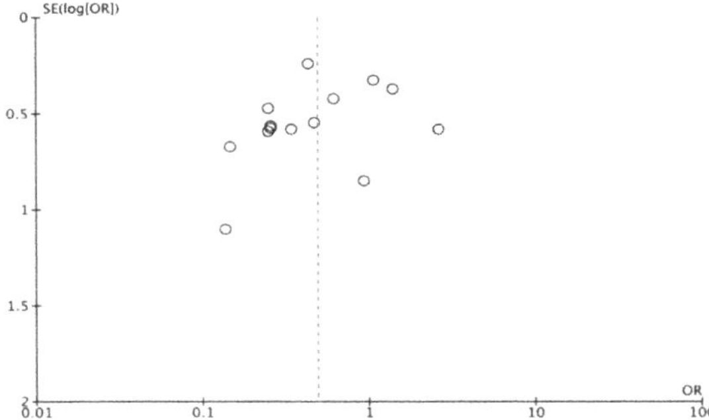

Figure A1. Funnel plot of urinary tract infection for early (<3 weeks) versus late (>3 weeks) stent removal.

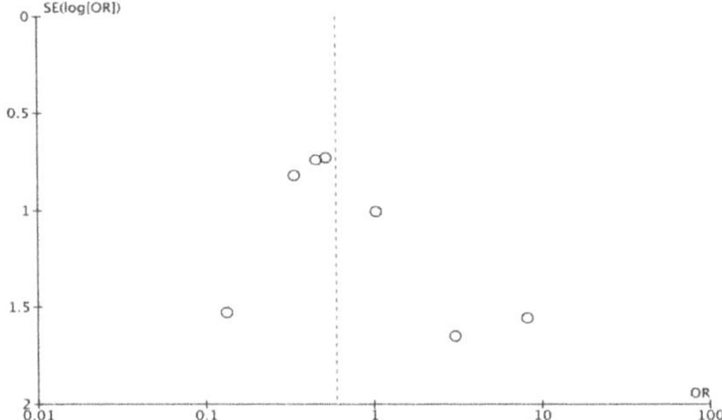

Figure A2. Funnel plot of urinary leakage for early (<3 weeks) versus late (>3 weeks) stent removal.

Study or Subgroup	Early stent removal Events	Total	Late stent removal Events	Total	Weight	Odds Ratio M–H, Random, 95% CI
Liu et al	0	52	0	51		Not estimable
Coskun et al	0	10	0	38		Not estimable
Soldano et al.	0	47	3	47	5.5%	0.13 [0.01, 2.66]
Gunawansa et al.	0	203	2	179	5.4%	0.17 [0.01, 3.66]
Dadkhah et al.	3	326	3	112	12.0%	0.34 [0.07, 1.70]
Asgari et al.	4	61	4	30	13.1%	0.46 [0.11, 1.97]
Verma et al.	3	52	6	57	13.3%	0.52 [0.12, 2.20]
Huang et al.	2	179	2	186	9.7%	1.04 [0.14, 7.46]
Lee et al.	6	26	3	26	12.7%	2.30 [0.51, 10.41]
Anil et al	1	50	0	50	4.9%	3.06 [0.12, 76.95]
Yuksel et al.	38	601	3	217	15.3%	4.81 [1.47, 15.76]
Patel et al.	3	79	1	126	8.1%	4.93 [0.50, 48.29]
Total (95% CI)		1686		1119	100.0%	1.01 [0.45, 2.27]
Total events	60		27			

Heterogeneity: Tau^2 = 0.74; Chi^2 = 16.97, df = 9 (P = 0.05); I^2 = 47%
Test for overall effect: Z = 0.03 (P = 0.98)

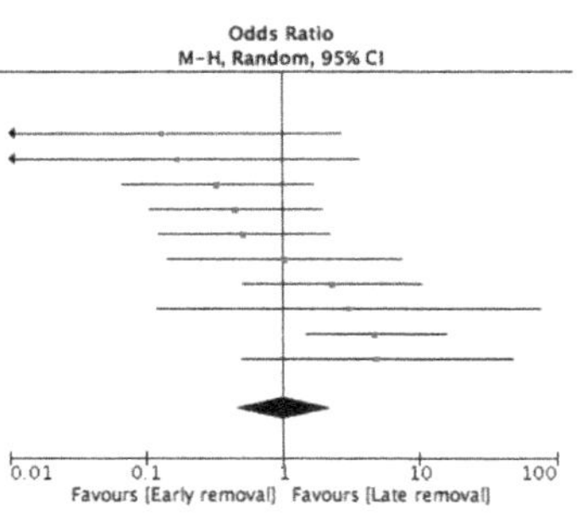

Figure A3. Forest plot of major urological complications for early (<3 weeks) versus late (>3 weeks) stent removal.

Table A1. Overview of the study characteristics.

Studies	Date of Patient Results	Timing of Stent Removal	Type of Stent	Living/Deceased Donor	Mean Age of Patients	Technique UNC	Technique of Stent Removal	Immunsupression Threapy	Prophylactic Antibiotics	Follow-Up
Yuksel et al. [23]	jan2014–jan2016	5–7 days	Double J-stent	100%/0%	40.7 y *	Lich-Gregoir	Cystoscopy	CNI + MMF + Cor	Yes *	NR
		8–14 days		"	43.5 y *		Cystoscopy		Until stent removal	
		15–21 days		"	41.5 y *		Cystoscopy			
		>22 days		"	41.9 y *		Cystoscopy			
Patel et al. [21]	may2010–nov2013	5 days	Double J stent	60.5%/39.5%	47.5 y *	Lich-Gregoir	Attached to UC	NR	Yes *	UTI: 3 months
		6 weeks		65.6%/34.4%	41.7 y *		Cystoscopy		6 months	MUC: 6 months
Sarier et al. [22]	jan2016–may2016	15–21 days	Double J-stent	100%/0%	45.14 y	Extravesical = Lich-Gregoir	Cystoscopy	CNI + Ster	Yes *	NR
		21–28 days		"	41.18 y		Cystoscopy			
		28–35 days		"	47.52 y		Cystoscopy			
Wingate et al. [8]	jan2010–jan2015	<3 weeks	Double J-stent	32/68% (5)	55.5 y (5)	NR	Attached to external string = suture	Tac+ MMF+ Pred + (Atg/Bas/Dac(6))	NR	9 months
		>3 weeks		"	"		Cystoscopy			
Liu et al. [20]	oct2010–march2015	7 days	Double J-stent	100%/0%	34.9 y	Lich-Gregoir	Attached to external sutures	CNI + MMF + Cor + Bas	Yes	3 months
		28 days		"	35.4 y		Cystoscopy		3 days post operative	
Dadkhah et al. [37]	may2011–march2012	10 days	Unspecified	100%/0%	40.5 y *	NR	NR	NR	NR	1 month
		20 days		"	40.4 y *					
		30 days		"	41.9 y *					
Asgari et al. [38]	may2011–march2012	10 days	Unspecified	100%/0%	41.4 y *	NR	NR	NR	NR	1 month
		20 days		"	38.0 y *					
		30 days		"	43.7 y *					
Gunawansa et al. [36] (1)	Jan2009–August2013	6 days	Unspecified	100%/0%	NR	NR	Attached to UC	NR	NR	16 (12–36) months
		28 days		"			Cystoscopy			
Soldano et al. [35] (2)	NR	5 days	Unspecified	NR	NR	NR	Attached to UC	NR	Yes	NR
		6 weeks					Cystoscopy			
Lee et al. [34] (3)	jan2011–aug2011	5 days	Unspecified	NR	NR	NR	Attached to UC	NR	Yes *	12 months
		6 weeks					Cystoscopy			
Huang et al. [33]	jan2009–dec2010	3 weeks	Double J-stent	0%/100%	42.8 y	NR	Cystoscopy	CNI + MMF + Pred	Yes	3 months
		6 weeks		"	43.5 y		Cystoscopy		First week post operative	
Indu et al. [31]	Jan 2007–Dec 2009	7 days	Double J stent	100%/0%	34.4y	Lich-Gregoir	NR	Cycl + Aza/ MMF + Pred + (Dac(6))	Yes*	6 months
		28 days		"	33.8 y)				6 months	
Coskun et al. [13]	nov2005–may2010	13–14 days	Double J stent	70%/30%	21–41 y	Lich-Gregoir	NR	NR	Yes*	14–49 months
		>20 days (4)		58%/42%	19–56 y				3 months	4–55 months
Verma et al. [32]	Jan 1996–June 1996	2 weeks	Double J stent	100%/0%	31.2 y	Lich-Gregoir	Cystoscopy	Cycl+ Aza + Pred	Yes*	NR
		4 weeks		"	33.8 y		Cystoscopy		3 months	

NR = not recorded, UNC = ureteroneocystostomy, LG = Lich–Gregoir, UC = urinary catheter, CNI = calcineurin inhibitors, MMF = mycophenolate mofetil, Cor = corticosteroids, Tac = Tacrolimus, Cyc = cyclosporine, Pred = prednisone, ATG = antithymocyte globulin, Bas = Basiliximab, Dac = Daclizumab, Aza = Azathioprine. (1) 20–30, 30–40, 40–50, 50–60 days, (2) including the non-stented population ($n = 99$). * Recorded that they both included children and adults; ^ Induction therapy; ʺ Specific type of prophylactic antibiotics.

Search string A

Embase.com	944	936
Medline Ovid	443	55
Web of Science	268	25
Cochrane CENTRAL	43	3
Google Scholar	100	24
Total	**1798**	**1043**

Embase.com 944

('kidney graft'/exp OR 'kidney transplantation'/exp OR (((kidney* OR renal*) NEAR/3 (graft* OR transplant* OR allograft* OR allotransplant* OR recipient*))):ab,ti) AND ('ureter stent'/exp OR (ureter/de AND stent/de) OR (((ureter* OR nephroureter* OR double-j OR jj OR j-j OR pigtail* OR urinar*) NEAR/3 stent*)):ab,ti) NOT ([animals]/lim NOT [humans]/lim)

Medline Ovid 443

(kidney transplantation/ OR kidney/tr OR (((kidney* OR renal*) ADJ3 (graft* OR transplant* OR allograft* OR allotransplant* OR recipient*))).ab,ti.) AND ((ureter/ AND stents/) OR (((ureter* OR nephroureter* OR double-j OR jj OR j-j OR pigtail* OR urinar*) ADJ3 stent*)).ab,ti.) NOT (exp animals/ NOT humans/)

Cochrane CENTRAL 43

(((((kidney* OR renal*) NEAR/3 (graft* OR transplant* OR allograft* OR allotransplant* OR recipient*))):ab,ti) AND ((((ureter* OR nephroureter* OR double-j OR jj OR j-j OR pigtail* OR urinar*) NEAR/3 stent*)):ab,ti)

Web of Science 268

TS=((((((kidney* OR renal*) NEAR/2 (graft* OR transplant* OR allograft* OR allotransplant* OR recipient*)))) AND ((((ureter* OR nephroureter* OR double-j OR jj OR j-j OR pigtail* OR urinar*) NEAR/2 stent*))) NOT ((animal* OR rat OR rats Or mouse OR mice OR murine) NOT (human* OR patient*))) AND DT=(article) AND LA=(English)

Google Scholar

"kidney|renal graft|transplantation|allograft|allotransplant|recipients"
"ureter|ureteral|nephroureteral|jj|pigtail|urinary stent|stents"|"j|double j stent|stents

References

1. Abecassis, M.; Bartlett, S.T.; Collins, A.J.; Davis, C.L.; Delmonico, F.L.; Friedewald, J.J.; Hays, R.; Howard, A.; Jones, E.; Leichtman, A.B.; et al. Kidney transplantation as primary therapy for end-stage renal disease: A National Kidney Foundation/Kidney Disease Outcomes Quality Initiative (NKF/KDOQITM) conference. *Clin. J. Am. Soc. Nephrol.* **2008**, *3*, 471–480. [CrossRef]
2. Lafranca, J.A.; Hesselink, D.A.; Dor, F.J.M.F. *Oxford Textbook of Urological Surgery*; Ploeg, R., Ed.; Oxford University Press: Oxford, UK, 2017.
3. Wolfe, R.A.; Ashby, V.B.; Milford, E.L.; Ojo, A.O.; Ettenger, R.E.; Agodoa, L.Y.; Held, P.J.; Port, F.K. Comparison of mortality in all patients on dialysis, patients on dialysis awaiting transplantation, and recipients of a first cadaveric transplant. *N. Engl. J. Med.* **1999**, *341*, 1725–1730. [CrossRef] [PubMed]
4. Rigg, K.M.; Proud, G.; Taylor, R.M. Urological complications following renal transplantation. A study of 1016 consecutive transplants from a single centre. *Transplant. Int.* **1994**, *7*, 120–126.
5. Kumar, A.; Verma, B.S.; Srivastava, A.; Bhandari, M.; Gupta, A.; Sharma, R. Evaluation of the urological complications of living related renal transplantation at a single center during the last 10 years: Impact of the Double-J* stent. *J. Urol.* **2000**, *164*, 657–660. [CrossRef]
6. Wilson, C.H.; Bhatti, A.A.; Rix, D.A.; Manas, D.M. Routine intraoperative ureteric stenting for kidney transplant recipients. *Cochrane Database Syst. Rev.* **2005**, *4*, CD004925.
7. Sansalone, C.V.; Maione, G.; Aseni, P.; Mangoni, I.; Soldano, S.; Minetti, E.; Radaelli, L.; Civati, G. Advantages of short-time ureteric stenting for prevention of urological complications in kidney transplantation: An 18-year experience. *Transplant. Proc.* **2005**, *37*, 2511–2515. [CrossRef] [PubMed]

8.   Wingate, J.T.; Brandenberger, J.; Weiss, A.; Scovel, L.G.; Kuhr, C.S. Ureteral stent duration and the risk of BK polyomavirus viremia or bacteriuria after kidney transplantation. *Transplant. Infect. Dis.* **2017**, *19*, 1. [CrossRef] [PubMed]

9.   Mangus, R.S.; Haag, B.W. Stented versus nonstented extravesical ureteroneocystostomy in renal transplantation: A metaanalysis. *Am. J. Transplant.* **2004**, *4*, 1889–1896. [CrossRef]

10.   Dominguez, J.; Clase, C.M.; Mahalati, K.; MacDonald, A.S.; McAlister, V.C.; Belitsky, P.; Kiberd, B.; Lawen, J.G. Is routine ureteric stenting needed in kidney transplantation? A randomized trial. *Transplantation* **2000**, *70*, 597–601. [CrossRef]

11.   Osman, Y.; Ali-El-Dein, B.; Shokeir, A.A.; Kamal, M.; El-Din, A.B. Routine insertion of ureteral stent in live-donor renal transplantation: Is it worthwhile? *Urology* **2005**, *65*, 867–871. [CrossRef] [PubMed]

12.   Tavakoli, A.; Surange, R.S.; Pearson, R.C.; Parrott, N.R.; Augustine, T.; Riad, H.N. Impact of Stents on Urological Complications and Health Care Expenditure in Renal Transplant Recipients: Results of a Prospective, Randomized Clinical Trial. *J. Urol.* **2007**, *177*, 2260–2264. [CrossRef] [PubMed]

13.   Coskun, A.K.; Harlak, A.; Ozer, T.; Eyitilen, T.; Yigit, T.; Demirbaş, S.; Uzar, A.İ.; Kozak, O.; Cetiner, S. Is removal of the stent at the end of 2 weeks helpful to reduce infectous or urologic complications after renal transplantation? *Transplant. Proc.* **2011**, *43*, 813–815. [CrossRef]

14.   Guvence, N.; Oskay, K.; Karabulut, I.; Ayli, D. Effects of ureteral stent on urologic complications in renal transplant recipients: A retrospective study. *Renal Fail.* **2009**, *31*, 899–903. [CrossRef]

15.   Ranganathan, M.; Akbar, M.; Ilham, M.A.; Chavez, R.; Kumar, N.; Asderakis, A. Infective Complications Associated with Ureteral Stents in Renal Transplant Recipients. *Transplant. Proc.* **2009**, *41*, 162–164. [CrossRef]

16.   Glazier, D.B.; Jacobs, M.G.; Lyman, N.W.; Whang, M.I.; Manor, E.; Mulgaonkar, S.P. Urinary tract infection associated with ureteral stents in renal transplantation. *Can. J. Urol.* **1998**, *5*, 462–466. [PubMed]

17.   Breda, A.; Olsburgh, J.; Budde, K.; Figueiredo, A.; LledóGarcía, E.; Regele, H. EAU Guidelines on Renal Transplantation 2014. Available online: https://www.uroweb.org/guideline/renal-transplantation/ (accessed on 1 June 2018).

18.   Parapiboon, W.; Ingsathit, A.; Disthabanchong, S.; Nongnuch, A.; Jearanaipreprem, A.; Charoenthanakit, C.; Jirasiritham, S.; Sumethkul, V. Impact of early ureteric stent removal and cost-benefit analysis in kidney transplant recipients: Results of a randomized controlled study. *Transplant. Proc.* **2012**, *44*, 737–739. [CrossRef]

19.   Ali Asgari, M.; Dadkhah, F.; Tara, S.A.; Argani, H.; Tavoosian, A.; Ghadian, A. Early Stent Removal After Kidney Transplantation: Is it Possible? *Nephrourol. Mon.* **2016**, *8*, e30598. [CrossRef]

20.   Liu, S.; Luo, G.; Sun, B.; Lu, J.; Zu, Q.; Yang, S.; Zhang, X.; Dong, J. Early Removal of Double-J Stents Decreases Urinary Tract Infections in Living Donor Renal Transplantation: A Prospective, Randomized Clinical Trial. *Transplant. Proc.* **2017**, *49*, 297–302. [CrossRef]

21.   Patel, P.; Rebollo-Mesa, I.; Ryan, E.; Sinha, M.D.; Marks, S.D.; Banga, N.; Macdougall, I.C.; Webb, M.C.; Koffman, G.; Olsburgh, J. Prophylactic Ureteric Stents in Renal Transplant Recipients: A Multicenter Randomized Controlled Trial of Early Versus Late Removal. *Am. J. Transplant.* **2017**, *17*, 2129–2138. [CrossRef] [PubMed]

22.   Sarier, M.; Demir, M.; Duman, I.; Yuksel, Y.; Demirbas, A. Evaluation of Ureteral Stent Colonization in Live-Donor Renal Transplant Recipients. *Transplant. Proc.* **2017**, *49*, 415–419. [CrossRef] [PubMed]

23.   Yuksel, Y.; Tekin, S.; Yuksel, D.; Duman, I.; Sarier, M.; Yucetin, L.; Kiraz, K.; Demirbas, M.; Kaya Furkan, A.; Aslan Sezer, M.; et al. Optimal Timing for Removal of the Double-J Stent After Kidney Transplantation. *Transplant. Proc.* **2017**, *49*, 523–527. [CrossRef]

24.   Thompson, E.R.; Hosgood, S.A.; Nicholson, M.L.; Wilson, C.H. Early versus late ureteric stent removal after kidney transplantation. *Cochrane Database Syst. Rev.* **2018**, *1*, CD011455. [CrossRef] [PubMed]

25.   Moher, D.; Liberati, A.; Tetzlaff, J.; Altman, D.G.; Group, P. Preferred reporting items for systematic reviews and meta-analyses: The PRISMA statement. *BMJ* **2009**, *339*, b2535. [CrossRef] [PubMed]

26.   Higgins, J.P.T.; Green, S. (Eds.) Cochrane Handbook for Systematic Reviews of Interventions Version 5.1.0 (updated March 2011). The Cochrane Collaboration. 2011. Available online: http://handbook.cochrane.org.

27.   Visser, I.J.; Van der Staaij, J.P.T.; Willicombe, M.; Muthusamy, A.; Lafranca, J.A.; Dor, F.J.M.F. Timing of Double-J stent Removal and Occurrence of Urological Complications: A Systematic Review and Meta-Analysis. PROSPERO 2018 CRD42018079867. Available online: http://www.crd.york.ac.uk/PROSPERO/display_record.php?ID=CRD42018079867 (accessed on 23 April 2019).

28. Bonkat, G.; Groschl, I.; Rieken, M.; Rentsch, C.A.; Wyler, S.; Gasser, T.C.; Widmer, A.F.; Bachmann, A. Microbial biofilm formation on ureteral stents in renal transplant recipients: Frequency and influence on short time functional outcome. *Eur. Urol. Suppl.* **2010**, *9*, 164. [CrossRef]

29. *GRADEpro GDT*; McMaster University: Hamilton, ON, Canada, 2015.

30. *Review Manager*; The Nordic Cochrane Centre: Copenhagen, Denmark, 2014.

31. Indu, K.N.; Lakshminarayana, G.; Anil, M.; Rajesh, R.; George, K.; Ginil, K.; Georgy, M.; Nair, B.; Sudhindran, S.; Appu, T.; et al. Is early removal of prophylactic ureteric stents beneficial in live donor renal transplantation. *Indian J. Nephrol.* **2012**, *22*, 275–279.

32. Verma, B.S.; Bhandari, M.; Srivastava, A.; Kapoor, R.; Kumar, A. Optimum duration of J.J. Stenting in live related renal transplantation. *Indian J. Urol.* **2002**, *19*, 54–57.

33. Huang, L.; Wang, X.; Ma, Y.; Wang, J.; Tao, X.; Liao, L.; Tan, J. A comparative study of 3-week and 6-week duration of double-j stent placement in renal transplant recipients. *Urol. Int.* **2012**, *89*, 89–92. [CrossRef] [PubMed]

34. Lee, G.; Herzig, J.; Crotty, C.; Shah, K.; Nicholson, M.L.; Hosgood, S.A. Comparison of early versus late ureteric stent removal after kidney transplantation. *Transplant. Int.* **2013**, *26*, 271.

35. Soldano, S.; Ali, A.; Pawelec, K.; Sammartino, C.; Sivaprakasam, R.; Puliatti, C.; Cacciola, R. Safety and potential benefits of early ureteric stent removal tied with urinary catheter after renal transplant. *Transplantation* **2014**, *98*, 638–639. [CrossRef]

36. Gunawansa, N.; Wijeyaratne, M.; Cassim, R.; Sahabandu, C. Early bedside removal versus delayed cystoscopic removal of ureteric stents following live donor renal transplantation: A randomized prospective study. *Transplant. Int.* **2015**, *28*, 118.

37. Dadkhah, F.; Yari, H.; Asgari, M.A.; Fallahnezhad, M.H.; Tavoosian, A.; Ghadian, A. Benefits and complications of removing ureteral stent based on the elapsed time after renal transplantation surgery. *Nephro-Urol. Mon.* **2016**, *8*, 2. [CrossRef] [PubMed]

38. Asgari, M.A.; Dadkhah, F.; Tara, S.A.; Argani, H.; Tavoosian, A.; Ghadian, A. Early stent removal after kidney transplantation: Is it possible? *Nephro-Urol. Mon.* **2016**, *8*, 2.

39. Thiel, K.; Wichmann, D.; Nadalin, S.; Ladurner, R.; Königsrainer, A. Urinary tract infection in renal transplant patients-what to do? *Transplant. Int.* **2013**, *26*, 284.

40. Mannu, G.S.; Bettencourt-Silva, J.H.; Gilbert, J. The ideal timing of ureteric stent removal in transplantation patients. *Transplant. Int.* **2014**, *27*, e96–e97. [CrossRef]

41. Raza, S.; Ghazanfar, A.; Alahmadi, I.; Alahdal, H.; Brockmann, J.; Broring, D.; Abassi, A.; Aleid, H. Impacts of ureteric stent removal timing on post renal transplant major urological complication. A single centre experience. *Transplantation* **2016**, *100*, S318.

42. Pleass, H.C.C.; Clark, K.R.; Rigg, K.M.; Reddy, K.S.; Forsythe, J.L.R.; Proud, G.; Taylor, R.M. Urologic complications after renal transplantation: A prospective randomized trial comparing different techniques of ureteric anastomosis and the use of prophylactic ureteric stents. *Transplant. Proc.* **1995**, *27*, 1091–1092.

43. Eschwege, P.; Blancher, P.; Bellamy, J.; Charpentier, B.; Jardin, A.; Benoit, G. Does the use of double J ureteral stents reduce stenosis and fistulas in renal transplantation. *Transplant. Proc.* **1995**, *27*, 2436. [PubMed]

44. Kumar, A.; Kumar, R.; Bhandari, M. Significance of routine JJ stenting in living related renal transplantation: A prospective randomised study. *Transplant. Proc.* **1998**, *30*, 2995–2997. [CrossRef]

45. Gedroyc, W.M.W.; Koffman, G.; Saunders, A.J.S. Ureteric obstruction in stented renal transplants. *Brit. J. Urol.* **1988**, *62*, 123–126. [CrossRef] [PubMed]

46. Mangus, R.S.; Haag, B.W.; Carter, C.B. Stented Lich-Gregoir ureteroneocystostomy: Case series report and cost-effectiveness analysis. *Transplant. Proc.* **2004**, *36*, 2959–2961. [CrossRef] [PubMed]

47. Thomalla, J.V.; Leapman, S.B.; Filo, R.S. The use of internalised ureteric stens in renal transplant recipients. *Brit. J. Urol.* **1990**, *66*, 363–368. [CrossRef] [PubMed]

48. Ooms, L.; Ijzermans, J.; Voor, I.; Holt, A.; Betjes, M.; Vos, M.; Terkivatan, T. Urinary Tract Infections After Kidney Transplantation: A Risk Factor Analysis of 417 Patients. *Ann. Transplant.* **2017**, *22*, 402–408. [CrossRef] [PubMed]

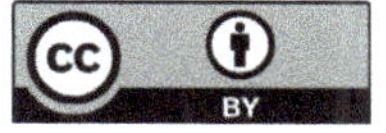

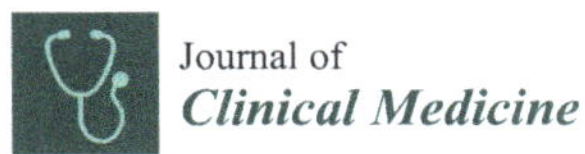

Journal of
Clinical Medicine

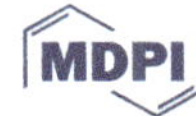

Article

Incidence and Mortality of Renal Cell Carcinoma after Kidney Transplantation: A Meta-Analysis

Api Chewcharat [1,2], Charat Thongprayoon [3,*], Tarun Bathini [4], Narothama Reddy Aeddula [5], Boonphiphop Boonpheng [6], Wisit Kaewput [7], Kanramon Watthanasuntorn [8], Ploypin Lertjitbanjong [8], Konika Sharma [8], Aldo Torres-Ortiz [9], Napat Leeaphorn [10], Michael A. Mao [11], Nadeen J. Khoury [12] and Wisit Cheungpasitporn [9]

[1] Department of Epidemiology, Harvard T.H. Chan School of Public Health, Boston, MA 02115, USA; api.che@hotmail.com

[2] Department of Internal Medicine, Faculty of Medicine, Chulalongkorn University, Bangkok 10300, Thailand

[3] Division of Nephrology and Hypertension, Mayo Clinic, Rochester, MN 55905, USA

[4] Department of Internal Medicine, University of Arizona, Tucson, AZ 85721, USA; tarunjacobb@gmail.com

[5] Division of Nephrology, Department of Medicine, Deaconess Health System, Evansville, IN 47747, USA; dr.anreddy@gmail.com

[6] Department of Internal Medicine, East Tennessee State University, Johnson City, TN 37614, USA; boonpipop.b@gmail.com

[7] Department of Military and Community Medicine, Phramongkutklao College of Medicine, Bangkok 10400, Thailand; wisitnephro@gmail.com

[8] Department of Internal Medicine, Bassett Medical Center, Cooperstown, NY 13326, USA; kanramon@gmail.com (K.W.); ploypinlert@gmail.com (P.L.); drkonika@gmail.com (K.S.)

[9] Division of Nephrology, Department of Medicine, University of Mississippi Medical Center, Jackson, MS 39216, USA; Aldo_t86@hotmail.com (A.T.-O.); wcheungpasitporn@gmail.com (W.C.)

[10] Department of Nephrology, Department of Medicine, Saint Luke's Health System, Kansas City, MO 64111, USA; napat.leeaphorn@gmail.com

[11] Division of Nephrology and Hypertension, Mayo Clinic, Jacksonville, FL 32224, USA; mao.michael@mayo.edu

[12] Department of Nephrology, Department of Medicine, Henry Ford Hospital, Detroit, MI 48202, USA; nadeenj.khoury@gmail.com

* Correspondence: charat.thongprayoon@gmail.com

Received: 31 March 2019; Accepted: 15 April 2019; Published: 17 April 2019

Abstract: Background: The incidence and mortality of renal cell carcinoma (RCC) after kidney transplantation (KTx) remain unclear. This study's aims were (1) to investigate the pooled incidence/incidence trends, and (2) to assess the mortality/mortality trends in KTx patients with RCC. Methods: A literature search was conducted using the MEDLINE, EMBASE and Cochrane databases from inception through October 2018. Studies that reported the incidence or mortality of RCC among kidney transplant recipients were included. The pooled incidence and 95% CI were calculated using a random-effect model. The protocol for this meta-analysis is registered with PROSPERO; no. CRD42018108994. Results: A total of 22 observational studies with a total of 320,190 KTx patients were enrolled. Overall, the pooled estimated incidence of RCC after KTx was 0.7% (95% CI: 0.5–0.8%, I^2 = 93%). While the pooled estimated incidence of de novo RCC in the native kidney was 0.7% (95% CI: 0.6–0.9%, I^2 = 88%), the pooled estimated incidence of RCC in the allograft kidney was 0.2% (95% CI: 0.1–0.4%, I^2 = 64%). The pooled estimated mortality rate in KTx recipients with RCC was 15.0% (95% CI: 7.4–28.1%, I^2 = 80%) at a mean follow-up time of 42 months after RCC diagnosis. While meta-regression analysis showed a significant negative correlation between year of study and incidence of de novo RCC post-KTx (slopes = −0.05, p = 0.01), there were no significant correlations between the year of study and mortality of patients with RCC (p = 0.50). Egger's regression asymmetry test was performed and showed no publication bias in all analyses. Conclusions: The overall estimated incidence of RCC after KTX was 0.7%. Although there has been a potential decrease in the incidence of RCC post-KTx, mortality in KTx patients with RCC has not decreased over time.

Keywords: malignancy; post-transplant malignancy; renal cell carcinoma; meta-analysis; kidney transplantation; transplantation; systematic reviews

---

1. Introduction

Kidney transplantation (KTx) is the renal replacement therapy of choice for the majority of patients with end-stage renal disease (ESRD) and it significantly improves survival and quality of life [1,2]. The long-term mortality rate is 48% to 82% lower in KTx recipients when compared to ESRD patients on the transplant waitlist [2,3]. However, due to immunosuppression, KTx patients are at a two-fold increased risk of developing malignancy in comparison to the general population [4–6]. Malignancies are among the top three leading causes of death in KTx recipients, following infection and cardiovascular complications [6].

Studies have demonstrated a higher incidence of renal cell carcinoma (RCC) among ESRD patients (0.3%) than its reported incidence in the general population (approximately 0.005%) [7,8]. Thus, the Clinical Practice Guidelines Committee of the American Society of Transplantation (AST) [9] has recommended RCC screening for high-risk candidates, such as ESRD patients on dialysis for more than 3 years [10]. Despite screening for RCC among KTx candidates, de novo RCC has been reported among KTx patients in both native kidneys [11–18], and transplanted kidneys [17,19,20]. However, the incidence and incidence trends of RCC among KTx patients remain unclear [11–42].

Thus, we performed a systematic review to (1) investigate the pooled incidence/incidence trends, and (2) assess the mortality/mortality trends in KTx patients with RCC.

2. Methods

2.1. Search Strategy and Literature Review

The protocol for this systematic review is registered with PROSPERO (International Prospective Register of Systematic Reviews; no. CRD42018108994). A systematic literature search of MEDLINE (1946 to October 2018), EMBASE (1988 to October 2018), and the Cochrane Database of Systematic Reviews (database inception to October 2018) was performed to assess (1) the pooled incidence/incidence trends, and (2) to assess the mortality/mortality trends in KTx patients with RCC. The systematic literature review was conducted independently by two investigators (C.T. and W.C) using a search strategy that consolidated the terms "kidney cancer" OR "renal cell carcinoma" AND "kidney transplantation" OR "renal transplantation" which is provided in the online Supplementary Data S1. The database searches were limited to English language articles only. A manual search for conceivably related studies using references of the included articles was also performed. This study was conducted using the Preferred Reporting Items for Systematic Reviews and Meta-Analysis (PRISMA) statement [43].

2.2. Selection Criteria

Eligible studies had to be clinical trials or observational studies (cohort, case-control, or cross-sectional studies) that reported the incidence or mortality of RCC among adult KTx recipients (age >/= 18 years old). Retrieved articles were individually reviewed for eligibility by two investigators (A.C. and C.T.). Discrepancies were addressed and solved by mutual consensus. Inclusion was not limited by the size of study.

2.3. Data Abstraction

A structured data collecting form was used to obtain the following information from each study: title, name of the first author, year of the study, publication year, country where the study was conducted, RCC definition, incidence of RCC, and mortality in KTx patients with RCC.

2.4. Statistical Analysis

Analyses were performed utilizing the Comprehensive Meta-Analysis 3.3 software (Biostat Inc, Englewood, NJ, USA). Adjusted point estimates from each study were consolidated by the generic inverse variance approach of DerSimonian and Laird, which designated the weight of each study based on its variance [44]. Given the possibility of between-study variance, we used a random-effect model rather than a fixed-effect model. Forest plots were constructed to visually evaluate the incidence and mortality of RCC among adult KTx recipients. Cochran's Q test and I^2 statistic were applied to determine the between-study heterogeneity. A value of I^2 of 0–25% represents insignificant heterogeneity, 26–50% low heterogeneity, 51–75% moderate heterogeneity and 76–100% high heterogeneity [45]. The presence of publication bias was assessed using the Egger test [46]. Funnel plots were created to evaluate for the presence or absence of publication bias.

3. Results

A total of 7815 potentially eligible articles were identified using our search strategy. After the exclusion of 7629 articles based on their title and abstract for clearly not fulfilling the inclusion criteria on the basis of type of article, patient population, study design, or outcome of interest, and 81 due to being duplicates, 105 articles were left for full-length review. Fifty-nine of them were excluded from the full-length review as they did not report the outcome of interest. Twenty-one articles were case reports and three articles were not in English. Thus, 22 cohort studies [11–20,23,28–36,38,39] with a total of 320,190 KTx patients were enrolled. The literature retrieval, review, and selection process are demonstrated in Figure 1. The characteristics of the included studies are presented in Table 1.

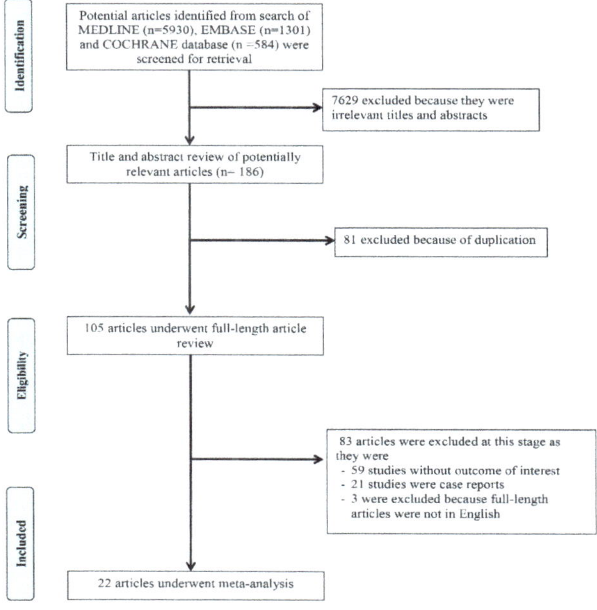

Figure 1. Outline of our search methodology.

Table 1. Main characteristics of studies included in the meta-analysis of incidence and mortality of renal cell carcinoma (RCC) after kidney transplantation (KTx) [11–20,23,28–36,38,39].

Study	Year	Type of Study	Number of Patients	Incidence of RCC	Follow-Up Time after Transplant	Time from Transplant to Cancer Diagnosis	Mortality of RCC	Quality Assessment
Hoshida et al. [11]	1997	Cohort	1744	15/1744	N/A	N/A	N/A	S4 C0 O3
Agraharkar et al. [12]	2004	Cohort	1739	6/1739	Mean 6.1 years	N/A	N/A	S4 C1 O3
Neuzillet et al. [13]	2004	Cohort	933	11/933	N/A	Mean 70.9 ± 49.4 (range 8–156) months	2/11 (1 died due to cancer)	S4 C0 O2
Moudouni et al. [14]	2006	Cohort	373	10/373	N/A	Mean 12.8 years Median 127 in patients treated with cyclosporine A and 114 months in patients not treated with cyclosporine A	1/10 (1 died due to cancer)	S4 C0 O3
Ianhez et al. [39]	2007	Cohort	1375	10/1375 9 in native kidney 1 in allograft kidney	N/A	N/A	3/10 (2 died due to myocardial infarction and one due to penile cancer)	S4 C0 O2
Schwarz et al. [38]	2007	Cohort	561	8/561 7 de novo in native kidney 1 de novo in allograft kidney	N/A	105.2 ± 62.39 months	N/A	S4C2O3
Tsai et al. [15]	2008	Cohort	3259	Touring group 15/215 kidney cancer Domestic group 4/321 kidney cancer	Touring group Mean 76.2 ± 48.1 months Domestic group Mean 81.5 ± 53.4 months	N/A	N/A	S4 C1 O3
Filocamo et al. [16]	2009	cohort	694	Native de novo 10/694	N/A	61.8 months (12–156 months)	3/10 (3 died due to cancer other than RCC)	S4 C1 O3
Leveridge et al. [17]	2010	cohort	3568	39/3568 native kidney 8/3568 allograft kidney	6.6 years	Native 10.6 years allograft 12.1 years	5 native died (not RCC cause), 1 allograft died due to cardiac cause	S4 C0 O3
Hwang et al. [18]	2011	Cohort	1695	7/1695	9.1 ± 6.9 years	Mean 11.8 ± 6.0 years	N/A	S4 C0 O3
Lee et al. [28]	2011	Cohort	2757	21/2757	N/A	Mean 119 (range 0–264) months	N/A	S4 C1 O2
Ploussard et al. [20]	2012	Cohort	2396	Allograft kidney 12/2396	N/A	Mean 13 (range 4–20) years	0/12	S4 C0 O3
Einollahi et al. [29]	2012	Cohort	12,525	6/12,525	N/A	Median 16 months	N/A	S4 C0 O3
Gigante et al. [30]	2012	Cohort	213	N/A	N/A	Mean 91 ± 82 months	6/213 due to RCC	S4 C0 O2

Table 1. *Cont.*

Study	Year	Type of Study	Number of Patients	Incidence of RCC	Follow-Up Time after Transplant	Time from Transplant to Cancer Diagnosis	Mortality of RCC	Quality Assessment
Tillou et al. [19]	2012	Cohort	41,806	Allograft kidney 79/41,806	N/A	Mean 131.7 (0.9–244) months	4/79	S4 C0 O3
Cheung et al. [31]	2012	Cohort	4895	26/4895	N/A	Median 4 (0.2–16.5) years	N/A	S4 C1 O3
Piselli et al. [32]	2013	Cohort	7217	31/7217	Median 5.2 years (2.9–7.8)	N/A	N/A	S4 C1 O3
Ryosaka et al. [33]	2015	Cohort	202	N/A	N/A	N/A	Solid-type renal cell carcinoma 2/17 Cystic-type renal cell carcinoma 2/27	S4 C0 O3
Kalil et al. [34]	2015	Cohort	115,845	Primary kidney transplant 514/109,224 Retransplant 43/6621	Mean 1st–4.6 years 2nd–3.7 years 3rd–2.9 years 4th–3.4 years	N/A	N/A	S4 C2 O3
Karami et al. [35]	2016	Cohort	116,208	683/116,208	Median 4.2 years (range 0.003–23.1)	N/A	N/A	S4 C0 O2
Takagi et al. [36]	2017	Cohort	42	N/A	N/A	Mean 86 ± 69 months	9/42 (5 died due to cancer)	S4 C0 O3
Cognard et al. [23]	2018	Cohort	143 with history of pre-transplant kidney cancer	13/143	Mean 5.6 ± 3.2 years	Mean 3 ± 2.3 years (range 45 days–7 years)	10/13 (9 died due to cancer)	S4 C0 O3

KTx, kidney transplantation; N/A, not available; RCC, renal cell carcinoma; S, C, O, selection, comparability, and outcome.

3.1. Incidence of RCC after KTx

Eighteen studies provided data on the incidence of RCC after KTx [11–20,28,29,31,32,34,35]. Overall, the pooled estimated incidence of RCC after KTx was 0.7% (95% CI: 0.5–0.8%, I^2 = 93%, Figure 2). While the pooled estimated incidence of de novo RCC in the native kidney was 0.7% (95% CI: 0.6–0.9%, I^2 = 88%, Figure 3A), the pooled estimated incidence of RCC in the allograft kidney was 0.2% (95% CI: 0.1–0.4%, I^2 = 64%, Figure 3B).

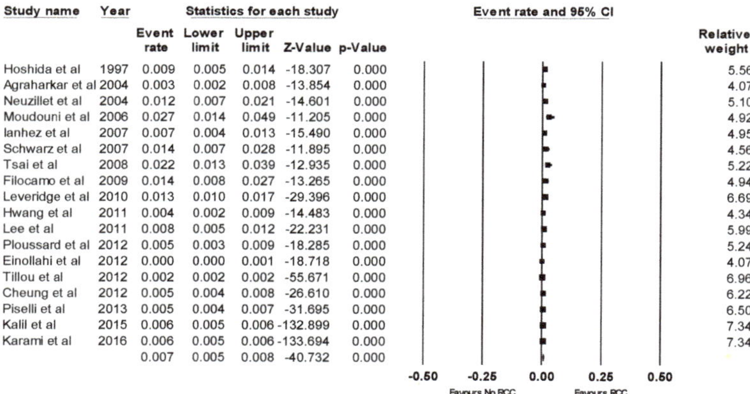

Figure 2. Forest plots of the included studies [11–20,28,29,31,32,34,35,38,39] assessing incidence rates of RCC after KTx. A diamond data marker represents the overall rate from each included study (square data marker) and 95% confidence interval.

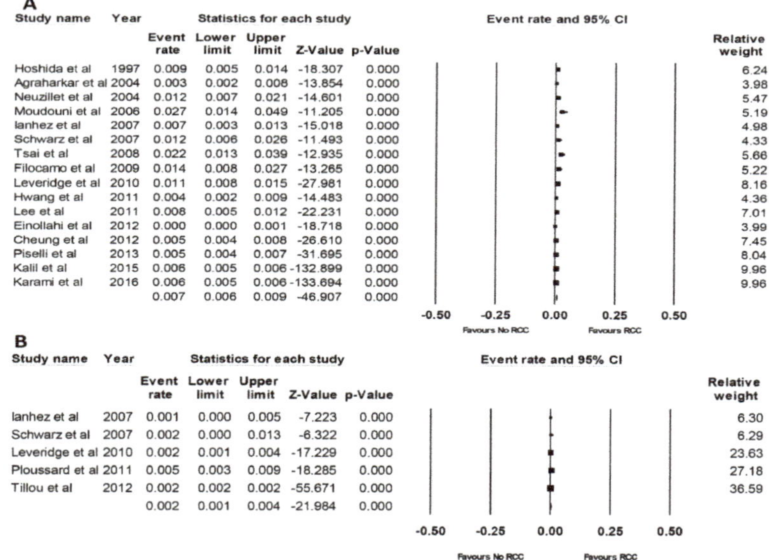

Figure 3. Forest plots of the included studies [11–18,28,29,31,32,34,35,38,39] assessing incidence rates of (**A**) de novo RCC in the native kidney and (**B**) RCC in the allograft kidney [17,19,20,38,39]. A diamond data marker represents the overall rate from each included study (square data marker) and 95% confidence interval.

Meta-regression showed a significant negative correlation between year of study and incidence of de novo RCC post-KTx (slopes = −0.05, *p* = 0.01, Figure 4).

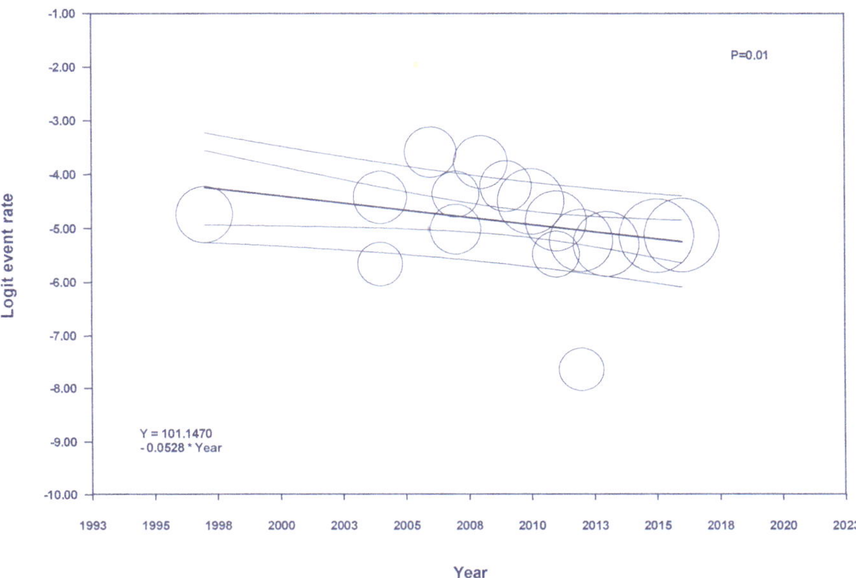

Figure 4. Meta-regression analyses showed a significant negative correlation between the year of study and incidence of de novo RCC post-KTx (slopes = −0.05, *p* = 0.01). The solid line represents the weighted regression line based on variance-weighted least squares. The inner and outer lines show the 95% confidence interval and prediction interval around the regression line. The circles indicate the log event rates in each study.

3.2. Mortality Rate in KTx Recipients with RCC

Eleven studies provided data the on mortality rate in KTx recipients with RCC [13,14,16,17,19,20,23,30,33,36,39]. Overall, the pooled estimated mortality rate in KTx recipients with RCC was 15.0% (95% CI: 7.4–28.1%, I^2 = 80%, Figure 5) at a mean follow-up time of 42 months after RCC diagnosis. The data on the incidence and mortality of recurrent RCC among KTx recipients with a previous history of RCC prior to KTX were limited. A prior study demonstrated an incidence of recurrent RCC after KTX of 9.1% with an associated 5-year survival of 41.7% [23]. Sensitivity analysis, excluding the study of recurrent RCC among KTx recipients with a previous history of RCC prior to KTX (23), demonstrated a pooled estimated mortality rate of 11.5% in KTx recipients with RCC (95% CI: 6.4–19.8%, I^2 = 67%).

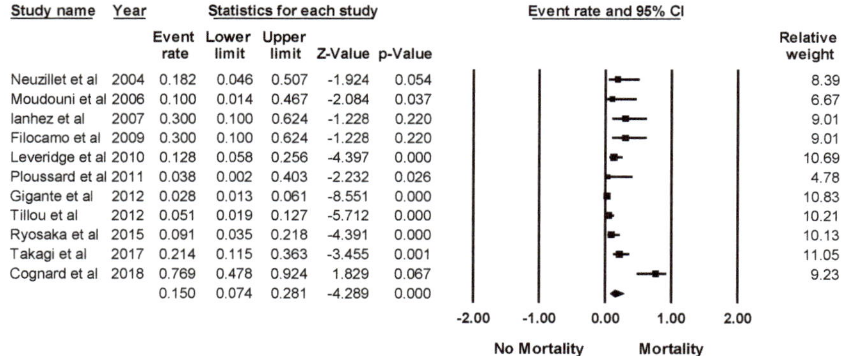

Figure 5. Forest plots of the included studies [13,14,16,17,19,20,23,30,33,36,39] assessing mortality rate in KTx recipients with RCC. A diamond data marker represents the overall rate from each included study (square data marker) and 95% confidence interval.

Meta-regression showed no significant correlations between the year of study and mortality of patients with RCC (p = 0.50, Figure 6). When meta-regression was performed excluding the study of recurrent RCC among KTx recipients with a previous history of RCC prior to KTX [30], there were still no significant correlations between the year of study and mortality of patients with RCC (p = 0.56, Figure 7).

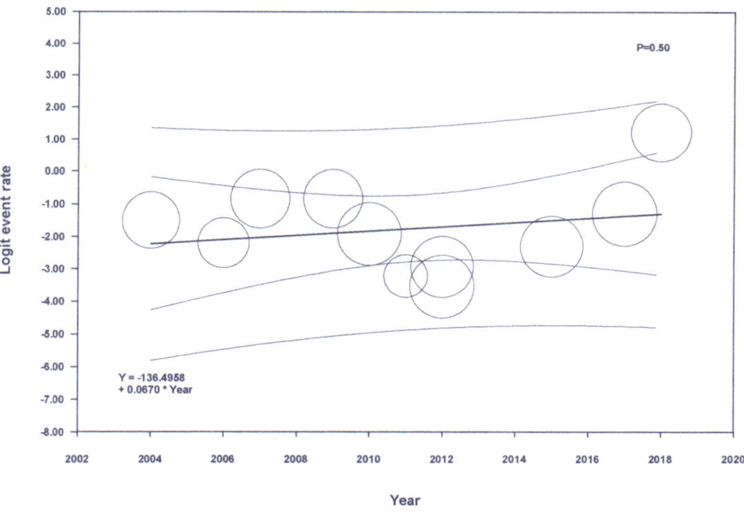

Figure 6. Meta-regression analyses showed no significant correlations between the year of study and mortality of patients with RCC (p = 0.50). The solid line represents the weighted regression line based on variance-weighted least-squares. The inner and outer lines show the 95% confidence interval and prediction interval around the regression line. The circles indicate the log event rates in each study.

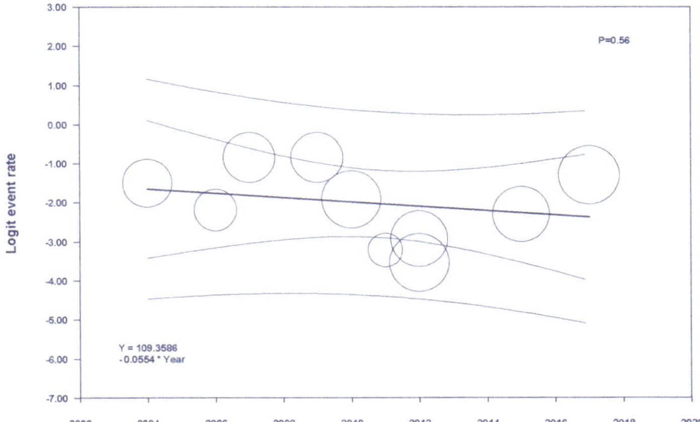

Figure 7. Meta-regression analyses, excluding the study of recurrent RCC among KTx recipients with a previous history of RCC prior to KTX, showed no significant correlations between the year of study and mortality of patients with RCC ($p = 0.56$). The solid line represents the weighted regression line based on variance-weighted least-squares. The inner and outer lines show the 95% confidence interval and prediction interval around the regression line. The circles indicate log event rates in each study.

3.3. Evaluation for Publication Bias

Funnel plots (Supplementary Figures S1 and S2) and Egger's regression asymmetry tests were performed to evaluate publication bias in the analysis evaluating the incidence and mortality of KTx recipients with RCC. There was no significant publication bias, with p-values of 0.58 and 0.54, respectively.

4. Discussion

In this systematic review, we found that RCC after KTx occurs with an incidence of 0.7%. RCC can occur in the native kidney with an incidence of 0.7% or in the allograft kidney with an incidence of 0.2%. Our findings also showed a statistically significant negative correlation between the incidence of RCC after KTx and study year, representing a potential decrease in the RCC incidence among KTx patients. However, mortality in KTx patients with RCC has not decreased over time.

Post-KTx malignancy is a common cause of death [5,6,47–51] and RCC is the most common solid-organ malignancy in this population [52,53]. Due to the increased risk of RCC among ESRD patients [7,8], the Clinical Practice Guidelines Committee of the AST has suggested RCC screening in ESRD patients on dialysis for longer than 3 years [9,10]. In addition, it is suggested that most KTx candidates with a history of RCC should wait at least 2 years from successful cancer treatment to KTx (unless candidates have only small localized incidental tumors, which may not require any waiting period) [54,55]. Candidates with large, invasive or symptomatic RCC may require a longer waiting period of 5 years [54,55]. Despite RCC screening prior to KTx, the findings from our study suggest that RCC can still occur post-KTx at a higher incidence (0.7%) than its reported incidence among ESRD patients (0.3%) [8]. In addition, studies have demonstrated that KTx recipients have a relative increased risk of five- to ten-fold for RCC compared with an age-matched general population, and that the majority of these tumors arise in the setting of acquired kidney cystic disease (AKCD) which develops with chronic renal failure [5,8,35,56–64]. Although RCC occurrence is more frequent in the native kidneys of KTx recipients, RCC can also occur in the renal allograft (incidence of 0.2%) [17,19,20].

While the exact etiology of the increased risk of RCC in KTx remains unclear, it is likely linked to the immunosuppressed state [4]. Reported risk factors for post-KTx RCC include older age, male sex, African descent, excess body weight, smoking, hypertension, history of acquired cystic kidney disease (ACKD), previous RCC prior to KTx, and longer pre-transplant dialysis duration [3,6,18,23,29,31,34,35,65–67]. Studies have shown that causes of ESRD before KTx may also affect the incidence of post-KTx RCC [14,32,35]. While KTx recipients with ESRD due to glomerulonephritis, hypertensive nephrosclerosis, and vascular diseases have been shown to have a higher incidence of post-KTx RCC, recipients with ESRD due to diabetic nephropathy carry a lower risk of post-KTx RCC [14,32,35,68]. KTx recipients are usually under intensified medical surveillance and the higher incidence of RCC among KTx recipients compared to general populations and ESRD patients might be due to detection bias. On the other hand, the lack of consensual RCC screening among KTx recipients may also have underestimated the exact incidence among the KTx patient population. Currently, there are no universal recommendations for RCC screening among KTx patients [3,22,69–72]. While the European Renal Best Practice (ERBP) guidelines recommend native kidney ultrasound as RCC screening in kidney transplant recipients, and the European Association of Urology (EAU) recommends an annual ultrasound of native kidneys and allografts for anyone with ACKD, previous RCC, or von Hippel–Lindau disease [3,71,72], the Kidney Disease Improving Global Outcomes (KDIGO) and AST guidelines for post-KTx care currently do not suggest universal screening for RCC among KTx recipients [22,69,70]. Thus, there are various RCC screening approaches for KTx recipients at different transplant centers. Many cases of RCC have been discovered during investigations for post-transplant erythrocytosis, elevated serum creatinine, hematuria, urinary infection, or incidentally from imaging for other indications [33,73–75]. The majority of studies with available data on surveillance programs performed screening for RCC post-KTx annually by ultrasonography of native and allograft kidneys. Among KTx recipients with ACKD, acquired multicystic dysplasia, or a prior history of RCC required more frequent screenings, every 6 months [16,17,19,20,28,36,76]. Given that the risk is greatest in the first year post-KTx and the majority of RCCs occur in the first 5 years after KTx [15,29,31,65,77], previous reports suggest that KTx recipients should routinely undergo ultrasonography to screen RCC on the native kidney during the first 30 days post-KTx and every 5 years afterwards in the absence of renal cysts, or every 2 years in the presence of renal cysts [65,77–79]. Our study's findings suggest the need for future studies to identify a cost-effective surveillance strategy for RCC among KTx recipients. This strategy would need to take into consideration both native and allograft kidneys, and differentiate KTx recipients with non-simple renal cysts [3,80].

Several limitations of our systematic review are worth mentioning. First, there are statistical heterogeneities in our meta-analysis. Potential sources for heterogeneities were the variations in the renal transplant recipient screening methods, patient characteristics, and differences in the immunosuppressive regimens used at various transplant centers, which may have affected the incidence of RCC and mortality rate in this population. Second, there is a lack of data from included studies on immunosuppressive regimens [81–85]. Mammalian target of rapamycin (mTOR) inhibitors have shown antineoplastic activities [86]. Although the effects of mTOR among KTx recipients have been shown mostly for non-melanoma skin cancer [87–89], future studies evaluating the effects of different immunosuppressive regimens on mortality in KTx patients with RCC are needed. Lastly, this is a meta-analysis of cohort studies and the data from population-based studies were limited. Thus, large population-based studies evaluating the incidence of RCC in KTx patients are required in the future.

In summary, the overall estimated incidence of RCC after KTX was 0.6%, with an associated high mortality rate in KTx recipients of 13.9%. Despite potential improvements in the post-KTx RCC incidence, the mortality in KTx patients with RCC has remained unchanged over time.

Supplementary Materials: The following are available online at http://www.mdpi.com/2077-0383/8/4/530/s1, Data S1: Search terms for systematic review; Figure S1: Funnel plot evaluating for publication bias evaluating incidence of KTx recipients with RCC; Figure S2: Funnel plot evaluating for publication bias evaluating mortality of KTx recipients with RCC.

Author Contributions: Conceptualization, A.C., C.T., W.K., M.A.M., N.J.K. and W.C.; Data curation, A.C. and C.T.; Formal analysis, C.T. and W.C.; Investigation, A.C., C.T. and W.C.; Methodology, A.C., T.B., B.B., W.K., P.L., N.L. and W.C.; Project administration, K.W. and K.S.; Resources, K.W. and K.S.; Software, K.W.; Supervision, T.B., N.R.A., B.B., W.K., A.T.-O., N.L., M.A., N.J. and W.C.; Validation, A.C., C.T., P.L. and W.C.; Visualization, T.B. and K.S.; Writing—original draft, A.C. and N.R.; Writing—review and editing, C.T., T.B., N.R.A., B.B., W.K., K.W., P.L., K.S., A.T.-O., N.L., M.A.M., N.J.K. and W.C.

Conflicts of Interest: The authors declare no conflict of interest.

References

1. Kaballo, M.A.; Canney, M.; O'Kelly, P.; Williams, Y.; O'Seaghdha, C.M.; Conlon, P.J. A comparative analysis of survival of patients on dialysis and after kidney transplantation. *Clin. Kidney J.* **2018**, *11*, 389–393. [CrossRef] [PubMed]
2. Wolfe, R.A.; Ashby, V.B.; Milford, E.L.; Ojo, A.O.; Ettenger, R.E.; Agodoa, L.Y.; Held, P.J.; Port, F.K. Comparison of mortality in all patients on dialysis, patients on dialysis awaiting transplantation, and recipients of a first cadaveric transplant. *N. Engl. J. Med.* **1999**, *341*, 1725–1730. [CrossRef] [PubMed]
3. Hickman, L.A.; Sawinski, D.; Guzzo, T.; Locke, J.E. Urologic malignancies in kidney transplantation. *Am. J. Transpl.* **2018**, *18*, 13–22. [CrossRef] [PubMed]
4. Engels, E.A.; Pfeiffer, R.M.; Fraumeni, J.F.; Jr Kasiske, B.L.; Israni, A.K.; Snyder, J.J.; Wolfe, R.A.; Goodrich, N.P.; Bayakly, A.R.; Clarke, C.A.; et al. Spectrum of cancer risk among US solid organ transplant recipients. *JAMA* **2011**, *306*, 1891–1901. [CrossRef] [PubMed]
5. Bennett, W.M.; Simonich, E.L.; Garre, A.M.; McEvoy, K.M.; Farinola, M.A.; Batiuk, T.D. Renal Cell Carcinoma in Renal Transplantation: The Case for Surveillance. *Transpl. Proc.* **2017**, *49*, 1779–1782. [CrossRef]
6. Briggs, J.D. Causes of death after renal transplantation. *Nephrol Dial. Transpl.* **2001**, *16*, 1545–1549. [CrossRef]
7. Dy, G.W.; Gore, J.L.; Forouzanfar, M.H.; Naghavi, M.; Fitzmaurice, C. Global Burden of Urologic Cancers, 1990. *Eur. Urol.* **2017**, *71*, 437–446. [CrossRef] [PubMed]
8. Kompotiatis, P.; Thongprayoon, C.; Manohar, S.; Cheungpasitporn, W.; Gonzalez Suarez, M.L.; Craici, I.M.; Mao, M.A.; Herrmann, S.M. Association between urologic malignancies and end-stage renal disease: A meta-analysis. *Nephrology* **2019**, *24*, 65–73. [CrossRef] [PubMed]
9. Kasiske, B.L.; Cangro, C.B.; Hariharan, S.; Hricik, D.E.; Kerman, R.H.; Roth, D.; Rush, D.N.; Vazquez, M.A.; Weir, M.R. The evaluation of renal transplantation candidates: Clinical practice guidelines. *Am. J. Transplant.* **2001**, *1* (Suppl. 2), 3–95.
10. Holley, J.L. Screening, diagnosis, and treatment of cancer in long-term dialysis patients. *Clin. J. Am. Soc. Nephrol.* **2007**, *2*, 604–610. [CrossRef] [PubMed]
11. Hoshida, Y.; Tsukuma, H.; Yasunaga, Y.; Xu, N.; Fujita, M.Q.; Satoh, T.; Ichikawa, Y.; Kurihara, K.; Imanishi, M.; Matsuno, T.; et al. Cancer risk after renal transplantation in Japan. *Int. J. Cancer* **1997**, *71*, 517–520. [CrossRef]
12. Agraharkar, M.L.; Cinclair, R.D.; Kuo, Y.F.; Daller, J.A.; Shahinian, V.B. Risk of malignancy with long-term immunosuppression in renal transplant recipients. *Kidney Int.* **2004**, *66*, 383–389. [CrossRef] [PubMed]
13. Neuzillet, Y.; Lay, F.; Luccioni, A.; Daniel, L.; Berland, Y.; Coulange, C.; Lechevallier, E. De novo renal cell carcinoma of native kidney in renal transplant recipients. *Cancer* **2005**, *103*, 251–257. [CrossRef] [PubMed]
14. Moudouni, S.M.; Lakmichi, A.; Tligui, M.; Rafii, A.; Tchala, K.; Haab, F.; Gattegno, B.; Thibault, P.; Doublet, J.D. Renal cell carcinoma of native kidney in renal transplant recipients. *BJU Int.* **2006**, *98*, 298–302. [CrossRef]
15. Tsai, M.K.; Yang, C.Y.; Lee, C.Y.; Yeh, C.C.; Hu, R.H.; Lee, P.H. De novo malignancy is associated with renal transplant tourism. *Kidney Int.* **2011**, *79*, 908–913. [CrossRef]
16. Filocamo, M.T.; Zanazzi, M.; Li Marzi, V.; Guidoni, L.; Villari, D.; Dattolo, E.; Nicita, G. Renal cell carcinoma of native kidney after renal transplantation: Clinical relevance of early detection. *Transpl. Proc.* **2009**, *41*, 4197–4201. [CrossRef] [PubMed]
17. Leveridge, M.; Musquera, M.; Evans, A.; Cardella, C.; Pei, Y.; Jewett, M.; Robinette, M.; Finelli, A. Renal cell carcinoma in the native and allograft kidneys of renal transplant recipients. *J. Urol.* **2011**, *186*, 219–223. [CrossRef]
18. Hwang, J.K.; Moon, I.S.; Kim, J.I. Malignancies after kidney transplantation: A 40-year single-center experience in Korea. *Transpl. Int.* **2011**, *24*, 716–721. [CrossRef] [PubMed]

19. Tillou, X.; Doerfler, A.; Collon, S.; Kleinclauss, F.; Patard, J.J.; Badet, L.; Barrou, B.; Audet, M.; Bensadoun, H.; Berthoux, E.; et al. De novo kidney graft tumors: Results from a multicentric retrospective national study. *Am. J. Transpl.* **2012**, *12*, 3308–3315. [CrossRef]

20. Ploussard, G.; Chambade, D.; Meria, P.; Gaudez, F.; Tariel, E.; Verine, J.; De Bazelaire, C.; Peraldi, M.N.; Glotz, D.; Desgrandchamps, F.; et al. Biopsy-confirmed de novo renal cell carcinoma (RCC) in renal grafts: A single-centre management experience in a 2396 recipient cohort. *BJU Int.* **2012**, *109*, 195–199. [CrossRef]

21. Scandling, J.D. Acquired cystic kidney disease and renal cell cancer after transplantation: Time to rethink screening? *Clin. J. Am. Soc. Nephrol.* **2007**, *2*, 621–622. [CrossRef]

22. Kasiske, B.L.; Vazquez, M.A.; Harmon, W.E.; Brown, R.S.; Danovitch, G.M.; Gaston, R.S.; Roth, D.; Scandling, J.D.; Singer, G.G. Recommendations for the outpatient surveillance of renal transplant recipients. American Society of Transplantation. *J. Am. Soc. Nephrol* **2000**, *11* (Suppl. 15), S1–S86. [PubMed]

23. Cognard, N.; Anglicheau, D.; Gatault, P.; Girerd, S.; Essig, M.; Hurault de Ligny, B.; Le Meur, Y.; Le Roy, F.; Garrouste, C.; Thierry, A.; et al. Recurrence of Renal Cell Cancer After Renal Transplantation in a Multicenter French Cohort. *Transplantation* **2018**, *102*, 860–867. [CrossRef] [PubMed]

24. EBPG Expert Group on Renal Transplantation. European best practice guidelines for renal transplantation. Section IV: Long-term management of the transplant recipient. IV.6. Cancer risk after renal transplantation. Solid organ cancers: Prevention and treatment. *Nephrol Dial. Transplant.* **2002**, *17* (Suppl. 4), 34–36.

25. Wiesel, M.; Carl, S.; Drehmer, I.; Hofmann, W.J.; Zeier, M.; Staehler, G. [The clinical significance of renal cell carcinoma in dialysis dependent patients in comparison with kidney transplant recipients]. *Urol. A* **1997**, *36*, 126–129. [CrossRef]

26. Gulanikar, A.C.; Daily, P.P.; Kilambi, N.K.; Hamrick-Turner, J.E.; Butkus, D.E. Prospective pretransplant ultrasound screening in 206 patients for acquired renal cysts and renal cell carcinoma. *Transplantation* **1998**, *66*, 1669–1672. [CrossRef]

27. Brunner, F.P.; Landais, P.; Selwood, N.H. Malignancies after renal transplantation: The EDTA-ERA registry experience. European Dialysis and Transplantation Association-European Renal Association. *Nephrol. Dial. Transplant.* **1995**, *10* (Suppl. 1), 74–80. [CrossRef] [PubMed]

28. Lee, H.H.; Choi, K.H.; Yang, S.C.; Han, W.K. Renal cell carcinoma in kidney transplant recipients and dialysis patients. *Korean J. Urol.* **2012**, *53*, 229–233. [CrossRef] [PubMed]

29. Einollahi, B.; Rostami, Z.; Nourbala, M.H.; Lessan-Pezeshki, M.; Simforoosh, N.; Nemati, E.; Pourfarziani, V.; Beiraghdar, F.; Nafar, M.; Pour-Reza-Gholi, F.; et al. Incidence of malignancy after living kidney transplantation: A multicenter study from iran. *J. Cancer* **2012**, *3*, 246–256. [CrossRef] [PubMed]

30. Gigante, M.; Neuzillet, Y.; Patard, J.J.; Tillou, X.; Thuret, R.; Branchereau, J.; Timsit, M.O.; Terrier, N.; Boutin, J.M.; Sallusto, F.; et al. Renal cell carcinoma (RCC) arising in native kidneys of dialyzed and transplant patients: Are they different entities? *BJU Int.* **2012**, *110*, E570–E573. [CrossRef] [PubMed]

31. Cheung, C.Y.; Lam, M.F.; Chu, K.H.; Chow, K.M.; Tsang, K.Y.; Yuen, S.K.; Wong, P.N.; Chan, S.K.; Leung, K.T.; Chan, C.K.; et al. Malignancies after kidney transplantation: Hong Kong renal registry. *Am. J. Transpl.* **2012**, *12*, 3039–3046. [CrossRef]

32. Piselli, P.; Busnach, G.; Citterio, F.; Richiardi, L.; Cimaglia, C.; Angeletti, C.; Doringhet, P.V.; Pozzetto, U.; Perrino, M.L.; Serraino, D. [Kidney transplant and cancer risk: An epidemiological study in Northern and Central Italy]. *Epidemiol. Prev.* **2008**, *32*, 205–211.

33. Ryosaka, M.; Ishida, H.; Takagi, T.; Shimizu, T.; Tanabe, K.; Kondo, T. Solid-type RCC originating from native kidneys in renal transplant recipients should be monitored cautiously. *Transpl. Int.* **2015**, *28*, 813–819. [CrossRef]

34. Kalil, R.S.; Lynch, C.F.; Engels, E.A. Risk of cancer in retransplants compared to primary kidney transplants in the United States. *Clin. Transpl.* **2015**, *29*, 944–950. [CrossRef]

35. Karami, S.; Yanik, E.L.; Moore, L.E.; Pfeiffer, R.M.; Copeland, G.; Gonsalves, L.; Hernandez, B.Y.; Lynch, C.F.; Pawlish, K.; Engels, E.A. Risk of Renal Cell Carcinoma Among Kidney Transplant Recipients in the United States. *Am. J. Transpl.* **2016**, *16*, 3479–3489. [CrossRef]

36. Takagi, T.; Kondo, T.; Okumi, M.; Ishida, H.; Tanabe, K. Differences in Clinical and Pathological Features of Renal Cell Carcinoma Between Japanese Patients After Kidney Transplantation and Those on Hemodialysis. *Ther. Apher. Dial.* **2017**, *21*, 133–138. [CrossRef]

37. Olsson, C.A. Renal cell carcinoma (RCC) arising in native kidneys of dialyzed and transplant patients: Are they different entities? *BJU Int.* **2012**, *110*, E574. [CrossRef]

38. Schwarz, A.; Vatandaslar, S.; Merkel, S.; Haller, H. Renal cell carcinoma in transplant recipients with acquired cystic kidney disease. *Clin. J. Am. Soc. Nephrol.* **2007**, *2*, 750–756. [CrossRef] [PubMed]
39. Ianhez, L.E.; Lucon, M.; Nahas, W.C.; Sabbaga, E.; Saldanha, L.B.; Lucon, A.M.; Srougi, M. Renal cell carcinoma in renal transplant patients. *Urology* **2007**, *69*, 462–464. [CrossRef] [PubMed]
40. Levine, E. Renal cell carcinoma in uremic acquired renal cystic disease: Incidence, detection, and management. *Urol Radiol* **1992**, *13*, 203–210. [CrossRef] [PubMed]
41. Doublet, J.D.; Peraldi, M.N.; Gattegno, B.; Thibault, P.; Sraer, J.D. Renal cell carcinoma of native kidneys: Prospective study of 129 renal transplant patients. *J. Urol.* **1997**, *158*, 42–44. [CrossRef]
42. Nie, H.; Wang, W.; Zhao, Y.; Zhang, X.; Xiao, Y.; Zeng, Q.; Zhang, C.; Zhang, L. New-Onset Diabetes After Renal Transplantation (NODAT): Is It a Risk Factor for Renal Cell Carcinoma or Renal Failure? *Ann. Transpl.* **2019**, *24*, 62–69. [CrossRef]
43. Moher, D.; Liberati, A.; Tetzlaff, J.; Altman, D.G. Preferred reporting items for systematic reviews and meta-analyses: The PRISMA statement. *PLoS Med.* **2009**, *6*, e1000097. [CrossRef]
44. DerSimonian, R.; Laird, N. Meta-analysis in clinical trials. *Controll. Clin. Trials* **1986**, *7*, 177–188. [CrossRef]
45. Higgins, J.P.; Thompson, S.G.; Deeks, J.J.; Altman, D.G. Measuring inconsistency in meta-analyses. *BMJ* **2003**, *327*, 557–560. [CrossRef]
46. Easterbrook, P.J.; Berlin, J.A.; Gopalan, R.; Matthews, D.R. Publication bias in clinical research. *Lancet* **1991**, *337*, 867–872. [CrossRef]
47. Penn, I. Primary kidney tumors before and after renal transplantation. *Transplantation* **1995**, *59*, 480–485. [CrossRef]
48. Kasiske, B.L.; Snyder, J.J.; Gilbertson, D.T.; Wang, C. Cancer after kidney transplantation in the United States. *Am. J. Transplant.* **2004**, *4*, 905–913. [CrossRef]
49. Pedotti, P.; Cardillo, M.; Rossini, G.; Arcuri, V.; Boschiero, L.; Caldara, R.; Cannella, G.; Dissegna, D.; Gotti, E.; Marchini, F.; et al. Incidence of cancer after kidney transplant: Results from the North Italy transplant program. *Transplantation* **2003**, *76*, 1448–1451. [CrossRef]
50. Bellini, M.I.; Gopal, J.P.; Hill, P.; Nicol, D.; Gibbons, N. Urothelial Carcinoma arising from the transplanted kidney: A single centre experience and literature review. *Clin. Transplant.* **2019**. [CrossRef]
51. Benoni, H.; Eloranta, S.; Ekbom, A.; Wilczek, H.; Smedby, K.E. Survival among solid organ transplant recipients diagnosed with cancer compared to nontransplanted cancer patients-A nationwide study. *Int. J. Cancer* **2019**. [CrossRef] [PubMed]
52. Vajdic, C.M.; McDonald, S.P.; McCredie, M.R.; van Leeuwen, M.T.; Stewart, J.H.; Law, M.; Chapman, J.R.; Webster, A.C.; Kaldor, J.M.; Grulich, A.E. Cancer incidence before and after kidney transplantation. *JAMA* **2006**, *296*, 2823–2831. [CrossRef] [PubMed]
53. Birkeland, S.A.; Lokkegaard, H.; Storm, H.H. Cancer risk in patients on dialysis and after renal transplantation. *Lancet* **2000**, *355*, 1886–1887. [CrossRef]
54. Knoll, G.; Cockfield, S.; Blydt-Hansen, T.; Baran, D.; Kiberd, B.; Landsberg, D.; Rush, D.; Cole, E. Canadian Society of Transplantation: Consensus guidelines on eligibility for kidney transplantation. *CMAJ* **2005**, *173*, S1–S25. [CrossRef] [PubMed]
55. Knoll, G.; Cockfield, S.; Blydt-Hansen, T.; Baran, D.; Kiberd, B.; Landsberg, D.; Rush, D.; Cole, E. Canadian Society of Transplantation consensus guidelines on eligibility for kidney transplantation. *CMAJ* **2005**, *173*, 1181–1184. [CrossRef] [PubMed]
56. Butler, A.M.; Olshan, A.F.; Kshirsagar, A.V.; Edwards, J.K.; Nielsen, M.E.; Wheeler, S.B.; Brookhart, M.A. Cancer incidence among US Medicare ESRD patients receiving hemodialysis, 1996–2009. *Am. J. Kidney Dis.* **2015**, *65*, 763–772. [CrossRef]
57. Zorbas, K.A.; Karhadkar, S.S.; Lau, K.N.; Di Carlo, A. Renal Cell Carcinoma in Kidney Transplant Candidates. *Transpl. Proc.* **2017**, *49*, 1312–1317. [CrossRef]
58. Tillou, X.; Guleryuz, K.; Doerfler, A.; Bensadoun, H.; Chambade, D.; Codas, R.; Devonec, M.; Dugardin, F.; Erauso, A.; Hubert, J.; et al. Nephron sparing surgery for De Novo kidney graft tumor: Results from a multicenter national study. *Am. J. Transpl.* **2014**, *14*, 2120–2125. [CrossRef]
59. Krisl, J.C.; Doan, V.P. Chemotherapy and Transplantation: The Role of Immunosuppression in Malignancy and a Review of Antineoplastic Agents in Solid Organ Transplant Recipients. *Am. J. Transpl.* **2017**, *17*, 1974–1991. [CrossRef] [PubMed]

60. Purdue, M.P.; Moore, L.E.; Merino, M.J.; Boffetta, P.; Colt, J.S.; Schwartz, K.L.; Bencko, V.; Davis, F.G.; Graubard, B.I.; Janout, V.; et al. An investigation of risk factors for renal cell carcinoma by histologic subtype in two case-control studies. *Int. J. Cancer* **2013**, *132*, 2640–2647. [CrossRef]
61. Ishikawa, I. Uremic acquired renal cystic disease. Natural history and complications. *Nephron* **1991**, *58*, 257–267. [CrossRef] [PubMed]
62. Ishikawa, I. Uremic acquired cystic disease of kidney. *Urology* **1985**, *26*, 101–108. [CrossRef]
63. Levine, E.; Slusher, S.L.; Grantham, J.J.; Wetzel, L.H. Natural history of acquired renal cystic disease in dialysis patients: A prospective longitudinal CT study. *Am. J. Roentgenol.* **1991**, *156*, 501–506. [CrossRef] [PubMed]
64. Matson, M.A.; Cohen, E.P. Acquired cystic kidney disease: Occurrence, prevalence, and renal cancers. *Medicine* **1990**, *69*, 217–226. [CrossRef] [PubMed]
65. Goh, A.; Vathsala, A. Native renal cysts and dialysis duration are risk factors for renal cell carcinoma in renal transplant recipients. *Am. J. Transplant. Off. J. Am. Soc. Transplant. Am. Soc. Transpl. Surg.* **2011**, *11*, 86–92. [CrossRef] [PubMed]
66. Moris, D.; Kakavia, K.; Argyrou, C.; Garmpis, N.; Bokos, J.; Vernadakis, S.; Diles, K.; Sotirchos, G.; Boletis, J.; Zavos, G. De Novo Renal Cell Carcinoma of Native Kidneys in Renal Transplant Recipients: A Single-center Experience. *Anticancer Res.* **2017**, *37*, 773–779. [CrossRef]
67. Chow, W.H.; Devesa, S.S. Contemporary epidemiology of renal cell cancer. *Cancer J.* **2008**, *14*, 288–301. [CrossRef]
68. Dhakal, P.; Giri, S.; Siwakoti, K.; Rayamajhi, S.; Bhatt, V.R. Renal Cancer in Recipients of Kidney Transplant. *Rare Tumors* **2017**, *9*, 6550. [CrossRef] [PubMed]
69. Kidney Disease: Improving Global Outcomes (KDIGO) Transplant Work Group. KDIGO clinical practice guideline for the care of kidney transplant recipients. *Am. J. Transplant.* **2009**, *9* (Suppl. 3), S1–S155. [CrossRef]
70. Bia, M.; Adey, D.B.; Bloom, R.D.; Chan, L.; Kulkarni, S.; Tomlanovich, S. KDOQI US commentary on the 2009 KDIGO clinical practice guideline for the care of kidney transplant recipients. *Am. J. Kidney Dis.* **2010**, *56*, 189–218. [CrossRef]
71. European Renal Best Practice Transplantation Guideline Development Group. ERBP Guideline on the Management and Evaluation of the Kidney Donor and Recipient. *Nephrol. Dial. Transplant.* **2013**, *28* (Suppl. 2), ii1–ii71.
72. Kalble, T.; Lucan, M.; Nicita, G.; Sells, R.; Burgos Revilla, F.J.; Wiesel, M. EAU guidelines on renal transplantation. *Eur. Urol.* **2005**, *47*, 156–166. [CrossRef]
73. Fuiano, G.; Zoccali, C.; Bertoni, E.; Bartolomeo, F.; Cambareri, F.; Salvadori, M.; Altieri, P.; Ponticelli, C.; Sandrini, S.; Schena, F.P.; et al. [Guidelines for ambulatory monitoring of kidney transplant patients. Adaptation of the Guidelines of the American Society of Transplantation (J Am Soc Nephrol 2000; 11 (S1): 86)]. *Giornale italiano di nefrologia Organo ufficiale della Societa italiana di nefrologia* **2004**, *21* (Suppl. 28), S11–S50.
74. Marinella, M.A. Hematologic abnormalities following renal transplantation. *Int. Urol. Nephrol.* **2010**, *42*, 151–164. [CrossRef] [PubMed]
75. Park, P.; Kim, W.Y.; Lee, J.B.; Choi, S.B.; Kim, W.B.; Choi, S.Y. Incidental renal cell carcinoma originating from a native kidney after en-bloc resection for adrenal carcinoma in a kidney transplant recipient. *Transpl. Proc.* **2014**, *46*, 637–639. [CrossRef] [PubMed]
76. Brennan, J.F.; Stilmant, M.M.; Babayan, R.K.; Siroky, M.B. Acquired renal cystic disease: Implications for the urologist. *Br. J. Urol.* **1991**, *67*, 342–348. [CrossRef]
77. Klatte, T.; Seitz, C.; Waldert, M.; de Martino, M.; Kikic, Z.; Bohmig, G.A.; Haitel, A.; Schmidbauer, J.; Marberger, M.; Remzi, M. Features and outcomes of renal cell carcinoma of native kidneys in renal transplant recipients. *BJU Int.* **2010**, *105*, 1260–1265. [CrossRef] [PubMed]
78. Muruve, N.A.; Shoskes, D.A. Genitourinary malignancies in solid organ transplant recipients. *Transplantation* **2005**, *80*, 709–716. [CrossRef]
79. Ljungberg, B.; Cowan, N.C.; Hanbury, D.C.; Hora, M.; Kuczyk, M.A.; Merseburger, A.S.; Patard, J.J.; Mulders, P.F.; Sinescu, I.C. EAU guidelines on renal cell carcinoma: The 2010 update. *Eur. Urol.* **2010**, *58*, 398–406. [CrossRef] [PubMed]
80. Israel, G.M.; Bosniak, M.A. An update of the Bosniak renal cyst classification system. *Urology* **2005**, *66*, 484–488. [CrossRef]

81. Kauffman, H.M.; Cherikh, W.S.; McBride, M.A.; Cheng, Y.; Hanto, D.W. Post-transplant de novo malignancies in renal transplant recipients: The past and present. *Transpl. Int. Off. J. Eur. Soc. Organ. Transplant.* **2006**, *19*, 607–620. [CrossRef] [PubMed]
82. Taylor, A.L.; Marcus, R.; Bradley, J.A. Post-transplant lymphoproliferative disorders (PTLD) after solid organ transplantation. *Crit. Rev. Oncol. Hematol.* **2005**, *56*, 155–167. [CrossRef]
83. Barrett, W.L.; First, M.R.; Aron, B.S.; Penn, I. Clinical course of malignancies in renal transplant recipients. *Cancer* **1993**, *72*, 2186–2189. [CrossRef]
84. Kliem, V.; Kolditz, M.; Behrend, M.; Ehlerding, G.; Pichlmayr, R.; Koch, K.M.; Brunkhorst, R. Risk of renal cell carcinoma after kidney transplantation. *Clin. Transplant.* **1997**, *11*, 255–258.
85. Sandock, D.S.; Seftel, A.D.; Resnick, M.I. A new protocol for the followup of renal cell carcinoma based on pathological stage. *J. Urol.* **1995**, *154*, 28–31. [CrossRef]
86. Kapoor, A. Malignancy in kidney transplant recipients. *Drugs* **2008**, *68* (Suppl. 1), 11–19. [CrossRef]
87. Opelz, G.; Unterrainer, C.; Susal, C.; Dohler, B. Immunosuppression with mammalian target of rapamycin inhibitor and incidence of post-transplant cancer in kidney transplant recipients. *Nephrol. Dial. Transpl.* **2016**, *31*, 1360–1367. [CrossRef] [PubMed]
88. Kao, C.C.; Liu, J.S.; Lin, M.H.; Hsu, C.Y.; Chang, F.C.; Lin, Y.C.; Chen, H.H.; Chen, T.W.; Hsu, C.C.; Wu, M.S. Impact of mTOR Inhibitors on Cancer Development in Kidney Transplantation Recipients: A Population-Based Study. *Transpl. Proc.* **2016**, *48*, 900–904. [CrossRef]
89. Karpe, K.M.; Talaulikar, G.S.; Walters, G.D. Calcineurin inhibitor withdrawal or tapering for kidney transplant recipients. *Cochrane Database Syst. Rev.* **2017**, *7*, CD006750. [CrossRef]

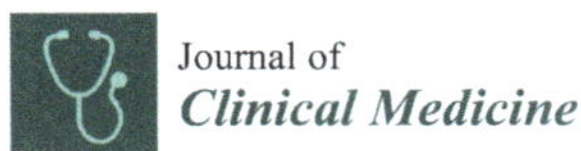
Journal of
Clinical Medicine

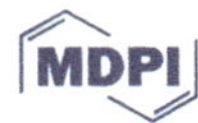

Article

Subarachnoid Hemorrhage in Hospitalized Renal Transplant Recipients with Autosomal Dominant Polycystic Kidney Disease: A Nationwide Analysis

Wisit Cheungpasitporn [1,*], Charat Thongprayoon [2], Patompong Ungprasert [3], Karn Wijarnpreecha [4], Wisit Kaewput [5], Napat Leeaphorn [6], Tarun Bathini [7], Fouad T. Chebib [2] and Paul T. Kröner [4]

[1] Division of Nephrology, Department of Medicine, University of Mississippi Medical Center, Jackson, MS 39216, USA

[2] Division of Nephrology and Hypertension, Mayo Clinic, Rochester, MN 55905, USA; charat.thongprayoon@gmail.com (C.T.); chebib.fouad@mayo.edu (F.T.C.)

[3] Clinical Epidemiology Unit, Department of Research and Development, Faculty of Medicine, Siriraj Hospital, Mahidol University, Bangkok 10700, Thailand; p.ungprasert@gmail.com

[4] Department of Medicine, Division of Gastroenterology and Hepatology, Mayo Clinic, Jacksonville, FL 32224, USA; karnjuve10@gmail.com (K.W.); thomaskroner@gmail.com (P.T.K.)

[5] Department of Military and Community Medicine, Phramongkutklao College of Medicine, Bangkok 10400, Thailand; wisitnephro@gmail.com

[6] Department of Nephrology, Department of Medicine, Saint Luke's Health System, Kansas City, MO 64111, USA; napat.leeaphorn@gmail.com

[7] Department of Internal Medicine, University of Arizona, Tucson, AZ 85721, USA; tarunjacobb@gmail.com

*   Correspondence: wcheungpasitporn@gmail.com

Received: 21 March 2019; Accepted: 15 April 2019; Published: 17 April 2019

Abstract: Background: This study aimed to evaluate the hospitalization rates for subarachnoid hemorrhage (SAH) among renal transplant patients with adult polycystic kidney disease (ADPKD) and its outcomes, when compared to non-ADPKD renal transplant patients. Methods: The 2005–2014 National Inpatient Sample databases were used to identify all hospitalized renal transplant patients. The inpatient prevalence of SAH as a discharge diagnosis between ADPKD and non-ADPKD renal transplant patients was compared. Among SAH patients, the in-hospital mortality, use of aneurysm clipping, hospital length of stay, total hospitalization cost and charges between ADPKD and non-ADPKD patients were compared, adjusting for potential confounders. Results: The inpatient prevalence of SAH in ADPKD was 3.8/1000 admissions, compared to 0.9/1000 admissions in non-ADPKD patients ($p < 0.01$). Of 833 renal transplant patients with a diagnosis of SAH, 30 had ADPKD. Five (17%) ADPKD renal patients with SAH died in hospitals compared to 188 (23.4%) non-ADPKD renal patients ($p = 0.70$). In adjusted analysis, there was no statistically significant difference in mortality, use of aneurysm clipping, hospital length of stay, or total hospitalization costs and charges between ADPKD and non-ADPKD patients with SAH. Conclusion: Renal transplant patients with ADPKD had a 4-fold higher inpatient prevalence of SAH than those without ADPKD. Further studies are needed to compare the incidence of overall admissions in ADPKD and non-ADPKD patients. When renal transplant patients developed SAH, inpatient mortality rates were high regardless of ADPKD status. The outcomes, as well as resource utilization, were comparable between the two groups.

Keywords: autosomal dominant polycystic kidney disease; epidemiology; hospitalization; kidney transplantation; subarachnoid hemorrhage

1. Introduction

Subarachnoid hemorrhage (SAH) is a major clinical problem worldwide, associated with a poor prognosis, long-term morbidity, and extremely high mortality [1–3]. In the United States, over 30,000 cases of SAH occur annually [4,5]. Although global SAH has decreased each year from 1960 through 2017 [6], approximately 30% to 50% of patients who developed SAH died at 60 days. Furthermore, over 30% of survivors subsequently suffered neurologic deficits post-SAH [1–4,7–9]. Major causes of SAH include ruptured intracranial aneurysm, cerebral arteriovenous malformation, and traumatic brain injury [6,10].

Among patients with autosomal dominant polycystic kidney disease (ADPKD), a disorder that affects the kidneys and other organs caused by mutations in PKD1 and PKD2, a wide spectrum of vascular abnormalities have been described including intracranial aneurysms (and dolichoectasias), thoracic aorta and cervicocephalic artery dissections, and coronary artery aneurysms [11,12]. Compared to the general population, the prevalence of intracranial aneurysms in ADPKD patients is approximately five times higher and is estimated at 4% to 22.5% [13–19]. Among ADPKD patients with a family history of SAH/intracranial aneurysms, the frequency is three to five times higher than the general population [12]. Thus, screening is recommended for intracranial aneurysms among ADPKD patients with (1) family or past medical history of intracranial aneurysm presence or rupture; (2) symptoms suggesting intracranial aneurysm; (3) occupations in which loss of consciousness may be fatal; (4) upcoming major elective surgery; and (5) patient subjective concern for possible intracranial aneurysm presence [20–22].

Despite the recommendation for intracranial aneurysm screening prior to major elective surgery, such screening for ADPKD patients is not consistently performed among all transplant centers in the USA during pre-transplant assessment for renal transplantation [23,24]. In addition, previously published studies on the increased risk of SAH after renal transplantation in patients with ADPKD have not yielded relevant information, or have been underpowered [25–31].

Thus, we conducted this study using a nationwide inpatient USA database to evaluate the hospitalization rates for SAH among renal transplant patients with ADPKD and its outcomes, when compared to non-ADPKD renal transplant patients.

2. Methods

2.1. Data Source

The 2005–2014 National Inpatient Sample (NIS) databases were used to conduct this retrospective cohort study. The NIS is the largest inpatient all-payer database that is publicly available in the US. This database was developed by the Agency for Healthcare Research and Quality (AHRQ) as part of its Healthcare Cost and Utilization Project (HCUP). The dataset for the studied years contains more than 78 million hospitalizations, which in itself is a 20% stratified sample of over 4000 non-federal acute care hospitals in 44 states of the United States, and is representative of 95% of hospitalizations nationwide. This dataset included codes for principal diagnosis, secondary diagnoses, and codes for procedures performed during the hospitalization.

2.2. Study Population

Initially, renal transplant patients were identified using the International Classification of Diseases, Ninth Revision, Clinical Modification (ICD-9-CM) codes of v42.0. The ADPKD status in this cohort was identified using the ICD-9-CM code 753.13. The associated diagnosis of SAH was identified using the ICD-9-CM code 430. Patients undergoing elective hospital admission or patients undergoing renal transplantation during the same admission were excluded from the analysis.

2.3. Variable Definition

Patient characteristics included age, gender, ethnicity, median income in patients' zip code, family history of stroke, and insurance type. Hospital characteristics included hospital region, teaching status, number of hospital beds, urban location, and weekend admission. The Healthcare Cost and Utilization Project (HCUP) divides the US into four census regions based on geographical location: Northeast, Midwest, South and West. The vital status at the end of hospitalization, length of hospital stay (LOS), and total hospitalization charges were abstracted from the database. To account for patient comorbidities, the Deyo adaptation of the Charlson Comorbidity Index was used, which was appropriate for the large database analysis [32].

2.4. Outcomes

The outcome for primary analysis was to determine the inpatient prevalence of SAH as a discharge diagnosis in renal transplant patients with ADPKD, compared to renal transplant patients without ADPKD. The outcomes for secondary analysis were to compare in-hospital mortality, the use of aneurysm clipping, length of hospital stay, and expenditures between ADPKD and non-ADPKD patients with SAH. Expenditures included total hospitalization charges and hospitalization costs. Total hospitalization charges represented the amount of financial resources that each hospital billed for providing its service for each patient, whereas hospitalization costs represented the amount of money spent by each hospital in providing the patient care. Hospitalization costs were calculated by multiplying the cost-to-charge ratios for the respective hospitals with the total hospitalization charges. Cost-to-charge ratios were provided by the Healthcare Cost and Utilization Project (HCUP) for each hospitalization in the database in order to enable this calculation. Since this study used datasets for 10 different calendar years, costs and charges were adjusted for inflation using the consumer price index and converting them to 2014 $USD equivalents.

2.5. Statistical Analysis

Discharge-level weights on the HCUP nationwide databases were used to estimate the total number of renal transplant patients that had an associated diagnosis of SAH. Descriptive statistics were used to identify the patient characteristics. Fisher's exact test was used to compare proportions. Students' *t*-test was used to compare means. A hybrid multivariate logistic regression model was built by first conducting a univariate regression analysis on variables that were identified from other studies as being relevant to the outcome. If these variables impacted the outcome in any direction with a p-value of <0.01, they were included in the multivariate logistic regression model. In multivariate logistic regression, odds ratios and means were adjusted for age, gender, insurance type, family history of stroke, the median income in patients' zip code, hospital region, urban location, number of hospital beds and teaching status. All statistical analyses were performed using STATA, Version 13 (StataCorp LP, College Station, TX, USA).

3. Results

3.1. Inpatient Prevalence of SAH as a Discharge Diagnosis

Out of 382,516,561 patients admitted to hospitals during the study period, 918,478 were identified as having had a history of renal transplant. ADPKD patients who underwent renal transplant had higher inpatient prevalence of SAH as a discharge diagnosis than non-ADPKD renal transplant patients (3.8 vs. 0.9 cases per 1000 discharges; $p < 0.01$).

3.2. Patient and Hospital Characteristics in SAH Patients

In total, 833 patients had an associated diagnosis of SAH. These included 30 ADPKD renal transplant patients and 803 non-ADPKD renal transplant patients. The ADPKD renal transplant patients were older, had higher comorbidity burden, and were more likely to be admitted to teaching hospitals than non-ADPKD renal patients. There was no significant difference in terms of weekend admission, the median income in patients' zip code, insurance type, hospital region, urban location, and number of hospital beds between the two cohorts (Table 1).

Table 1. Patient and hospital characteristics.

Patient Characteristics	Non-ADPKD ($n = 803$)	ADPKD ($n = 30$)	p-Value
Mean age (years)	53.4	58.9	<0.01
Female gender (%)	491 (61.2%)	18 (59.1%)	0.7
Ethnicity			
Caucasian	522 (65%)	21 (70%)	
African American	112 (14%)	3 (10%)	0.02
Hispanic	145 (18%)	5 (18%)	
Other	24 (3%)	1 (2%)	
Weekend admission	193 (24%)	5 (18%)	0.17
Income in zip code			
$1–37,999	217 (27%)	6 (21%)	
$38,000–47,999	208 (26%)	8 (28%)	0.36
$48,000–63,999	193 (24%)	7 (22%)	
>$64,000	185 (23%)	9 (29%)	
Insurance			
Medicare	313 (39%)	9 (29%)	
Medicaid	104 (13%)	4 (13%)	0.28
Private	321 (40%)	14 (48%)	
Self-Pay	64 (8%)	3 (10%)	
Charlson score			
0	0 (0%)	0 (0%)	
1–2	586 (73%)	13 (42%)	<0.01
>3	214 (27%)	17 (58%)	
Hospital Region			
Northeast	145 (18%)	6 (19%)	
Midwest	177 (22%)	7 (23%)	0.15
South	297 (37%)	8 (25%)	
West	185 (23%)	10 (33%)	
Urban Location	779 (97%)	29 (98%)	0.39
Hospital Number of Beds			
Small	48 (6%)	2 (6%)	
Medium	145 (18%)	4 (14%)	0.64
Large	610 (76%)	24 (80%)	
Hospital Teaching Status	602 (75%)	26 (88%)	<0.01

ADPKD, adult polycystic kidney disease.

3.3. Mortality

A total of 5 (17%) ADPKD renal transplant patients with SAH died in hospitals compared to 188 (23.4%) non-ADPKD renal transplant patients ($p = 0.70$). Similarly, in adjusted analysis, there was no difference in in-hospital mortality between the two groups, with an adjusted odds ratio (aOR) of 0.87 (95% confidence interval (CI) 0.12–6.23; $p = 0.89$) (Table 2).

Table 2. Outcomes and procedures of ADPKD and non-ADPKD patients with SAH.

Outcome	Adjusted OR	95% CI	*p*-Value
Mortality	0.87	(0.12–6.23)	0.89
Procedure	**Adjusted OR**	**95% CI**	**_p_-Value**
Aneurysm clipping	2.02	0.28–14.81	0.49

3.4. Use of Aneurysm Clipping

Ten (33.0%) ADPKD renal transplant patients with SAH underwent aneurysm clipping, compared to 137 (17.1%) non-ADPKD renal transplant patients ($p = 0.32$). On adjusted analysis, the use of aneurysm clipping in ADPKD renal transplant patients was not significantly higher than non-ADPKD renal transplant patients (aOR: 2.02; 95% CI 0.28–14.81; $p = 0.49$) (Table 2).

3.5. Hospital Length of Stay

The mean LOS in ADPKD renal transplant patients with SAH was 9.8 days, compared to 8.9 days in the non-ADPKD renal transplant SAH patients. Although the mean additional LOS in ADPKD renal transplant patients with SAH was 3.0 days shorter than non-ADPKD renal transplant patients with SAH, this was not statistically significant (95% CI: −10.1–4.1, $p = 0.41$) on adjusted analysis (Table 3).

Table 3. Hospital length of stay and expenditure differences between ADPKD and non-ADPKD patients with SAH.

Additional Expenditures	Mean Difference	95% CI	*p*-Value
Hospital length of stay (days)	−3.0	−10.1–4.1	0.41
Total hospitalization cost	−$1086	−$22,548–$20,376	0.92
Total hospitalization charge	−$14,944	−$73,293–$43,404	0.62

3.6. Total Hospitalization Costs and Charges

The mean hospital cost for ADPKD renal transplant patients with SAH was $ 30,519, while the mean hospital cost for non-ADPKD renal transplant patients with SAH was $ 33,526 ($p = 0.04$). Although the ADPKD renal transplant patients with SAH had a mean hospital cost $ 1086 lower than the non-ADPKD renal transplant patients, the difference was not statistically significant (95% CI: −22,548–20,376, $p = 0.92$) on adjusted analysis (Table 3).

The mean total hospitalization charge for ADPKD renal transplant patients with SAH was $ 85,682, while the mean total hospitalization charges for non-ADPKD renal transplant patients with SAH was $ 112,514. Although ADPKD renal transplant patients with SAH had a mean hospitalization charge $ 14,944 lower than the non-ADPKD renal transplant patients, this was not statistically significant (95% CI: −73,293–43,404, $p = 0.62$) on adjusted analysis (Table 3).

4. Discussion

In this study utilizing the USA Nationwide Inpatient Sample database, we demonstrated that renal transplant patients with ADPKD had a 4-fold higher inpatient prevalence of SAH than those without ADPKD. When renal transplant patients developed SAH, the inpatient mortality rate was high (around 20 to 30%), regardless of ADPKD status. In addition, the use of aneurysm clipping for SAH and hospital LOS were comparable among renal transplant patients with and without ADPKD.

In the previous analysis using USA Renal Data System registry data, Lentine et al. reported a decreased risk of SAH in renal transplant patients when compared to end-stage renal disease (ESRD) patients on the transplant waiting list [33]. Additionally, among ESRD patients on dialysis, it has been shown that ADPKD is associated with an increased risk of SAH [34,35]. Despite an overall reduction in SAH risk after renal transplantation [33], our study demonstrates a higher relative frequency of SAH among ADPKD patients compared to those without ADPKD and aims to raise awareness that SAH remains an important concern in the post-transplantation population.

The risk of intracranial aneurysms among ADPKD patients increased with age [36,37] and its prevalence is substantially increased after 45 years of age, especially among ADPKD Caucasian patients [38]. The average age of patients with ADPKD and ESRD is greater than 45 years [34,35,38]. However, intracranial aneurysm screening during pre-transplant evaluation for renal transplantation was a requirement for some but not all transplant centers in the USA, despite recommendation for intracranial aneurysm screening prior to major elective surgery [23,24]. Furthermore, a very recent study by Flahault et al. including 495 ADPKD patients suggested that systematic screening was cost-effective and provided a gain of 0.68 quality-adjusted life years compared to targeted screening in only those with a familial history of intracranial aneurysms [21]. The investigators concluded that intracranial aneurysm screening could be proposed to all ADPKD patients regardless of family history of stroke [21].

In our study involving renal transplanted patients, after adjusting for potential confounders including family history of stroke, the relative frequency of SAH among ADPKD patients remained significantly higher compared to those without ADPKD. This may suggest potential development of SAH in renal transplant patients with ADPKD, regardless of family history of stroke. When patients develop SAH, the mortality rate is high regardless of renal transplant status [27,33,39–41]. In our study, nearly 25% of renal transplant patients with SAH died during hospital admission. After adjusting for potential confounders, we found no differences in in-hospital mortality, rate of aneurysm clipping, hospital LOS, hospital costs and total hospitalization charges among ADPKD and non-ADPKD renal transplant patients with SAH.

Several limitations of this study must be acknowledged. Firstly, although the utilization of the NIS database enables an assessment of inpatient relative frequency and burden of SAH in renal transplant patients in the USA, potential inaccuracies in ICD-9-CM coding are significant limitations to our study. Secondly, the data relating to types of mutation among ADPKD patients were limited in this study. Since patients with *PKD2*-associated ADPKD usually develop ESRD at an older age compared to renal-transplanted ADPKD patients (mean age: 79.7 vs. 58.9 years) [22,42,43], it is likely that our study represents the outcomes of SAH among renal transplant patients with *PKD1*-associated ADPKD. Thirdly, this is an analysis of an inpatient USA database and, thus, it does not consider the broader USA outpatient renal transplant population nor the renal transplant population in other countries. Because of the nature of the NIS database, our study included only inpatient renal transplant patients and might be subject to selection bias. Without knowing the total number of all ADPKD and non-ADPKD renal transplant patients, the overall admission rates for any reasons cannot be calculated. Fourthly, although the findings of our study highlight the burden of SAH in ADPKD renal transplant patients, it cannot be concluded that screening all ADPKD patients prior to renal transplantation is cost-effective. Nevertheless, physicians should take into account the risk of SAH among ADPKD renal transplant patients. Furthermore, the practice of intracranial aneurysm screening in ADPKD patients might vary between hospitals. However, information regarding the practice of intracranial aneurysm screening was not available in our study. Lastly, given the administrative nature of the dataset, it was not possible to investigate the effects of medication, such as immunosuppressants, on economic burden and mortality among ADPKD and non-ADPKD renal transplant patients with SAH.

5. Conclusions

In conclusion, in this study using the USA Nationwide Inpatient Sample database, we demonstrate higher inpatient relative frequency of SAH among ADPKD renal transplant patients when compared with non-ADPKD renal transplant patients. In-hospital mortality due to SAH among renal transplant patients was high, regardless of ADPKD status. The use of aneurysm clipping for SAH and hospital length of stay were comparable between ADPKD renal transplant patients and those without ADPKD.

Author Contributions: Conceptualization, W.C., N.L., F.T.C. and P.T.K.; Data curation, P.T.K.; Investigation, W.C., C.T., W.K. and P.T.K.; Methodology, W.C., C.T., P.U., K.W., T.B., F.T.C. and P.T.K.; Project administration, W.C. and P.U.; Resources, P.T.K.; Software, P.T.K.; Supervision, N.L., F.T.C. and P.T.K.; Validation, W.C. and P.T.K.; Visualization, N.L.; Writing—original draft, W.C. and C.T.; Writing—review & editing, P.U., K.W., W.K., N.L., T.B., F.T.C. and P.T.K.

Conflicts of Interest: The authors declare no conflict of interest.

References

1. Macdonald, R.L.; Schweizer, T.A. Spontaneous subarachnoid haemorrhage. *Lancet* **2017**, *389*, 655–666. [CrossRef]
2. van Gijn, J.; Kerr, R.S.; Rinkel, G.J. Subarachnoid haemorrhage. *Lancet* **2007**, *369*, 306–318. [CrossRef]
3. Vivancos, J.; Gilo, F.; Frutos, R.; Maestre, J.; Garcia-Pastor, A.; Quintana, F.; Roda, J.M.; Ximenez-Carrillo, A.; Diez Tejedor, E.; Fuentes, B.; et al. Clinical management guidelines for subarachnoid haemorrhage. Diagnosis and treatment. *Neurologia* **2014**, *29*, 353–370. [CrossRef]
4. D'Souza, S. Aneurysmal subarachnoid hemorrhage. *J. Neurosurg. Anesthesiol.* **2015**, *27*, 222–240. [CrossRef]
5. Diringer, M.N.; Zazulia, A.R. Aneurysmal subarachnoid hemorrhage: Strategies for preventing vasospasm in the intensive care unit. *Semin. Respir. Crit. Care Med.* **2017**, *38*, 760–767.
6. Etminan, N.; Chang, H.S.; Hackenberg, K.; de Rooij, N.K.; Vergouwen, M.D.I.; Rinkel, G.J.E.; Algra, A. Worldwide incidence of aneurysmal subarachnoid hemorrhage according to region, time period, blood pressure, and smoking prevalence in the population: A systematic review and meta-analysis. *JAMA Neurol.* **2019**. [CrossRef] [PubMed]
7. Lantigua, H.; Ortega-Gutierrez, S.; Schmidt, J.M.; Lee, K.; Badjatia, N.; Agarwal, S.; Claassen, J.; Connolly, E.S.; Mayer, S.A. Subarachnoid hemorrhage: Who dies, and why? *Crit. Care* **2015**, *19*, 309. [CrossRef]
8. Kaptain, G.J.; Lanzino, G.; Kassell, N.F. Subarachnoid haemorrhage: Epidemiology, risk factors, and treatment options. *Drugs Aging* **2000**, *17*, 183–199. [CrossRef] [PubMed]
9. Cahill, J.; Calvert, J.W.; Zhang, J.H. Mechanisms of early brain injury after subarachnoid hemorrhage. *J. Cereb. Blood Flow Metab.* **2006**, *26*, 1341–1353. [CrossRef] [PubMed]
10. Kirkpatrick, P.J. Subarachnoid haemorrhage and intracranial aneurysms: What neurologists need to know. *J. Neurol. Neurosurg. Psychiatry* **2002**, *73*, 28–33.
11. Graf, S.; Schischma, A.; Eberhardt, K.E.; Istel, R.; Stiasny, B.; Schulze, B.D. Intracranial aneurysms and dolichoectasia in autosomal dominant polycystic kidney disease. *Nephrol. Dial. Transplant.* **2002**, *17*, 819–823. [CrossRef] [PubMed]
12. Rossetti, S.; Harris, P.C. The genetics of vascular complications in autosomal dominant polycystic kidney disease (ADPKD). *Curr. Hypertens Rev.* **2013**, *9*, 37–43. [CrossRef] [PubMed]
13. Vlak, M.H.; Algra, A.; Brandenburg, R.; Rinkel, G.J. Prevalence of unruptured intracranial aneurysms, with emphasis on sex, age, comorbidity, country, and time period: A systematic review and meta-analysis. *Lancet Neurol.* **2011**, *10*, 626–636. [CrossRef]
14. Chapman, A.B.; Rubinstein, D.; Hughes, R.; Stears, J.C.; Earnest, M.P.; Johnson, A.M.; Gabow, P.A.; Kaehny, W.D. Intracranial aneurysms in autosomal dominant polycystic kidney disease. *N. Engl. J. Med.* **1992**, *327*, 916–920. [CrossRef]
15. Schievink, W.I.; Torres, V.E.; Piepgras, D.G.; Wiebers, D.O. Saccular intracranial aneurysms in autosomal dominant polycystic kidney disease. *J. Am. Soc. Nephrol.* **1992**, *3*, 88–95.
16. Xue, C.; Zhou, C.C.; Wu, M.; Mei, C.L. The clinical manifestation and management of autosomal dominant polycystic kidney disease in china. *Kidney Dis.* **2016**, *2*, 111–119. [CrossRef]
17. Niemczyk, M.; Gradzik, M.; Fliszkiewicz, M.; Kulesza, A.; Golebiowski, M.; Paczek, L. Natural history of intracranial aneurysms in autosomal dominant polycystic kidney disease. *Neurol. Neurochir. Pol.* **2017**, *51*, 476–480. [CrossRef] [PubMed]
18. Lee, V.W.; Dexter, M.A.; Mai, J.; Vladica, P.; Lopez-Vargas, P.; Rangan, G.K. Kha-cari autosomal dominant polycystic kidney disease guideline: Management of intracranial aneurysms. *Semin. Nephrol.* **2015**, *35*, 612–617. [CrossRef] [PubMed]
19. Gieteling, E.W.; Rinkel, G.J. Characteristics of intracranial aneurysms and subarachnoid haemorrhage in patients with polycystic kidney disease. *J. Neurol.* **2003**, *250*, 418–423. [CrossRef]

20. Kanaan, N.; Devuyst, O.; Pirson, Y. Renal transplantation in autosomal dominant polycystic kidney disease. *Nat. Rev. Nephrol.* **2014**, *10*, 455–465. [CrossRef]

21. Flahault, A.; Trystram, D.; Nataf, F.; Fouchard, M.; Knebelmann, B.; Grunfeld, J.P.; Joly, D. Screening for intracranial aneurysms in autosomal dominant polycystic kidney disease is cost-effective. *Kidney Int.* **2018**, *93*, 716–726. [CrossRef]

22. Chebib, F.T.; Torres, V.E. Autosomal dominant polycystic kidney disease: Core curriculum 2016. *Am. J. Kidney Dis.* **2016**, *67*, 792–810. [CrossRef]

23. Mosconi, G.; Persici, E.; Cuna, V.; Pedone, M.; Tonioli, M.; Conte, D.; Ricci, A.; Feliciangeli, G.; La Manna, G.; Nanni Costa, A.; et al. Renal transplant in patients with polycystic disease: The Italian experience. *Transplant. Proc.* **2013**, *45*, 2635–2640. [CrossRef]

24. Patel, M.S.; Kandula, P.; Wojciechowski, D.; Markmann, J.F.; Vagefi, P.A. Trends in the management and outcomes of kidney transplantation for autosomal dominant polycystic kidney disease. *J. Transplant.* **2014**, *2014*, 675697. [CrossRef]

25. Aull-Watschinger, S.; Konstantin, H.; Demetriou, D.; Schillinger, M.; Habicht, A.; Horl, W.H.; Watschinger, B. Pre-transplant predictors of cerebrovascular events after kidney transplantation. *Nephrol. Dial. Transplant.* **2008**, *23*, 1429–1435. [CrossRef] [PubMed]

26. Abedini, S.; Holme, I.; Fellstrom, B.; Jardine, A.; Cole, E.; Maes, B.; Holdaas, H. Cerebrovascular events in renal transplant recipients. *Transplantation* **2009**, *87*, 112–117. [CrossRef]

27. Oliveras, A.; Roquer, J.; Puig, J.M.; Rodriguez, A.; Mir, M.; Orfila, M.A.; Masramon, J.; Lloveras, J. Stroke in renal transplant recipients: Epidemiology, predictive risk factors and outcome. *Clin. Transplant.* **2003**, *17*, 1–8. [CrossRef]

28. Adams, H.P., Jr.; Dawson, G.; Coffman, T.J.; Corry, R.J. Stroke in renal transplant recipients. *Arch. Neurol.* **1986**, *43*, 113–115. [CrossRef]

29. Pirson, Y.; Christophe, J.L.; Goffin, E. Outcome of renal replacement therapy in autosomal dominant polycystic kidney disease. *Nephrol. Dial. Transplant.* **1996**, *11*, 24–28. [CrossRef]

30. Wijdicks, E.F.; Torres, V.E.; Schievink, W.I.; Sterioff, S. Cerebral hemorrhage in recipients of renal transplantation. *Mayo Clin. Proc.* **1999**, *74*, 1111–1112. [CrossRef] [PubMed]

31. Martinez-Vila, E.; Quiroga, J. Neurological complications after transplants: Cerebrovascular complications. *Rev. Neurol.* **1995**, *23*, 79–86.

32. Deyo, R.A.; Cherkin, D.C.; Ciol, M.A. Adapting a clinical comorbidity index for use with ICD-9-cm administrative databases. *J. Clin. Epidemiol.* **1992**, *45*, 613–619. [CrossRef]

33. Lentine, K.L.; Rocca Rey, L.A.; Kolli, S.; Bacchi, G.; Schnitzler, M.A.; Abbott, K.C.; Xiao, H.; Brennan, D.C. Variations in the risk for cerebrovascular events after kidney transplant compared with experience on the waiting list and after graft failure. *Clin. J. Am. Soc. Nephrol.* **2008**, *3*, 1090–1101. [CrossRef]

34. Yoo, D.J.; Agodoa, L.; Yuan, C.M.; Abbott, K.C.; Nee, R. Risk of intracranial hemorrhage associated with autosomal dominant polycystic kidney disease in patients with end stage renal disease. *BMC Nephrol.* **2014**, *15*, 39. [CrossRef]

35. Rivera, M.; Gonzalo, A.; Gobernado, J.M.; Orte, L.; Quereda, C.; Ortuno, J. Stroke in adult polycystic kidney disease. *Postgra. Med. J.* **1992**, *68*, 735–738. [CrossRef]

36. Xu, H.W.; Yu, S.Q.; Mei, C.L.; Li, M.H. Screening for intracranial aneurysm in 355 patients with autosomal-dominant polycystic kidney disease. *Stroke* **2011**, *42*, 204–206. [CrossRef]

37. Rozenfeld, M.N.; Ansari, S.A.; Shaibani, A.; Russell, E.J.; Mohan, P.; Hurley, M.C. Should patients with autosomal dominant polycystic kidney disease be screened for cerebral aneurysms? *AJNR Am. J. Neuroradiol.* **2014**, *35*, 3–9. [CrossRef]

38. Niemczyk, M.; Gradzik, M.; Niemczyk, S.; Bujko, M.; Golebiowski, M.; Paczek, L. Intracranial aneurysms in autosomal dominant polycystic kidney disease. *AJNR Am. J. Neuroradiol.* **2013**, *34*, 1556–1559. [CrossRef]

39. Rincon, F.; Mayer, S.A. The epidemiology of intracerebral hemorrhage in the united states from 1979 to 2008. *Neurocrit. Care* **2013**, *19*, 95–102. [CrossRef]

40. An, S.J.; Kim, T.J.; Yoon, B.W. Epidemiology, risk factors, and clinical features of intracerebral hemorrhage: An update. *J. Stroke* **2017**, *19*, 3–10. [CrossRef]

41. Tatlisumak, T.; Cucchiara, B.; Kuroda, S.; Kasner, S.E.; Putaala, J. Nontraumatic intracerebral haemorrhage in young adults. *Nat. Rev. Neurol.* **2018**, *14*, 237–250. [CrossRef] [PubMed]

42. Chebib, F.T.; Perrone, R.D.; Chapman, A.B.; Dahl, N.K.; Harris, P.C.; Mrug, M.; Mustafa, R.A.; Rastogi, A.; Watnick, T.; Yu, A.S.L.; et al. A practical guide for treatment of rapidly progressive adpkd with tolvaptan. *J. Am. Soc. Nephrol.* **2018**, *29*, 2458–2470. [CrossRef] [PubMed]
43. Chebib, F.T.; Torres, V.E. Recent advances in the management of autosomal dominant polycystic kidney disease. *Clin. J. Am. Soc. Nephrol.* **2018**. [CrossRef] [PubMed]

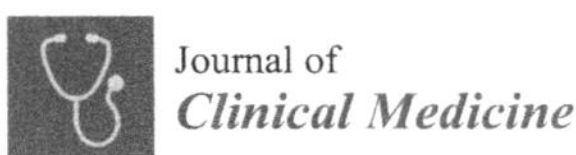

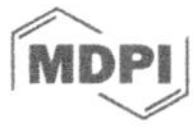

Journal of
Clinical Medicine

Article

Epidemiology, Risk Factors, and Outcomes of Opportunistic Infections after Kidney Allograft Transplantation in the Era of Modern Immunosuppression: A Monocentric Cohort Study

Philippe Attias [1,†], Giovanna Melica [2,†], David Boutboul [3,4], Nathalie De Castro [5], Vincent Audard [1,6], Thomas Stehlé [1,6], Géraldine Gaube [2], Slim Fourati [7,8], Françoise Botterel [7,8,9], Vincent Fihman [7,8,9], Etienne Audureau [10], Philippe Grimbert [1,6,11] and Marie Matignon [1,6,*]

[1] AP-HP (Assistance Publique-Hôpitaux de Paris), Nephrology and Renal Transplantation Department, Groupe Hospitalier Henri-Mondor/Albert-Chenevier, 94010 Créteil, France; philippe.attias@aphp.fr (P.A.); vincent.audard@aphp.fr (V.A.); thomas.stehle@aphp.fr (T.S.); philippe.grimbert@aphp.fr (P.G.)

[2] AP-HP (Assistance Publique-Hôpitaux de Paris), Infectious Disease Department, Groupe Hospitalier Henri-Mondor/Albert Chenevier, 94010 Créteil, France; giovanna.melica@aphp.fr (G.M.); geraldine.gaube@aphp.fr (G.G.)

[3] AP-HP (Assistance Publique-Hôpitaux de Paris), Clinical Immunology Department, Hôpital Saint Louis, 75010 Paris, France; david.boutboul@aphp.fr

[4] INSERM U967 HIPI, Université Paris Diderot, 75012 Paris, France

[5] AP-HP (Assistance Publique-Hôpitaux de Paris), Infectious Disease Department, Hôpital Saint Louis, 75010 Paris, France; nathalie.de-castro@aphp.fr

[6] Université Paris-Est-Créteil, (UPEC), DHU (Département Hospitalo-Universitaire) VIC (Virus-Immunité-Cancer), IMRB (Institut Mondor de Recherche Biomédicale), Equipe 21, INSERM U 955, 94010 Créteil, France

[7] AP-HP (Assistance Publique-Hôpitaux de Paris, Clinical Microbiology Department, Virology, Bacteriology and Infection Control Units, 94010 Créteil, France; slim.fourati@aphp.fr (S.F.); francoise.botterel@aphp.fr (F.B.); vincent.fihman@aphp.fr (V.F.)

[8] Université Paris-Est-Créteil (UPEC), DHU (département hospitalo-universitaire) VIC (virologie immunité cancer), IMRB (Institut Mondor de Recherche Biomédicale), INSERM U955, équipe 18, 94010 Créteil, France

[9] EA Dynamyc, Université Paris Est Créteil– Ecole vétérinaire de Maison Alfort, F-94000 Créteil, France

[10] Université Paris-Est-Créteil, UPEC, DHU (Département Hospitalo-Universitaire) A-TVB, IMRB (Institut Mondor de Recherche Biomédicale)- EA 7376 CEpiA (Clinical Epidemiology And Ageing Unit), 94010 Créteil, France; etienne.audureau@aphp.fr

[11] AP-HP, CIC-BT 504, 94010 Créteil, France

* Correspondence: marie.matignon@aphp.fr; Tel.: +33-1-49-81-44-51; Fax: +33-1-49-81-24-52

† P.A. and G.M. contributed equally to this work.

Received: 13 March 2019; Accepted: 22 April 2019; Published: 30 April 2019

Abstract: Epidemiology of opportunistic infections (OI) after kidney allograft transplantation in the modern era of immunosuppression and the use of OI prevention strategies are poorly described. We retrospectively analyzed a single-center cohort on kidney allograft adult recipients transplanted between January 2008 and December 2013. The control group included all kidney recipients transplanted in the same period, but with no OI. We analyzed 538 kidney transplantations (538 patients). The proportion of OI was 15% (80 and 72 patients). OI occurred 12.8 (6.0–31.2) months after transplantation. Viruses were the leading cause ($n = 54$, (10%)), followed by fungal ($n = 15$ (3%)), parasitic ($n = 6$ (1%)), and bacterial ($n = 5$ (0.9%)) infections. Independent risk factors for OI were extended criteria donor (2.53 (1.48–4.31), $p = 0.0007$) and BK viremia (6.38 (3.62–11.23), $p < 0.0001$). High blood lymphocyte count at the time of transplantation was an independent protective factor (0.60 (0.38–0.94), $p = 0.026$). OI was an independent risk factor for allograft loss (2.53 (1.29–4.95), $p = 0.007$) but not for patient survival. Post-kidney transplantation OIs were mostly viral and occurred beyond one year after transplantation. Pre-transplantation lymphopenia and extended criteria donor are independent risk factors for OI, unlike induction therapy, hence the need to adjust immunosuppressive regimens to such transplant candidates.

Keywords: kidney transplantation; opportunistic infection; allograft survival; BK virus nephropathy

1. Introduction

Kidney allograft recipients are exposed to a broad range of infectious pathogens that give rise to infections with unusual and more severe presentations [1]. Opportunistic infections (OIs) include infections caused by uncommon pathogens and those caused by common pathogens but with unusual and more severe forms [2]. The reported incidence of OIs is variable, from 10% to 25% [3,4]. Currently, prevention strategies against cytomegalovirus (CMV), herpes simplex viruses (HSV), and *Pneumocystis* spp. are recommended and result in a significant reduction of post-transplantation OIs [5] and 50% decrease in the risk of death due to infectious causes. However, infections remain the most common cause of non-cardiovascular deaths (15–20%) [5,6].

After solid-organ transplantation (SOT), OIs flourish in the first 12 months boosted by the immunosuppressive status [2] since less than 20% of SOT recipients receive no induction therapy and up to 60% of kidney transplant recipients receive a T-cell depleting agent [7,8]. Anti-thymocyte globulin primarily induces rapid, profound, and long-lasting depletion of T-lymphocytes in peripheral blood and lymphoid organs, and apparently it does not spare B-cell and NK cell populations [9,10]. Thanks to such therapies, patient and kidney allograft survival after kidney transplantation have markedly improved and acute allograft rejection has decreased [11–13]. On the other hand, one could argue that the long duration of immunosuppression might be the culprit for the increased incidence of OIs.

The epidemiology of OIs after SOT was previously described in two large cohorts on transplant recipients. The first one was conducted 10 years ago and included SOT recipients treated with alemtuzumab [4]. They showed that receiving lung or intestinal transplants was independent risk factors for OIs [4]. Published in the era of modern immunosuppression and after the wide use of prevention strategies, the second study included abdominal SOT recipients (kidney, pancreas, and liver), hence the heterogeneous patient profiles and immunosuppressive regimens [3]. The authors highlighted the delayed onset of OIs where most infections occurred after six months without any impact on recipient's survival and graft function [3]. A recent pediatric cohort on kidney allograft recipients has confirmed the absence of impact of viral OIs (CMV, Epstein Barr virus (EBV), and BK virus (BKV)) on kidney allograft survival [14]. In other studies on kidney allograft recipients, only selected OIs, secondary to specific pathogens (*Nocardia, Aspergillus, Cryptococcus neoformans*), have been reported [15–17].

Given the lack of clinical and epidemiological data on OIs after kidney allograft transplantation, we conducted a large monocentric cohort study on all kidney allograft recipients in our center to analyze the epidemiology of OIs and their impact on kidney recipient survival and allograft function.

2. Materials and Methods

2.1. Study Design and Patients

We conducted a single center retrospective cohort enrolling all adult kidney allograft recipients registered between January 2008 and December 2013. We excluded cases with primary allograft non-function happening within seven days after transplantation. Expanded criteria donor (ECD) was defined as donors older than 60 years or between 50 and 60 years, with two of the three following criteria: (i) hypertension; (ii) pre-retrieval serum creatinine > 1.50 mg/dL; and (iii) cerebrovascular cause of brain death [18]. Glomerular filtration rate was estimated (eGFR) using MDRD formula [19].

Acute rejection episodes were classified according to updated Banff classification [20]. Allograft loss was considered if eGFR was below 15 mL/min/1.73 m^2. All recipients were followed at least one year after transplantation unless death or graft loss occurred earlier.

2.2. Infectious Prophylaxis

The management for CMV prophylaxis followed international recommendations [21]. Prophylaxis involved the administration of oral valganciclovir to high (D+/R-) and intermediate (R+ treated with thymoglobulin) risk patients. Duration of prophylaxis was 6 months in high risk patients and 3 months in intermediate ones.

Participants with past history of tuberculosis were treated with isoniazid for three months after transplantation. *Pneumocystis jirovecii* prophylaxis included trimethoprim-sulfamethoxazole (400 mg) or pentacarinat aerosol for 12 months after transplantation and till CD4 count dropped to <200/μL.

2.3. Opportunistic Infections

OIs were defined according to current literature [1] and international guidelines [22,23]. All episodes were retrospectively and blindly validated (review of all medical reports without the patient name and the final conclusion (clinical and biological data) of infections that happened in kidney-transplant recipients included in the study) by an infectious disease specialist part of the study group. The following OIs were considered:

-Bacteria: *Mycobacterium* sp., *Listeria monocytogenes* and *Nocardia* sp.

-Virus: CMV, active replication of HSV, Varicella-Zoster virus (VZV), Human Herpes Virus-8 (HHV8), BKV, Norovirus, and JC virus.

We included BKV infection, as BK virus, highly seroprevalent in humans, appears to cause clinical disease only in immunocompromised patients and almost all after kidney transplantation (tubulointerstitial nephritis called BKV-induced nephropathy directly related to plasma viral load) [24]. In our center, during the first year after kidney transplantation, BK viruria tests were performed at 1, 2, 3, 6, 9, and 12 months. BK viremia was checked once BK viruria was positive. If BK viruria (associated with BK viremia or not) was positive, a blood test was performed every two weeks.

We also considered Kaposi sarcoma, as one of the four types was organ transplant-associated and usually regresses with reduction in immunosuppression [25].

-Fungi: Candida spp, Cryptococcus spp., invasive molds, and *Pneumocystis jirovecii*.

-Parasites: Toxoplasma gondii, Microsporidium sp, Cryptosporidium sp, Leishmania sp.

2.4. Endpoints

Clinical endpoints were an OI episode, death, and allograft loss. Recipients with at least one episode of OI were compared with the control group which included all other kidney allograft recipients engrafted at the same time period.

2.5. Statistical Analysis

Continuous variables are presented as mean (± Standard Deviation (SD)) or median (Interquartile Range (IQR)). Categorical variables are presented as counts (%). Baseline donor, recipient, and kidney transplant characteristics were compared between OI and control groups using Student *t*-test or Wilcoxon test for continuous variables, and Chi-2 or Fisher's exact tests for categorical variables, as appropriate. Time-to-event survival analyses were conducted to determine predictors of OI occurrence, patient overall survival, and allograft survival. Survival curves were plotted using Kaplan–Meier method and logrank tests to assess significance upon group comparison. Time varying Cox proportional hazard models were built for each endpoint, and hazard ratios (HR) along with their 95% confidence intervals (95% CI) were calculated. Factors yielding $p < 0.2$ in the univariate analyses were then considered in the multivariate analyses' models, using a stepwise backward approach by sequentially removing variables not significant at $p < 0.1$ until the final model was reached. Variables with available repeated data over time were entered both as time-fixed (value at the time of transplantation) and as time-varying (all available time points) variables into the Cox model. No imputation of missing data was done. Competing risk survival analysis (e.g., Fine–Gray methodology) cannot be directly applied on time-varying variables, therefore only results from Cox models are reported for allograft survival. All tests were two-tailed, and the significance level was reached with *p* value < 0.05. The analysis was performed using Stata SE v15.1 (College Station, TX, USA).

3. Results

3.1. Whole Cohort

A flow-chart of the study population is presented in Figure 1. Between January 2008 and December 2013, 557 kidney transplantations were performed in 557 patients (*n*), of whom 19 showed early primary allograft non-function. Overall, only 538 transplantations in 538 patients were included. Mean age was 52 ± 14 years. Mean follow-up was 55 ± 24 months. At the end of follow-up period, patient survival was 88% with 65 deaths, allograft survival was 87% with 72 allograft losses, and mean eGFR was 48 ± 20 mL/min/1.73 m². Tables 1 and 2 described the whole cohort.

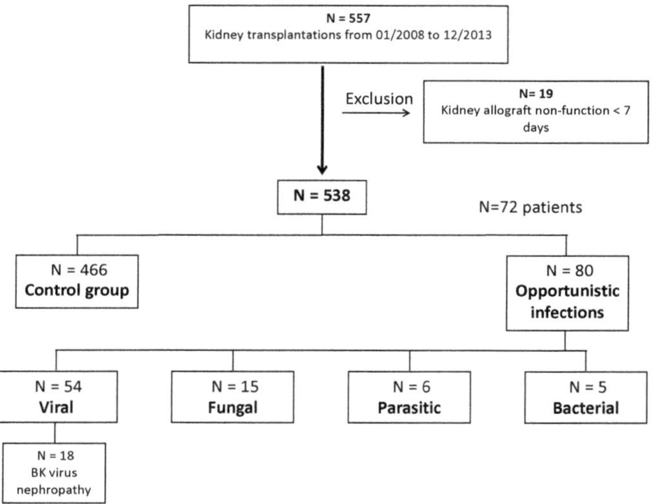

Figure 1. Flow chart of the study population. Between January 2008 and December 2013, 557 kidney transplantations were performed in *n* = 557 patients. Nineteen patients were excluded because of primary allograft non-function within the first week after transplantation. The final cohort included 538 transplantations in 538 patients.

Table 1. Baseline characteristics of the patients included in the study.

Variables	Whole Cohort $n = 538$ (100%)	Opportunistic Infections Group $n = 72$ (13%)	Control Group $n = 466$ (87%)	*p*-Value
Recipients characteristics				
Age, years, mean (SD)	52 ± 14	55 ± 15	51 ± 13	0.06
Sex, Female, *n* (%)	200 (37)	25 (35)	175 (38)	0.64
Initial nephropathy				
Glomerulopathy, *n* (%)	140 (26)	17 (24)	123 (26)	0.62
Unknown, *n* (%)	104 (19)	15 (21)	89 (19)	0.73
Diabetes Mellitus, *n* (%)	88 (16)	12 (17)	76 (16)	0.94
Hypertension, *n* (%)	54 (10)	8 (11)	46 (10)	0.75
Chronic interstitial nephropathy, *n* (%)	32 (6)	7 (10)	25 (5)	0.15
Genetic, *n* (%)	78 (15)	6(8)	72 (15)	0.11
Urologic, *n* (%)	29 (5)	6 (8)	23 (5)	0.23
Other, *n* (%)	13 (3)	2(3)	12 (3)	1.00
Diabetes before transplantation, *n*(%)	120 (22)	16 (22)	104 (22)	0.97
Dialysis, *n* (%)	488 (91)	67 (93)	421 (90)	0.46
Hemodialysis, *n* (%)	448 (83)	387 (83)	61 (85)	0.72
HIV +, *n* (%)	25 (5)	4 (6)	21 (5)	0.69
HCV +, *n* (%)	38 (7)	5 (7)	33 (7)	0.97
CMV +, *n* (%)	443 (82)	58 (81)	385 (83)	0.67
Donor characteristics				
Living donor, *n* (%)	43 (8)	3 (4)	40 (9)	0.20
Extended criteria donor, *n* (%)	245 (46)	48 (67)	197 (42)	0.0001
Age, years, mean (SD)	55 ± 16	59 ± 14	54 ± 16	0.02
eGFR, mL/min/1.73 m^2, median (IQR)	80 (58–103)	72 (56–94)	81 (58–103)	0.26
CMV +, *n* (%)	291 (54)	39 (54)	252 (54)	0.99
Sensitization risk factors				
Former kidney transplantation, *n* (%)	39 (7)	6 (8)	33 (7)	0.70
Anti-HLA antibodies, *n* (%)	285 (53)	38 (53)	247 (53)	0.93
Donor specific anti-HLA antibodies, *n* (%)	77 (14)	7 (10)	70 (15)	0.23
Kidney transplant characteristics				
Cold ischemia time, hours, median (IQR)	16 (12–20)	16 (13–20)	16 (12–20)	0.50
Immunosuppressive therapy				
Induction, *n* (%)	521 (97)	72 (100)	449 (96)	0.10
Basiliximab, *n* (%)	265 (49)	39 (54)	226 (48)	0.37
Antithymocyte globulin, *n* (%)	257 (48)	34 (47)	223 (48)	0.92
Rituximab, *n* (%)	47 (9)	6 (8)	41 (9)	0.90
Intravenous immunoglobulins, *n* (%)	89 (16)	9 (13)	80 (17)	0.32
Maintenance				
Calcineurin inhibitors, *n* (%)	534 (99)	72 (100)	462 (99)	0.43
Mycophenolate mofetil, *n* (%)	538 (100)	72 (100)	466 (100)	1.00
Steroids, *n* (%)	537 (99,8)	71 (99)	466 (100)	0.13
Belatacept	6 (1)	0 (0)	6 (1)	0.33
Combined transplant				
Heart, *n* (%)	4 (1)	1 (1)	3 (1)	0.67
Pancreas, *n* (%)	10 (2)	1 (1)	9 (2)	0.67
Liver, *n* (%)	19 (3)	4 (6)	15 (3)	0.67
White blood cells at the time of transplantation				
Leucocytes (G/L), median (IQR)	6.3 (5.2–7.9)	6.3 (5.3–8.2)	6.3 (5.2–7.8)	0.66
Neutrophils (G/L), median (IQR)	4.2 (3.1–5.4)	4.6 (3.2–6.2)	4.1 (3.0–5.4)	0.17
Lymphocytes (G/L), median (IQR)	1.3 (1.0–1.7)	1.2 (0.9–1.6)	1.3 (1.0–1.8)	0.04
CD4 T-cells (/µL), median (IQR)	525 (373–704)	493 (340–637)	526 (389–704)	0.15
CD4 T-cells (%), median (IQR)	45.1 (37.8–52.9)	46.1 (37.2–52.3)	45.1 (38.0–53.0)	0.51
CD8 T-cells (/µL), median (IQR)	312 (200–451)	284 (242–411)	314 (198–466)	0.79
CD8 T-cells (%), median (IQR)	26.9 (20.3–33.0)	27.7 (23.6–36.7)	26.6 (19.8–32.7)	0.11

Table 2. Follow-up of the patients included in the study.

Variables	Whole Cohort $n = 538$ (100%)	Opportunistic Infections Group $n = 72$ (13%)	Control Group $n = 466$ (87%)	*p*-Value
New onset diabetes after transplantation, *n* **(%)**	34 (6)	5 (7)	29 (6)	0.82
Acute rejection, *n* **(%)**	136 (25)	23 (32)	113 (24)	0.19
T-cell mediated, *n* (%)	87 (16)	15 (21)	72 (16)	0.54
Antibody-mediated, *n* (%)	34 (6)	6 (8)	28 (6)	0.54
Mixed, *n* (%)	15 (3)	2 (3)	13 (3)	0.54
Time from transplantation, months (median, IQR)	5 (2–18)	7 (3–35)	4 (2–14)	0.14
Before opportunistic infection, *n* (%)	127 (24)	15 (21)	112 (24)	0.66
Viral Infections				
BK viruria	163 (30)	26 (36)	137 (29)	0.25
Time from transplantation, months (median, IQR)	6 (3–17)	7 (3–12)	6 (3–21)	0.83
Before opportunistic infection, *n* (%)	149 (28)	16 (22)	133 (28)	0.32
BK viremia	58 (11)	22 (31)	36 (8)	0.0001
Time from transplantation, months (median, IQR)	5 (3–8)	6 (3–12)	4 (3–6)	0.14
Before opportunistic infection, *n* (%)				
CMV viremia	178 (33)	30 (42)	148 (32)	0.10
Time from transplantation, CMV viremia (months, median, IQR)	4 (2–7)	5 (2–11)	3 (2–7)	0.22
Before opportunistic infection, *n* (%)	161 (30)	17 (24)	144 (31)	0.27
12-month follow-up				
eGFR mL/min/1.73 m^2 (median, IQR)	48 (36–60)	41 (31–53)	48 (37–61)	0.003
Allograft loss, *n* (%)	19 (4)	5 (7)	14 (3)	0.09
Time from transplantation, months (median, IQR)	7 (5–11)	10 (7–11)	6 (3–10)	0.252
Death, *n* (%)	16 (3)	3 (4)	13 (3)	0.52
Time from transplantation, months (median, IQR)	6 (2–9)	6 (5–7)	5 (2–9)	0.95
Last follow-up				
Time from transplantation, months (median, IQR)	52 (38–75)	48 (34–68)	53 (38–77)	0.045
eGFR mL/min/1.73 m^2 (median, IQR)	45 (36–60)	38 (29–52)	46 (34–62)	0.0009
Allograft loss, *n* (%)	68 (13)	13 (18)	55 (12)	0.14
Time from transplantation, months (median, IQR)	34 (13–54)	31 (110–48)	34 (14–55)	0.81
Death, *n* (%)	65 (12)	10 (14)	55 (12)	0.64
Time from transplantation, months (median, IQR)	34 (13–51)	29.9 (6–51)	34 (14–55)	0.58

3.2. Opportunistic Infections

Eighty OI episodes were reported in 15% of patients ($n = 72$). The median time to post-transplantation OI was 12.8 (6.0–31.2) months, and in 39 patients (48.8%), OI occurred over the first post-transplantation year.

Viruses were the leading cause of OI episodes, $n = 54$ (68%), representing 10% of the whole cohort. Median time to viral OI onset was 14 (7–31) months after transplantation. Of those viral OIs, we recorded 21 (39%) shingles (4%-whole cohort), 18 (33%) BKV nephropathy (BKVN) (3%-whole cohort), 6 (11%) Kaposi sarcoma (1%-whole cohort), 3 (6%) CMV disease (0.5%-whole cohort), 3 (6%) norovirus gastroenteritis (0.5%-whole cohort), and 1 (2%) of each of the following: JC virus causing progressive multifocal leukoencephalopathy (PML) (0.2%-whole cohort), VZV retinitis (0.2%-whole cohort), and HSV-1 esophagitis (0.2%-whole cohort).

Fungal infections were the second most common OIs, registered in 15 patients (19%) (3%-whole cohort), in the first 6 (2–25) months after transplantation, which is significantly earlier than viral infections ($p = 0.04$). We counted five (33%) invasive candidiasis (0.9%-whole cohort), four (27%) invasive aspergillosis (IA) (0.7%-whole cohort), three (20%) cryptococcosis (0.5%-whole cohort), two (13%) *Pneumocystosis* pneumonia (PCP) (0.3%-whole cohort), and one (7%) disseminated *Trichophyton Rubrum* infection (0.2%-whole cohort).

Among the six (7%) parasitic infections (1%-whole cohort) occurring 16 (5–23) months after transplantation, four were cryptosporidiosis (0.7%-whole cohort) and two microsporidiosis with gastrointestinal involvement (0.3%-whole cohort). Finally, five (6%) bacterial infections (0.9%-whole cohort) were described, of which two (40%) were tuberculosis (0.3%-whole cohort), two (40%) were nocardiosis (0.3%-whole cohort), and one (20%) was disseminated atypical mycobacteria infection (0.15%-whole cohort). Time to post-transplantation infection was 11 (9–34) months. Seven (10%) recipients had more than one post-transplantation OI episode.

The comparison between OI and control groups is shown in Tables 1 and 2. Donors were significantly older in OI group than in control group ($p = 0.02$), with a similar statistical trend in recipients ($p = 0.056$). At the time of transplantation, blood lymphocytes count was significantly lower in OI group ($p = 0.04$). Numbers and percentages of CD4 and CD8 T-cells were similar in both groups; the same was found for the immunosuppressive treatments after transplantation (induction and maintenance).

The estimated GFR in OIs group was significantly lower than in control group at any given time (i.e., at 12-months or last available follow-up data). Acute rejection incidence and CMV viremia were similar in both groups. At the end of follow-up, event rates, allograft loss, and time to death after transplantation were similar in both groups.

In time-to-event analysis, the univariate risk factors for OIs after kidney transplantation (Table 3) were older recipient age (HR 1.02 (1–1.04), $p = 0.03$), older donor age (1.02 (1.01–1.04), $p = 0.02$), and ECD (2.76 (1.68–4.54), $p < 0.0001$). Higher CD4+ T-cells during follow-up and higher blood lymphocyte count at the time of transplantation were protective factors against OI (0.31 (0.11–0.83) and 0.61 (0.40–0.95), respectively). At the time of transplant, blood lymphocytes count was significantly lower in patients with OI (Table 1 (OI) Median 1.2 (IQR 0.9–1.6) vs. (Controls) 1.3 (1.0–1.8); $p = 0.04$) while CD4/CD8 numbers (%) were similar in both groups (Table 1) or using time-to-event analysis (Table 3). Induction and maintenance immunosuppressive regimens, acute rejection episode, and CMV viremia were not OI risk factors.

Independent risk factors for OI according to multivariate analysis were ECD (2.53 (1.48–4.31), $p = 0.0007$), and BK viremia (6.38 (3.62–11.23), $p < 0.0001$). High blood lymphocyte count at the time of transplantation was an independent protective risk factor (0.60 (0.38–0.94), $p = 0.026$). The multivariable analysis conducted only on patients with available pre-transplantation CD4 T-cell counts ($n = 456$) showed that ECD (2.92 (1.62–5.27), $p = 0.0004$) and BK viremia (5.11 (2.72–9.57), $p < 0.0001$) were independent risk factors for OI. In contrast, a higher CD4 T-cell percentage during follow-up (time-varying variable) (0.98 (0.96–0.99), $p = 0.015$) and, to a lesser extent, a higher lymphocyte count at the time of transplantation (0.68 (0.44–1.07), $p = 0.09$) were independent protective factors.

Table 3. Opportunistic infection risk factors, univariate analysis.

Variables	Whole Cohort			With No BK Virus Nephropathy		
	HR	95% CI	p-Value	HR	95% CI	p-Value
Recipient characteristics						
Female	0.88	0.54–1.43	0.60	0.97	0.56–1.69	0.91
Age at transplantation	1.02	1.00–1.04	0.03	1.03	1.01–1.06	0.003
Dialysis	1.76	0.64–4.83	0.27	2.71	0.66–1.11	0.17
Hemodialysis	1.21	0.62–2.37	0.57	1.32	0.59–2.92	0.50
HIV+	0.95	0.30–3.03	0.94	1.30	0.41–4.18	0.66
CMV+	0.90	0.50–1.61	0.72	0.95	0.48–1.89	0.88
HCV+	1.01	0.41–2.51	0.98	1.09	0.39–3.01	0.87
Initial nephropathy						
Hypertension	1.11	0.53–2.31	0.78	1.53	0.72–3.25	0.27
Unknown origin	1.13	0.64–2.00	0.68	1.23	0.65–2.35	0.52
Diabetes	1.11	0.60–2.07	0.73	1.00	0.47–2.11	0.99
Genetic	0.48	0.21–1.12	0.09	0.54	0.21–1.35	0.19
Glomerulopathy	0.91	0.53–1.57	0.74	0.76	0.39–1.47	0.41
Tubular and interstitial	1.64	0.71–3.78	0.25	1.85	0.74–4.65	0.19
Urologic	1.56	0.68–3.60	0.30	1.39	0.50–3.86	0.52
Other	1.03	0.25–4.20	0.97	*	*	*
Diabetes before transplantation	1.02	0.57–1.81	0.95	0.91	0.45–1.82	0.78
Donor characteristics						
Age	1.02	1.01–1.04	0.01	1.03	1.01–1.05	0.002
Expanded Criteria Donor	2.76	1.68–4.54	<0.0001	3.74	2.03–6.90	<0.0001
eGFR	1.00	0.99–1.00	0.31	1.00	0.99–1.00	0.41
Living donor	0.47	0.15–1.49	0.20	0.20	0.03–1.48	0.12
CMV+	1.00	0.63–1.60	0.99	1.05	0.61–1.80	0.86
Sensitization risk factors						
Anti HLA antibodies	0.99	0.62–1.59	0.98	0.97	0.56–1.66	0.90
Former kidney transplantation	1.02	0.41–2.54	0.96	1.10	0.40–3.04	0.86
Donor specific anti-HLA antibodies	0.69	0.32–1.51	0.36	0.39	0.12–1.25	0.11
Combined Transplants						
Pancreas	0.69	0.10–5.00	0.72	0.92	0.13–6.65	0.93
Liver	1.87	0.68–5/12	0.23	1.90	0.59–6.09	0.28
Heart	*	*	*	*	*	*

* data non analyzed.

Table 3. *Cont.*

Variables	Whole Cohort			With No BK Virus Nephropathy		
	HR	95% CI	*p*-Value	HR	95% CI	*p*-Value
Kidney Transplant Characteristics						
Cold ischemia time	1.02	0.99–1.05	0.28	1.03	0.99–1.07	0.18
Induction Immunosuppressive regimen						
Basiliximab	1.21	0.76–1.93	0.43	1.51	0.87–2.61	0.15
Antithymocyte globulin	1.01	0.63–1.61	0.96	0.84	0.48–1.45	0.52
Intravenous Immunoglobulin	0.74	0.37–1.48	0.39	0.42	0.15–1.16	0.09
Rituximab	1.03	0.44–2.37	0.95	0.45	0.11–1.83	0.26
Maintenance immunosuppressive regimen						
Calcineurin inhibitors	*	*	*	*	*	*
Mycophenolate Mophetil	*	*	*	*	*	*
Steroids	*	*	*	*	*	*
Belatacept	*	*	*	*	*	*
White blood cells at the time of transplantation						
Leucocytes (/1000)	1.01	0.92–1.11	0.84			
Neutrophils (/1000)	1.05	0.95–1.15	0.37			
Lymphocytes (/1000)	0.61	0.40–0.95	0.028			
TCD4 cells (/1000)	0.34	0.08–1.38	0.13			
TCD4 cells (%)	0.98	0.96–1.01	0.25			
TCD8 cells (/1000)	1.28	0.31–5.24	0.73			
TCD8 cells (%)	1.02	1.00–1.05	0.06			
White blood cells as time-varying variables during follow-up						
Leucocytes (/1000)	0.94	0.84–1.05	0.28	0.89	0.78–1.02	0.09
Neutrophils (/1000)	0.98	0.87–1.10	0.72	0.92	0.79–1.07	0.28
Lymphocytes (/1000)	0.74	0.50–1.11	0.15	0.70	0.43–1.13	0.14
TCD4 cells (/1000)	0.31	0.11–0.83	0.02	0.45	0.15–1.33	0.15
TCD4 cells (%)	0.97	0.95–0.99	0.004	0.98	0.96–1.00	0.11
TCD8 cells (/1000)	0.70	0.23–2.10	0.52	0.90	0.27–2.98	0.86
TCD8 cells (%)	1.01	0.99–1.03	0.42	1.00	0.98–1.02	0.94
Follow up						
CMV viremia before OI	1.29	0.76–2.18	0.34	1.53	0.85–2.76	0.16
BK viruria before OI	1.94	1.15–3.28	0.01	0.34	0.12–0.96	0.04
Acute rejection before OI	1.48	0.83–2.63	0.19	1.38	0.70–2.71	0.35
High calcineurin inhibitors level in the month before OI	2.06	0.97–4.35	0.06	3.87	1.53–9.80	0.004
Mycophenolate Mofetil at the time of OI	1.134	0.45–2.83	0.79	0.41	0.10–1.78	0.24
mTOR at the time of OI	0.49	0.15–1.56	0.23	0.56	0.17–1.80	0.33

* data non analyzed.

3.3. Patients and Allograft Survival

In OI group, patient survival was significantly lower than in control group (Figure 2a, p = 0.009). After OI episode, 10 patients (14%) died, of whom three (30%) deaths were related to an OI episode (one PML, one PCP, and one IA). Other causes of death included cardio-vascular disease (n = 3), hemorrhagic shock (n = 1), traumatism (n = 1), bacterial infections (n = 1), and neoplasia (n = 1). OI was not an independent risk factor for death as shown by the multivariable analysis (Table 4). OI lost its statistical significance after multivariable adjustment for recipient age at transplantation, TCD8 cells (/1000) during follow-up, neutrophils (/1000) during follow-up, HCV+ status, former kidney transplantation and diabetes. Consequently, and in accordance with our statistical analysis strategy (section #2), OI was left out of Table 4 showing only results from the final multivariable model after a stepwise backward approach was applied.

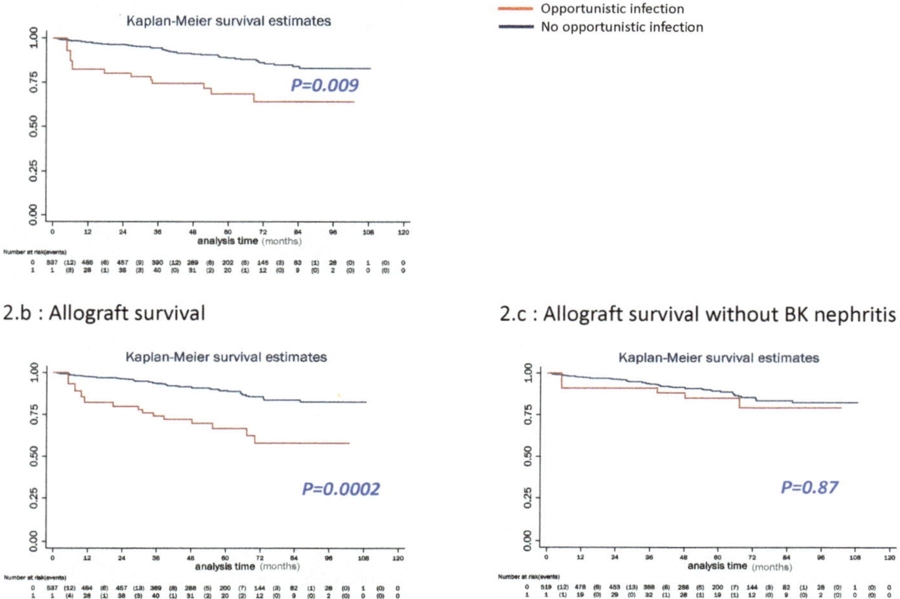

Figure 2. Patient, allograft, and event-free survival in both groups (Kaplan–Meier survival analysis): (**a**) in OI group, patient survival was significantly lower than in control group (p = 0.009); (**b**) allograft survival was significantly lower in OI group (p = 0.0002); and (**c**) allograft survival without BK virus nephropathy was not significantly lower in OI group (p = 0.87).

Table 4. Patient and allograft survival independent risk factors (time varying Cox model).

Patient Overall Survival			
Variables	**HR**	**95% CI**	***p*-Value**
Recipient age at transplantation	1.08	1.05–1.11	<0.0001
TCD8 cells (/1000), time-varying during follow-up	0.26	0.07–1.01	0.052
Neutrophils (/1000), time-varying during follow-up	1.12	0.99–1.27	0.08
HCV+	3.02	1.39–6.55	0.005
Former kidney transplantation	3.18	1.35–7.50	0.008
Diabetes	1.83	1.04–3.22	0.04
Allograft survival			
Variables	**HR**	**95% CI**	***p*-Value**
Donor age	1.02	1.00–1.04	0.03
TCD4 cells (/1000), time-varying during follow-up	0.23	0.08–0.67	0.007
Acute rejection before opportunistic infection	3.28	1.93–5.57	<0.0001
Opportunistic infection episode	2.53	1.29–4.95	0.007
Donor specific anti-HLA antibodies before transplantation	1.92	0.97–3.78	0.06
CMV+ donor	1.83	1.05–3.19	0.03
Diabetes	1.97	1.15–3.39	0.014

Allograft survival was significantly lower in OI group (Figure 2b, $p = 0.0002$). After OI episode, allograft loss occurred in 13 (18%) patients, around 31 (5–63) months after transplantation. Causes of allograft loss were five (38%) BKVN, five (38%) chronic allograft dysfunction, two (16%) refractory acute rejection, and one (8%) unknown cause. OI episode was an independent risk factor for allograft loss with HR = 2.53 (1.29–4.95) ($p = 0.007$) (Table 4).

3.4. Analysis Excluding BKVN

As BKVN is well-known to cause a chronic destructive infection [24], we performed another analysis excluding BKVN events (Table 3). ECD and low blood lymphocytes count at the time of transplantation remained the two independent risk factors for OI episode (4.09 (2.06–8.09), $p < 0.0001$ and 0.64 (0.38–1.06), $p = 0.08$, respectively). OI was not found to be a risk factor for allograft loss ($p = 0.87$; Figure 2c and Table S1).

4. Discussion

We present here the results of a monocentric cohort analysis conducted on more than 500 kidney allograft recipients. We showed that, in the era of modern immunosuppression and the wide use of infectious disease prophylactic strategies, OIs occurred more than one year after transplantation and that pre-transplantation lymphopenia was an independent risk factor for OI episode, which was not the case for induction therapy. Moreover, OIs were an independent risk factor for allograft loss but had no effect on patient survival.

Although OIs are well defined in the setting of HIV [23], no classification of post-SOT OIs is currently available [2]. However, we tried in our work to carefully apply the current OI definitions on post-SOT settings taking into account the standardized immunosuppressive regimen and the type of SOT. On this point, former studies on allograft recipients were quite heterogenous concerning the infections considered and the type of SOT [3,4,14]. To our knowledge, no study evaluating the risk factors for OIs versus more severe common infections in engrafted patients has been published. Therefore, no conclusion regarding physiopathology and risk factors is available. In our cohort, we used HIV classification to define OI updated with BKVN, an immunosuppression-induced infection after kidney transplantation [23,24]. This selection process allowed us to provide reliable data on incidence and spectrum of OI after kidney transplantation and could be routinely used by clinicians to customize the prevention strategies to the patient condition.

OI proportion in our cohort was significantly lower than the most recently published incidence rate of around 25% [3]. Several explanations may account for this low incidence. First, the post-transplantation CMV, PCP, and bacterial prophylaxis strategies we use in our center are in fulfilment with the international recommendations (e.g., trimethoprim-sulfamethoxazole for Nocardia) [5,21]. Secondly, the immunocompromised recipients were exposed to a lower level of CNI, a strategy previously described to significantly decrease OI incidence [26]. At last, solid-organs failure before transplantation induced variable degrees of immune suppression. For instance, liver cirrhosis is associated with dysfunction of the defensive mechanisms against infections and higher incidence of sepsis [27] unlike end-stage renal failure [28]. Therefore, fungal infections risk is lower after kidney transplantation compared with other SOT populations [29].

Thus, we updated the description of post- kidney transplantation OIs to align it with the new strategies of immunosuppressive therapy. In our cohort, the incidence of CMV disease was significantly lower than previously described, probably because of the application of the regularly-updated prevention recommendations [2]. However, viral infections remained the first cause of OIs, mainly cutaneous shingles and BKVN. No prevention strategy is currently recommended for shingles. BKVN is clearly problematic after kidney transplantation since it thrives in immune suppression status, has a great impact on kidney allograft survival, and there is no curative treatment for it [24]. IA incidence is also lower in our cohort [29], whereas other OIs incidence was in the previously described range [16] after kidney transplantation.

Interestingly, time to OI onset was long, more than one year after transplantation. The latest review has reported a peak of OI at 6–12 months after transplantation [2]. Again, prevention strategies could probably postpone post-transplantation infections onset. However, post-transplantation fungal infection developed significantly earlier as in former studies, which confirmed that those infections flourish by the peak of immunosuppression [29]. No prevention strategy is currently recommended for those infections as well as PCP.

Thereafter, we aimed to identify independent risk factors for post-kidney transplantation OI. We found that ECD and low pre-transplantation lymphocyte count were independent risk factors; the type of induction immunosuppressive treatments and the recipient age were not. In kidney allograft recipients, older donor age, irrespective of recipient age, increases the rate of acute allograft rejection and infections [30,31]. The underlying immune system seems to be more important than immunosuppressive therapy. Aged transplanted mice could have an impaired anti-infectious response with accumulation of memory CD4+ T-cells and reduced Th1 anti-donor immune response [32,33]. These immunological effects could significantly decrease anti-infectious response in recipients transplanted from ECD. High CD4+ T-cells count was significantly a protective factor, but there was no effect of CD8+ T-cells count while CD4/ CD8 numbers (%) at the time of transplant were similar in both groups. The total count in lymphocytes had a superior predictive value for OI than the separate levels of CD4/CD8. However, the study population for analyses on CD4/CD8 was slightly decreased due to missing information on these variables, thus possibly resulting in a moderate loss of statistical power. High late stage differentiated CD28+CD57+CD4+ T-cells rates at the time of transplantation is independently associated with a decreased risk of OI [28]. Analysis of naive CD4+ T-cells remains to be determined since such phenotype has been associated with a high risk of infection in patients with common variable immunodeficiency [34]. Surprisingly, immunosuppressive induction using depletive monoclonal agents was not associated with OI incidence. Comparing the risk of infection with depletive and non-depletive therapies yielded controversial data although the most recent work shows that thymoglobulin was not associated with higher infection risk [35–37]. Almost all of our patients were treated with induction therapy. No induction therapy in immunocompromised kidney allograft recipients could be an option [38]. Whether the absence of induction could be associated with a significantly lower incidence of OI need to be elucidated.

How lymphopenia before transplant could influence OI occurring more than one year after transplantation remains unknown. Again, the wide use of prophylaxis (trimethoprim-sulfamethoxazole and valganciclovir) prevents early infection (mostly PCP, Nocardia, and CMV disease). Considering late infection, we believed that lymphopenia before transplantation could be a cumulative effect of immunosuppressive therapies in older patients.

Our data confirm that OI is not an independent risk factor for death [3,4]. In a recent large Finnish cohort, OI rarely caused deaths after kidney transplantation, but the most common cause of infection-related mortality was common bacterial infections, e.g. septicemia and pneumonia [6]. The lack of OI-related effect on mortality compared with the role of common bacterial infections needs deeper analyses of causes and risk factors for common infections; this should enable us to adjust prevention strategies to different contexts. Additionally, recent data suggest that infections could be the first cause of death after transplantation [39].

Finally, in our cohort, OI was an independent risk factor for allograft loss only if BKVN episodes were considered. The negative impact of BKVN on kidney allograft survival is well-documented [24]. Thus, in one of the analyses, we excluded BKVN from OI episodes and found no impact on kidney allograft survival on the long-term [3]. To decrease BKVN, only m-TOR inhibitors based immunosuppressive combination showed a significant effect, thus should be considered in all patient with standard immunologic risk [40].

Our study presents limits. The first one is being a single center study and retrospective. These results must be confirmed in a prospective multicentric cohort. However, the single center study implies only one way to manage immunosuppression after transplantation. The second one is that we performed an overview of OI without considering specific prognosis of each infection.

In conclusion, our study showed that, in the era of modern immunosuppression and the wide use of infection prophylactic regimens, OIs occurred later, more than one year after kidney transplantation and were mainly viral. Pre-transplantation lymphopenia and ECD were the two independent risk factors for OI, hence the need for customized immunosuppressive regimen in such transplant candidates. BKVN incidence remained high with a clear negative impact on allograft survival. In low-risk recipients, m-TOR based immunosuppressive therapy is the only prophylaxis to prevent BKVN and should be considered more widely. Two more issues need to be further studied: the specific role of pre-transplantation leucocytes subpopulation especially naive T-cells, and the difference between OI and common infections which have been described as the main cause of patient death after kidney transplantation.

Supplementary Materials: The following are available online at http://www.mdpi.com/2077-0383/8/5/594/s1, Table S1: Allograft survival risk factors univariable analysis.

Author Contributions: Conceptualization, P.A., G.M., D.B., N.D.C., and M.M.; Methodology, G.M., E.A., and M.M.; Software, E.A.; Validation, all authors; Formal Analysis, P.A., G.M., D.B., E.A., M.M., and P.G.; Investigation, P.A., G.M., and M.M.; Resources, M.M.; Data Curation, V.A., T.S., S.F., G.G., F.B., and V.F.; Writing—Original Draft Preparation, P.A., G.M., and M.M.; Writing—Review and Editing: P.A., G.M., D.B., V.F., S.F., M.M., and P.G.; Visualization, G.M.; and Supervision, M.M.

Conflicts of Interest: The authors declare no conflict of interest. The results presented in this paper have not been published previously in whole or part, except in abstract format.

Abbreviations

ABMR	antibody-mediated rejection
ATG	antithymocyte globulin
BKV	BK virus
BKVN	BK virus nephropathy
CMV	cytomegalovirus
CNI	Calcineurin inhibitor
DGF	delayed graft function
DSA	donor specific antibodies
EBV	Epstein Barr virus
ECD	expanded criteria donor
eGFR	estimated glomerular filtration rate
HIV	Human immunodeficiency virus
HSV	herpes simplex virus
HHV8	Human Herpes virus-8
IQR	interquartile range
IA	invasive aspergillosis
M	month
MDRD	modified diet of renal disease
N	number
OIs	opportunistic infections
PML	progressive multifocal leukoencephalopathy
PCP	Pneumocystosis pneumonia
SD	standard deviation
TCMR	T-cell-mediated rejection
VZV	varicella-zoster virus

References

1. Fishman, J.A. Infection in solid-organ transplant recipients. *N. Engl. J. Med.* **2007**, *357*, 2601–2614. [CrossRef] [PubMed]
2. Fishman, J.A. Opportunistic infections–coming to the limits of immunosuppression? *Cold Spring Harb. Perspect. Med.* **2013**, *3*, a015669. [CrossRef] [PubMed]
3. Helfrich, M.; Dorschner, P.; Thomas, K.; Stosor, V.; Ison, M.G. A retrospective study to describe the epidemiology and outcomes of opportunistic infections after abdominal organ transplantation. *Transpl. Infect. Dis.* **2017**, *19*. [CrossRef]
4. Peleg, A.Y.; Husain, S.; Kwak, E.J.; Silveira, F.P.; Ndirangu, M.; Tran, J.; Shutt, K.A.; Shapiro, R.; Thai, N.; Abu-Elmagd, K.; et al. Opportunistic infections in 547 organ transplant recipients receiving alemtuzumab, a humanized monoclonal CD-52 antibody. *Clin. Infect. Dis.* **2007**, *44*, 204–212. [CrossRef]
5. Group KDIGOKTW. KDIGO clinical practice guideline for the care of kidney transplant recipients. *Am. J. Transplant.* **2009**, *9* (Suppl. 3), S1–S155. [CrossRef]
6. Kinnunen, S.; Karhapää, P.; Juutilainen, A.; Finne, P.; Helanterä, I. Secular Trends in Infection-Related Mortality after Kidney Transplantation. *Clin. J. Am. Soc. Nephrol.* **2018**, *13*, 755–762. [CrossRef] [PubMed]
7. Matas, A.J.; Smith, J.M.; Skeans, M.A.; Thompson, B.; Gustafson, S.K.; Schnitzler, M.A.; Stewart, D.E.; Cherikh, W.S.; Wainright, J.L.; Snyder, J.J.; et al. OPTN/SRTR 2012 Annual Data Report: Kidney. *Am. J. Transplant.* **2014**, *14* (Suppl. 1), 11–44. [CrossRef]
8. Yeung, M.Y.; Gabardi, S.; Sayegh, M.H. Use of polyclonal/monoclonal antibody therapies in transplantation. *Expert Opin. Biol. Ther.* **2017**, *17*, 339–352. [CrossRef] [PubMed]
9. Mohty, M. Mechanisms of action of antithymocyte globulin: T-cell depletion and beyond. *Leukemia* **2007**, *21*, 1387–1394. [CrossRef] [PubMed]
10. Zand, M.S.; Vo, T.; Huggins, J.; Felgar, R.; Liesveld, J.; Pellegrin, T.; Bozorgzadeh, A.; Sanz, I.; Briggs, B.J. Polyclonal rabbit antithymocyte globulin triggers B-cell and plasma cell apoptosis by multiple pathways. *Transplantation* **2005**, *79*, 1507–1515. [CrossRef]

11. Wolfe, R.A.; Roys, E.C.; Merion, R.M. Trends in organ donation and transplantation in the United States, 1999–2008. *Am. J. Transplant.* **2010**, *10 (4 Pt 2)*, 961–972. [CrossRef]

12. Hill, P.; Cross, N.B.; Barnett, A.N.; Palmer, S.C.; Webster, A.C. Polyclonal and monoclonal antibodies for induction therapy in kidney transplant recipients. *Cochrane Database Syst. Rev.* **2017**, *1*, CD004759. [CrossRef]

13. Organ Procurement and Transplantation Network and Scientific Registry of Transplant Recipients 2010 data report. *Am. J. Transplant.* **2012**, *12* (Suppl. 1), 1–156. [CrossRef]

14. Jordan, C.L.; Taber, D.J.; Kyle, M.O.; Connelly, J.; Pilch, N.W.; Fleming, J.; Meadows, H.B.; Bratton, C.F.; Nadig, S.N.; McGillicuddy, J.W.; et al. Incidence, risk factors, and outcomes of opportunistic infections in pediatric renal transplant recipients. *Pediatr. Transplant.* **2016**, *20*, 44–48. [CrossRef] [PubMed]

15. López-Medrano, F.; Fernández-Ruiz, M.; Silva, J.T.; Carver, P.L.; van Delden, C.; Merino, E.; Pérez-Saez, M.J.; Montero, M.; Coussement, J.; de Abreu Mazzolin, M.; et al. Multinational case-control study of risk factors for the development of late invasive pulmonary aspergillosis following kidney transplantation. *Clin. Microbiol. Infect.* **2018**, *24*, 192–198. [CrossRef] [PubMed]

16. Lebeaux, D.; Freund, R.; van Delden, C.; Guillot, H.; Marbus, S.D.; Matignon, M.; Van Wijngaerden, E.; Douvry, B.; De Greef, J.; Vuotto, F.; et al. Outcome and Treatment of Nocardiosis After Solid Organ Transplantation: New Insights from a European Study. *Clin. Infect. Dis.* **2017**, *64*, 1396–1405. [CrossRef]

17. Singh, N.; Dromer, F.; Perfect, J.R.; Lortholary, O. Cryptococcosis in solid organ transplant recipients: Current state of the science. *Clin. Infect. Dis.* **2008**, *47*, 1321–1327. [CrossRef]

18. Port, F.K.; Bragg-Gresham, J.L.; Metzger, R.A.; Dykstra, D.M.; Gillespie, B.W.; Young, E.W.; Delmonico, F.L.; Wynn, J.J.; Merion, R.M.; Wolfe, R.A.; et al. Donor characteristics associated with reduced graft survival: An approach to expanding the pool of kidney donors. *Transplantation* **2002**, *74*, 1281–1286. [CrossRef]

19. Levey, A.S.; Eckardt, K.U.; Tsukamoto, Y.; Levin, A.; Coresh, J.; Rossert, J.; De Zeeuw, D.; Hostetter, T.H.; Lameire, N.; Eknoyan, G. Definition and classification of chronic kidney disease: A position statement from Kidney Disease: Improving Global Outcomes (KDIGO). *Kidney Int.* **2005**, *67*, 2089–2100. [CrossRef] [PubMed]

20. Loupy, A.; Haas, M.; Solez, K.; Racusen, L.; Glotz, D.; Seron, D.; Nankivell, B.J.; Colvin, R.B.; Afrouzian, M.; Akalin, E.; et al. The Banff 2015 Kidney Meeting Report: Current Challenges in Rejection Classification and Prospects for Adopting Molecular Pathology. *Am. J. Transplant.* **2017**, *17*, 28–41. [CrossRef]

21. Kotton, C.N.; Kumar, D.; Caliendo, A.M.; Huprikar, S.; Chou, S.; Danziger-Isakov, L.; Humar, A. The Transplantation Society International CMV Consensus Group. The Third International Consensus Guidelines on the Management of Cytomegalovirus in Solid-organ Transplantation. *Transplantation* **2018**, *102*, 900–931. [CrossRef] [PubMed]

22. Humar, A.; Michaels, M. Monitoring AIWGoID. American Society of Transplantation recommendations for screening, monitoring and reporting of infectious complications in immunosuppression trials in recipients of organ transplantation. *Am. J. Transplant.* **2006**, *6*, 262–274. [CrossRef] [PubMed]

23. 1993 revised classification system for HIV infection and expanded surveillance case definition for AIDS among adolescents and adults. *MMWR Recomm. Rep.* **1992**, *41*, 1–19.

24. Nankivell, B.J.; Renthawa, J.; Sharma, R.N.; Kable, K.; O'Connell, P.J.; Chapman, J.R. BK Virus Nephropathy: Histological Evolution by Sequential Pathology. *Am. J. Transplant.* **2017**, *17*, 2065–2077. [CrossRef]

25. Penn, I. Kaposi's sarcoma in transplant recipients. *Transplantation* **1997**, *64*, 669–673. [CrossRef]

26. Ekberg, H.; Bernasconi, C.; Tedesco-Silva, H.; Vítko, S.; Hugo, C.; Demirbas, A.; Acevedo, R.R.; Grinyó, J.; Frei, U.; Vanrenterghem, Y.; et al. Calcineurin inhibitor minimization in the Symphony study: Observational results 3 years after transplantation. *Am. J. Transplant.* **2009**, *9*, 1876–1885. [CrossRef]

27. Fagiuoli, S.; Colli, A.; Bruno, R.; Craxì, A.; Gaeta, G.B.; Grossi, P.; Mondelli, M.U.; Puoti, M.; Sagnelli, E.; Stefani, S.; et al. Management of infections pre- and post-liver transplantation: Report of an AISF consensus conference. *J. Hepatol.* **2014**, *60*, 1075–1089. [CrossRef]

28. Crepin, T.; Carron, C.; Roubiou, C.; Gaugler, B.; Gaiffe, E.; Simula-Faivre, D.; Ferrand, C.; Tiberghien, P.; Chalopin, J.M.; Moulin, B.; et al. ATG-induced accelerated immune senescence: Clinical implications in renal transplant recipients. *Am. J. Transplant.* **2015**, *15*, 1028–1038. [CrossRef]

29. López-Medrano, F.; Fernández-Ruiz, M.; Silva, J.T.; Carver, P.L.; van Delden, C.; Merino, E.; Pérez-Saez, M.J.; Montero, M.; Coussement, J.; de Abreu Mazzolin, M.; et al. Clinical Presentation and Determinants of Mortality of Invasive Pulmonary Aspergillosis in Kidney Transplant Recipients: A Multinational Cohort Study. *Am. J. Transplant.* **2016**, *16*, 3220–3234. [CrossRef]

30. Tullius, S.G.; Milford, E. Kidney allocation and the aging immune response. *N. Engl. J. Med.* **2011**, *364*, 1369–1370. [CrossRef]

31. Meier-Kriesche, H.U.; Ojo, A.O.; Hanson, J.A.; Kaplan, B. Exponentially increased risk of infectious death in older renal transplant recipients. *Kidney Int.* **2001**, *59*, 1539–1543. [CrossRef]

32. Tesar, B.M.; Du, W.; Shirali, A.C.; Walker, W.E.; Shen, H.; Goldstein, D.R. Aging augments IL-17 T-cell alloimmune responses. *Am. J. Transplant.* **2009**, *9*, 54–63. [CrossRef]

33. Denecke, C.; Bedi, D.S.; Ge, X.; Kim, I.K.; Jurisch, A.; Weiland, A.; Habicht, A.; Li, X.C.; Tullius, S.G. Prolonged graft survival in older recipient mice is determined by impaired effector T-cell but intact regulatory T-cell responses. *PLoS ONE* **2010**, *5*, e9232. [CrossRef]

34. Mouillot, G.; Carmagnat, M.; Gérard, L.; Garnier, J.L.; Fieschi, C.; Vince, N.; Karlin, L.; Viallard, J.F.; Jaussaud, R.; Boileau, J.; et al. B-cell and T-cell phenotypes in CVID patients correlate with the clinical phenotype of the disease. *J. Clin. Immunol.* **2010**, *30*, 746–755. [CrossRef] [PubMed]

35. Hellemans, R.; Hazzan, M.; Durand, D.; Mourad, G.; Lang, P.; Kessler, M.; Charpentier, B.; Touchard, G.; Berthoux, F.; Merville, P.; et al. Daclizumab Versus Rabbit Antithymocyte Globulin in High-Risk Renal Transplants: Five-Year Follow-up of a Randomized Study. *Am. J. Transplant.* **2015**, *15*, 1923–1932. [CrossRef] [PubMed]

36. Brennan, D.C.; Schnitzler, M.A. Long-term results of rabbit antithymocyte globulin and basiliximab induction. *N. Engl. J. Med.* **2008**, *359*, 1736–1738. [CrossRef]

37. Thomusch, O.; Wiesener, M.; Opgenoorth, M.; Pascher, A.; Woitas, R.P.; Witzke, O.; Jaenigen, B.; Rentsch, M.; Wolters, H.; Rath, T.; et al. Rabbit-ATG or basiliximab induction for rapid steroid withdrawal after renal transplantation (Harmony): An open-label, multicentre, randomised controlled trial. *Lancet* **2016**, *388*, 3006–3016. [CrossRef]

38. Hellemans, R.; Bosmans, J.L.; Abramowicz, D. Induction Therapy for Kidney Transplant Recipients: Do We Still Need Anti-IL2 Receptor Monoclonal Antibodies? *Am. J. Transplant.* **2017**, *17*, 22–27. [CrossRef]

39. Colvin, M.; Smith, J.M.; Hadley, N.; Skeans, M.A.; Carrico, R.; Uccellini, K.; Lehman, R.; Robinson, A.; Israni, A.K.; Snyder, J.J.; et al. OPTN/SRTR 2016 Annual Data Report: Heart. *Am. J. Transplant.* **2018**, *18* (Suppl. 1), 291–362. [CrossRef]

40. Pascual, J.; Berger, S.P.; Witzke, O.; Tedesco, H.; Mulgaonkar, S.; Qazi, Y.; Chadban, S.; Oppenheimer, F.; Sommerer, C.; Oberbauer, R.; et al. Everolimus with Reduced Calcineurin Inhibitor Exposure in Renal Transplantation. *J. Am. Soc. Nephrol.* **2018**, *29*, 1979–1991. [CrossRef]

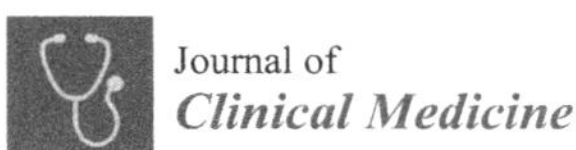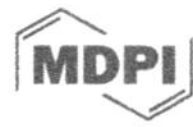

Journal of
Clinical Medicine

Article

Higher Incidence of BK Virus Nephropathy in Pediatric Kidney Allograft Recipients with Alport Syndrome

Young Hoon Cho [1], Hye Sun Hyun [1,2], Eujin Park [1,3], Kyung Chul Moon [4], Sang-Il Min [5], Jongwon Ha [5,6], Il-Soo Ha [1], Hae Il Cheong [1], Yo Han Ahn [1,7,*,†] and Hee Gyung Kang [1,*,†]

[1] Department of Pediatrics, Seoul National University College of Medicine and Seoul National University Hospital, Seoul 03080, Korea; tccyh@hanmail.net (Y.H.C.); inthy@naver.com (H.S.H.); eujinpark@hallym.or.kr (E.P.); ilsooha@snu.ac.kr (I.-S.H.); cheonghi@snu.ac.kr (H.I.C.)
[2] Department of Pediatrics, St. Vincent's Hospital, College of Medicine, The Catholic University College of Korea, Seoul 06591, Korea
[3] Department of Pediatrics, Kangnam Sacred Heart Hospital, Hallym University College of Medicine, Seoul 07441, Korea
[4] Department of Pathology, Seoul National University College of Medicine, Seoul 03080, Korea; blue7270@gmail.com
[5] Department of Surgery, Seoul National University College of Medicine, Seoul 03080, Korea; surgenmsi@gmail.com (S.-I.M.); jwhamd@snu.ac.kr (J.H.)
[6] Transplantation Research Institute, Seoul National University College of Medicine, Seoul 03080, Korea
[7] Department of Pediatrics, Seoul National University Bundang Hospital, Seongnam 13620, Korea
* Correspondence: yhahn@snubh.org (Y.H.A.); kanghg@snu.ac.kr (H.G.K.); Tel.: +82-31-787-7294 (Y.H.A.); +82-2-2072-0658 (H.G.K.)
† These authors equally contributed to this article.

Received: 7 March 2019; Accepted: 8 April 2019; Published: 11 April 2019

Abstract: A retrospective review was performed to assess the risk factors and outcomes of BK virus infection and nephropathy (BKVN), an early complication in pediatric kidney allograft recipients. The study investigated the incidence, risk factors, and clinical outcomes of BK viremia and BKVN in a Korean population of pediatric patients who received renal transplantation from 2001–2015 at the Seoul National University Hospital. BKVN was defined as biopsy-proven BKVN or plasma BK viral loads >10,000 copies/mL for >3 weeks. BK viremia was defined as a BK viral load >100 copies/mL in blood. Among 168 patients assessed for BK virus status, 30 patients (17.9%) tested positive for BK viremia at a median of 12.6 months after transplantation. BKVN was diagnosed in six patients (3.6%) at a median of 13.4 months after transplantation. Three of the six BKVN patients had Alport syndrome ($p = 0.003$), despite this disease comprising only 6% of the study population. Every patient with BK viremia and Alport syndrome developed BKVN, while only 11.1% of patients with BK viremia progressed to BKVN in the absence of Alport syndrome. Multivariate analysis revealed that Alport syndrome was associated with BKVN development (hazard ratio 13.2, $p = 0.002$). BKVN treatment included the reduction of immunosuppression, leflunomide, and intravenous immunoglobulin. No allografts were lost in the two years following the diagnosis of BKVN. In summary, the incidence of BKVN in pediatric kidney allograft recipients was similar to findings in previous reports, but was higher in patients with underlying Alport syndrome.

Keywords: BK virus; BK virus nephropathy; kidney allograft; transplantation; Alport syndrome; children

---

1. Introduction

BK virus (BKV) is a polyomavirus that resides in the urogenital tract as a latent infection [1]. The seroprevalence of BKV in the first decade of life is 90% or higher [1,2], implying that most primary infections occur during childhood. In immunocompromised patients, reactivation of a latent infection is frequently observed [1,3] as BK virus nephropathy (BKVN) or hemorrhagic cystitis [1,4]. While hemorrhagic cystitis frequently develops in patients with hematologic stem cell transplantation, BKVN is essentially a complication of kidney transplantation [2,5]. BKVN has recently gained clinical significance with the introduction of potent immunosuppressive agents. The prevalence of BKVN in adult kidney allograft recipients is 1% to 10% [2,5,6] and has been reported to be 2% to 8% in pediatric renal transplant recipients [7,8]. BKVN is considered to be an early complication of kidney transplantation that often occurs in the first year of transplantation; 95% of BKVN develops within two years of transplantation according to the organization Kidney Disease: Improving Global Outcomes (KDIGO), but it may develop as late as in the fifth year [9–11]. Importantly, after BKVN is diagnosed, over 15% of patients are expected to lose their allograft kidney within one year [9].

Risk factors for BKVN in kidney allograft recipients include older age, male sex, ethnicity (non-African American), increased number of human leukocyte antigen (HLA) mismatches, prolonged cold-ischemia time, ureteral stent placement, immunosuppression induction with anti-thymocyte globulin, tacrolimus- and/or mycophenolate mofetil-based maintenance immunosuppression, and prior rejection history [3,12]. The most important risk factor for BKVN is considered to be the degree of immunosuppression [12]. However, risk factors for BKVN in children have not yet been studied sufficiently. In a retrospective cohort study of children, a seronegative status for BKV in recipients was associated with BKVN [13].

To gain a better understanding of BKVN in pediatric kidney transplantation recipients, the clinical characteristics and risk factors for BK virus infection and BKVN in pediatric kidney allograft recipients was assessed in this study.

2. Methods

2.1. Study Population and Ethics

We retrospectively reviewed the medical records of all pediatric kidney allograft recipients who underwent transplantation at the Seoul National University Hospital between January 2001 and July 2015. Clinical findings until July 2018 were assessed. This study was approved by the Institutional Review Board of the Seoul National University Hospital (IRB no. 1808-156-967) and was conducted in accordance with the Declaration of Helsinki.

2.2. Immunosuppression

The immunosuppression protocol of the Seoul National University Hospital consisted of steroids, tacrolimus, and mycophenolate mofetil. Methylprednisolone was administered as a 10 mg/kg intravenous bolus dose at the time of surgery and was tapered gradually to a maintenance dose of prednisolone 0.3 mg/kg by one month after transplantation. In patients with a low risk of rejection, prednisolone was discontinued by one year after transplantation. The tacrolimus target trough level was 8–12 ng/mL for up to three months, 6–8 ng/mL until six months, and 4–6 ng/mL thereafter. From 2001 to 2008, basiliximab was used as an induction therapy for high-risk patients with a transplanted kidney from a deceased donor or a high number of HLA mismatches. After 2008, all patients received basiliximab induction therapy.

2.3. BK Viremia and BKVN

BK virus DNA in the plasma of patients was tested by polymerase chain reaction (PCR) to detect the large T antigen of BKV (BKV ELITe kit, ELITechGroup, Puteaux, France). BK viral load quantification became available as of June 2008 and thereafter BK viral load of >100 copies/mL was considered as BK viremia. In principle, since 2008, BK viremia was screened every month for three months after transplantation, then every three months for one year, and then every year up to five years. BK virus was additionally screened in patients with an unexplained acute rise in serum creatinine or in patients receiving acute rejection treatment. Upon detection, BK viremia was followed every month. Persisting BK virus PCR loads over 10,000 copies/mL for >3 weeks was categorized as presumptive BKVN, as described previously [6]. Presumptive BKVN and pathologically proven BKVN were collectively categorized as BKVN to assess the risk factors for BKVN in this study. Histologic grading of BKVN was classified according to the criteria of the University of Maryland, USA [14].

2.4. Statistical Analysis

SPSS version 23.0 (SPSS, Armonk, NY, USA) was used for data analysis. Categorical variables were analyzed using the Pearson chi-square test or Fisher exact test and continuous variables were compared using the *t*-test or Mann–Whitney U test. All values were reported as a median (range). To assess risk factors for BKVN, univariate analysis was performed using the Kaplan–Meier test with the log-rank test and multivariate analysis was done using the Cox proportional hazards model. Factors with a value of $p < 0.25$ in the univariate analysis were included in the multivariate analysis. A value of $p < 0.05$ was considered statistically significant.

3. Results

A total of 195 patients younger than 20 years underwent allograft kidney transplantation between January 2001 and July 2015, and of these, 168 were tested for BK virus by PCR more than once (Table 1). BK viremia was positive in 30 patients (17.9%, 30/168) at 12.6 months (0.4–73.1 months) after transplantation (Figure 1). BKVN was diagnosed in six patients (3.6%, 6/168, BKVN group) at 13.4 months (3.9–60.0 months) after transplantation, with a BK viral titer at first detection of 46,508 copies/mL (16,924–289,699 copies/mL) at 10.9 months (1.5–60.0 months) and 306,277 copies/mL (41,914–10,165,852 copies/mL) at the peak at 14.2 months (4.3–60.3 months). The BK viral titer in the 24 patients with BK viremia but not BKVN (only-BK viremia group) was 437 copies/mL (119–6794 copies/mL) at first detection at 12.6 months (0.4–73.1 months) after kidney transplantation, and increased to 561 copies/mL (123–42,288 copies/mL) copies/mL at 15.3 months (0.4–73.7 months).

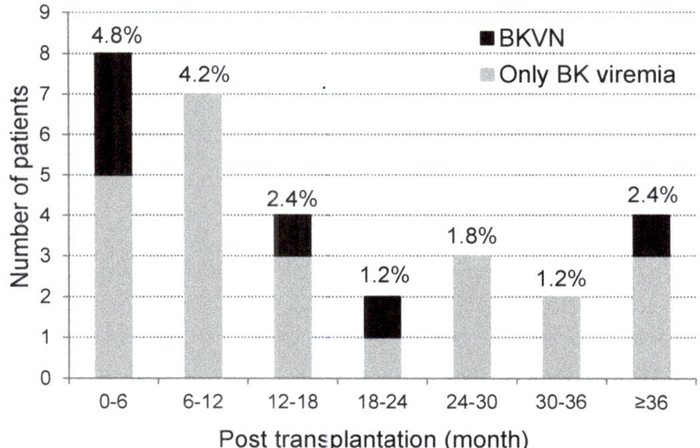

Figure 1. Onset of BK viremia after kidney transplantation. Values are represented as number of patients (% of total subject population).

Table 1. Baseline characteristics of patients with or without BK virus nephropathy.

Characteristic	BKVN (*n* = 6)	Non-BKVN (*n* = 162)	Total (*n* = 168)	*p*-Value
Sex, M:F	3:3	98:64	101:67	0.684
Recipient age at transplant, years	13.9 (7.7–18.9)	13.2 (1.5–19.9)	13.3 (1.5–19.9)	0.587
Primary kidney disease				
Glomerulopathy	5 (83.3)	85 (52.5)	90 (53.6)	0.282
CAKUT	0	36 (22.2)	36 (21.4)	
Other	1	41 (25.3)	42 (25.0)	
Alport syndrome	3 (50.0)	7 (4.3)	10 (6.0)	0.003
Donor type				
Deceased donor	3 (50.0)	63 (38.9)	66 (39.3)	0.681
Living donor	3 (50.0)	99 (61.1)	102 (60.7)	
Recipient age at transplant, years				
0 to <7	0	28 (17.3)	28 (16.7)	0.285
7 to <13	2 (33.3)	52 (32.1)	54 (32.1)	
≥13	4 (66.7)	82 (50.6)	86 (51.2)	
HLA mismatch				
0–2	0	35 (21.6)	35 (20.8)	0.578
3–4	6 (100)	112 (69.1)	118 (70.2)	
5–6	0	15 (9.3)	15 (8.9)	
Acute cellular rejection	4/6 (66.7)	95/151 (62.9)	99/157 (63.1)	1.000
Immunosuppression				
MMF	6	162	168	1.000
Tac	6	161 (99.4)	167 (99.4)	1.000
BSX	6	131 (80.9)	137 (81.5)	0.594
ATG	0	9 (5.6)	9 (5.4)	1.000
Transplant year				
2001–2008	0	47 (29.0)	47 (28.0)	0.187
2009–2015	6	115 (71.0)	121 (72.0)	
CMV infection	3/5 (60)	60/131 (45.8)	63/136 (46.3)	0.663
EBV infection	1/4 (25)	70/132 (53.0)	71/136 (52.2)	0.348
Pneumocystis jirovecii pneumonia	0	6 (3.7)	6 (3.6)	1.000
PTLD	0	8 (4.9)	8 (4.8)	1.000
Comorbidity				
Hypertension	2 (33.3)	27 (16.7)	29 (17.3)	0.277
Cardiovascular disease [1]	0	8 (4.9)	8 (4.8)	1.000
Diabetes mellitus	0	9 (5.6)	9 (5.4)	1.000
Dyslipidemia	0	10 (6.2)	10 (6.0)	1.000
Neurological disorder [2]	0	14 (8.6)	14 (8.3)	1.000
Liver disease [3]	1 (16.7)	7 (4.3)	8 (4.8)	0.257
Cancer except PTLD	0	1 (0.6)	1(0.6)	1.000
Mortality	0	2 (1.2)	2 (1.2)	1.000

[1] Cardiomyopathy, myocarditis, congenital heart defect, and myocardial infarction. [2] Developmental delay, congenital malformations of the nervous system, and epilepsy. [3] Hepatitis, fatty liver, congenital hepatic fibrosis, and liver cirrhosis. Values are expressed as numbers (%) and median (range). Abbreviations: BKVN: BK virus nephropathy; CAKUT: congenital anomalies of the kidney and the urinary tract; HLA: human leukocyte antigen; MMF: mycophenolate mofetil; Tac: tacrolimus; BSX: basiliximab; ATG: anti-thymocyte globulin; CMV: cytomegalovirus; EBV: Epstein–Barr virus; PTLD: post-transplant lymphoproliferative disease.

3.1. Risk Factors for BKVN and BK Viremia

To assess the risk factors for BKVN, the BKVN group (*n* = 6) and the remaining patients—including the BK viremia group and those who had not shown BK viremia (*n* = 162, non-BKVN group, Table 1)—were compared. There were no statistically significant differences in sex, age at transplant, primary kidney disease, donor source, HLA mismatch, induction with polyclonal or monoclonal antibody, prior acute rejection, and Epstein–Barr virus or cytomegalovirus infection. None of the BKVN patients had a ureteral stent placed after kidney transplantation. Interestingly, as a primary kidney disease of their native kidneys, Alport syndrome was significantly more common in the BKVN group compared to the non-BKVN group (50% vs. 4.3%, *p* = 0.003). Multivariate analysis using Cox proportional analysis also showed that Alport syndrome was a significant risk factor for BKVN (Table 2).

Table 2. Risk factors for BK virus nephropathy.

Factors	Univariate	Multivariate [1]	
	p-Value	Hazard Ratio (95% CI)	*p*-Value
Alport syndrome	<0.001	13.204 (2.662–65.502)	0.002
HLA mismatch ≥3	0.206	NS	0.984
Basiliximab	0.224	NS	0.975
Transplant year, 2009–2015	0.108	NS	0.976

[1] Factors with a value of $p < 0.25$ in the univariate analysis were included in the multivariate analysis. Abbreviations: CI: confidence interval; NS: not significant; HLA: human leukocyte antigen.

Comparison of the BK viremia group and non-BK viremia group revealed that basiliximab induction therapy and transplant in the years after 2008 were significantly higher in the BK viremia group than in the non-BK viremia group (Table S1). Multivariable Cox hazards regression analysis showed that induction with basiliximab was a significant risk factor for the development of BK viremia (Table S2).

Comparison between the BKVN group and the non-BKVN BK viremia group (BK viremia-only group) revealed no significant differences between the two groups, except for BK viral load and Alport syndrome (Table S3).

3.2. Clinical Course of BKVN

Among the six patients in the BKVN group, four had pathologically-proven BKVN and the remaining two presented with presumptive BKVN. BKVN was managed with the reduction of immunosuppressive medications, intravenous immunoglobulin, leflunomide, ciprofloxacin, or cidofovir (Table 3). Three of the six patients had a pathological diagnosis of acute rejection along with BKVN on an allograft kidney biopsy, and were also treated with intravenous methylprednisolone.

After a 2.2–8.3-year follow-up, no patients experienced graft loss, but impairment of renal function was evident (median estimated glomerular filtration rate 39.9 (range, 20.7–56.9) mL/min/1.73 m^2). BK viremia was only cleared in three patients over a median of 20.5 months (range, 16.6–89.9 months) after the first detection of viremia.

Table 3. The clinical course of patients with BKVN.

Patient No.	Sex/Age at BKVN (yr)	Primary Disease	Transplant Year/Donor Type	Onset of Viremia after KT	Initial Level [1] (Copies/mL)	Peak Level [2] (Copies/mL)	Biopsy Grade	Treatment	Follow up after BKVN	Time to Viremia Clearance
1	F/8.0	ATN	2009/D	1.5 mo	16,924	10,165,852	B1	Reduction of IS, IVIG, leflunomide	8.3 yr	89.9 mo
2	F/20.6	Alport	2010/D	60.3 mo	289,699	289,699	B3	Reduction of IS, IVIG, leflunomide	3.0 yr	No
3	M/13.1	Alport	2010/L	24.0 mo	41,914	41,914	B1	Reduction of IS, IVIG, leflunomide	6.4 yr	No
4	M/15.0	Alport	2014/L	15.9 mo	68,919	2,266,980	B1	Reduction of IS, IVIG, leflunomide, ciprofloxacin, cidofovir	2.2 yr	No
5	F/16.8	FSGS	2014/L	4.6 mo	51,102	322,854	ND	Reduction of IS, leflunomide, ciprofloxacin	3.8 yr	16.6 mo
6	M/19.5	FSGS	2015/D	6.0 mo	25,555	62,481	ND	Reduction of IS, leflunomide	2.4 yr	20.5 mo

[1] The value of BK virus load when BK viremia was first detected. [2] The highest value of BK virus load. Abbreviations: BKVN: BK virus nephropathy; S-Cr: serum creatinine; ATN: acute tubular necrosis; VUR: vesicoureteral regurgitation; FSGS: focal segmental glomerulosclerosis; D: deceased; L: living; ND: not done; IS: immunosuppressant; IVIG: intravenous immunoglobulin; mo: months; yr: year.

3.3. Alport Syndrome and BKVN

Although Alport syndrome comprised 6% of the study population (10 of 168 patients), as the primary disease of the native kidneys it accounted for 50% of BKVN patients. The prevalence of BK viremia was 30% (3 of 10 patients) for Alport syndrome, and all BK viremia in patients with Alport syndrome progressed to BKVN, whereas BK viremia was found in 17.1% of the remaining patients (other than Alport syndrome as their primary disease, 27 of 158 patients), and only 11.1% of those with BK viremia progressed to BKVN. In addition, BK viremia was detected relatively late in patients with Alport syndrome at 16, 24, and 60 months after transplantation (Table 3), and the initial viral load was higher, with a median 68,919 copies/mL (versus 4773 copies/mL in others with BK viremia, $p = 0.001$). BK viremia did not resolve in these patients, despite treatment for more than 2.2 years. BKVN-free survival curves of individuals with Alport syndrome and other patient groups also showed significant differences (Kaplan–Meier analysis, log-rank test $p < 0.001$, Figure 2).

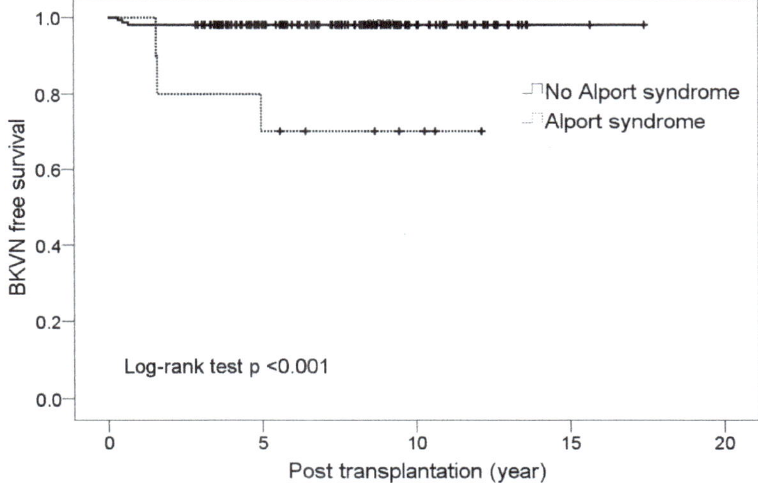

Figure 2. Kaplan–Meier curves indicating progression to BK virus nephropathy after renal transplantation.

4. Discussion

In our study, the prevalence of BK viremia was 17.8% in pediatric kidney allograft recipients, which was similar to that shown in previous studies in adults (11% to 25%) [4,11,15] and pediatric kidney recipients (21%) [16]. The prevalence of BKVN in our pediatric kidney transplantation recipients was 3.6%, which was similar to the 4.6% reported by the North American Pediatric Renal Trials and Collaborative Studies registry [8]. BK viremia was observed immediately following kidney transplantation (0.4 months) in a minority of patients, but most cases occurred sometime after the surgery. This suggested that most patients may have contracted BKV from their peers, as primary infections of BK virus usually occur in childhood [17]. However, the pre-donation BKV status of donors had not been assessed at Seoul National University Hospital until recently, and therefore data was unavailable to help assess the source of the BK virus infection. Interestingly, all patients with BKVN received their allograft kidney after 2009 and were older than seven years; however, neither of these parameters were statistically significant, likely due to the small size of the study population. Nevertheless, regarding why BKVN only occurred after 2009, it was speculated that: (1) BK monitoring was more aggressive after 2009, as was the availability of BK viremia quantitation protocols, and (2) immunosuppression became more potent with the awareness of antibody-mediated rejection associated with insufficient immunosuppression. BKVN in individuals older than seven years may reflect the timing of primary infection or a selection bias resulting from the small pool of younger recipients.

In this study, previously known risk factors in the adult population such as older age and type of immunosuppression were not identified as risk factors for BK viremia and BKVN. This was likely due to the relatively homogenous population in the study, as the Korean pediatric population evaluated mostly underwent induction treatment with monoclonal antibodies and maintenance treatment with tacrolimus and mycophenolate mofetil. Male sex and an increased number of HLA mismatches were not significant factors in this population, although there were no BKVN patients with zero HLA mismatches. Data relative to ischemia time was not available in this study, but the distribution of donor types did not differ between the groups, implying that ischemia time was not associated with BKVN in this population. Ureteral stent placement was previously indicated as a significant risk factor for BKVN [12], but in this study, no BKVN patients were subjected to ureteral stent placement. Acute rejection was more common in the BK viremia group and in the BKVN group compared with the BK viremia-free group, but there was no statistically significant difference either. While previous studies showed that the primary cause of end-stage renal disease was not a risk factor for BKVN in children [8,13,18], in this study population, Alport syndrome was a risk factor for BKVN. Alport syndrome is caused by a genetic defect in type IV collagen which comprises basement membranes. It is a rare hereditary disorder with an incidence of 1 in 50,000 persons [19], but it is relatively common in the pediatric population as a cause of end-stage renal disease compared to the adult population. Although Alport syndrome has not been previously reported to be a risk factor for BKVN, a study of kidney transplantations in Australia and New Zealand from 1965 to 2010 reported that BKVN ($n = 6$) was found only in the group with Alport syndrome, and not in the group without Alport syndrome in a group of 243 patients [20].

Thus, the question arises: how can the finding that Alport syndrome is a risk factor of BKVN be explained? Interestingly, BKVN developed in every patient with BK viremia if the patient had Alport syndrome, while only one-tenth of patients with BK viremia progressed to BKVN (3 of 27) when Alport syndrome patients were excluded. Hence, it is speculated that tubular cells in Alport syndrome patients might be more prone to BK virus propagation, possibly because of the defective distal tubular basement membrane [21]. The gradual repopulation of recipient cells in the allograft kidney has been documented previously [22]; therefore, the vulnerability of individuals with Alport syndrome might appear gradually, which might explain the delayed occurrence of BKVN. Alternatively, BK viremia screening might not be performed sufficiently early in these patients, resulting in the propagation of BKV irrespective of immunosuppression, and later the development of BKVN. Nonetheless, further study with larger populations is necessary to validate the notion that Alport syndrome is a risk factor for BKVN.

Screening for BK viremia is recommended for the prevention and early detection of BKVN [11]. Guidelines recommend screening for BK viremia regularly (every month for three to six months after transplantation, then every three months for one or two years, and then every year up to five years) with creatinine elevation and after acute rejection treatment [10]. Considering that Alport syndrome was a significant risk factor for BKVN in this study, a more meticulous screening for Alport syndrome patients is recommended, and for a longer period after kidney transplantation [23]. When BK viremia is detected from screening, it is recommended that immunosuppression be reduced [24,25]. In this study, by reducing immunosuppression, most cases of BK viremia resolved and did not progress to BKVN. Once BKVN is diagnosed, there are a few treatment options available in addition to the reduction of immunosuppression [2,6,10], with intravenous immunoglobulin treatment, fluoroquinolone, cidofovir, and leflunomide being reported as partially effective [26]. Most of our BKVN patients were treated with these methods and no allografts were lost. Nevertheless, neither allograft renal function of BKVN patients nor eradication of BK viremia was satisfactory, as both persisted in three patients with Alport syndrome.

A shortcoming of this study is that it was a retrospective study of a small patient population. Immunosuppression protocols have changed over time, and this factor could not be controlled well. In addition, not all the cases of BKVN were confirmed by an allograft kidney biopsy. Nonetheless, considering the pediatric focus of the study, the population size was appreciable, and a relatively good outcome of BKVN was evident with the application of aggressive treatment.

5. Conclusions

The incidence of BKVN was 3.6% in pediatric kidney allograft recipients at Seoul National University Hospital, and BKVN was associated with the underlying disease, Alport syndrome. Following aggressive treatment, no BKVN cases resulted in the loss of an allograft kidney for over two years. Further study with a larger population is necessary to validate the notion that Alport syndrome is a risk factor for BKVN.

Supplementary Materials: The following are available online at http://www.mdpi.com/2077-0383/8/4/491/s1. Table S1: Baseline characteristics of patients with and without BK viremia, Table S2: Risk factors for BK viremia, Table S3: Comparison between the BKVN group and only-BK viremia groups.

Author Contributions: Conceptualization, Y.H.C., H.S.H., E.P., K.C.M., S.-I.M., J.H., I.-S.H., H.I.C., Y.H.A., and H.G.K.; Methodology, Y.H.C., I.-S.H., H.I.C., Y.H.A., and H.G.K.; Formal analysis, Y.H.C. and Y.H.A.; Investigation, Y.H.C., H.S.H., and E.P.; Data curation, H.S.H, E.P., K.C.M., S.-I.M.; Writing—original draft preparation, Y.H.C. and H.G.K.; Writing—review and editing, Y.H.A. and H.G.K.; Visualization, Y.H.C. and Y.H.A.; Supervision, J.H., I.-S.H., H.I.C., Y.H.A., and H.G.K.

Conflicts of Interest: The authors declare no conflict of interest.

References

1. Reploeg, M.D.; Storch, G.A.; Clifford, D.B. BK virus: A clinical review. *Clin. Infect. Dis.* **2001**, *33*, 191–202. [CrossRef] [PubMed]

2. Hirsch, H.H.; Randhawa, P. BK polyomavirus in solid organ transplantation. *Am. J. Transplant.* **2013**, *13*, 179–188. [CrossRef] [PubMed]

3. Randhawa, P.; Brennan, D.C. BK virus infection in transplant recipients: An overview and update. *Am. J. Transplant.* **2006**, *6*, 2000–2005. [CrossRef] [PubMed]

4. Herman, J.; Van Ranst, M.; Snoeck, R.; Beuselinck, K.; Lerut, E.; Van Damme-Lombaerts, R. Polyomavirus infection in pediatric renal transplant recipients: Evaluation using a quantitative real-time PCR technique. *Pediatr. Transplant.* **2004**, *8*, 485–492. [CrossRef]

5. Hirsch, H.H.; Steiger, J. Polyomavirus BK. *Lancet Infect. Dis.* **2003**, *3*, 611–623. [CrossRef]

6. Hirsch, H.H.; Brennan, D.C.; Drachenberg, C.B.; Ginevri, F.; Gordon, J.; Limaye, A.P.; Mihatsch, M.J.; Nickeleit, V.; Ramos, E.; Randhawa, P.; et al. Polyomavirus-associated nephropathy in renal transplantation: Interdisciplinary analyses and recommendations. *Transplantation* **2005**, *79*, 1277–1286. [CrossRef]

7. Acott, P.D.; Hirsch, H.H. BK virus infection, replication, and diseases in pediatric kidney transplantation. *Pediatr. Nephrol.* **2007**, *22*, 1243–1250. [CrossRef]

8. Smith, J.M.; Dharnidharka, V.R.; Talley, L.; Martz, K.; McDonald, R.A. BK virus nephropathy in pediatric renal transplant recipients: An analysis of the North American Pediatric Renal Trials and Collaborative Studies (NAPRTCS) registry. *Clin. J. Am. Soc. Nephrol.* **2007**, *2*, 1037–1042. [CrossRef]

9. Ramos, E.; Drachenberg, C.B.; Papadimitriou, J.C.; Hamze, O.; Fink, J.C.; Klassen, D.K.; Drachenberg, R.C.; Wiland, A.; Wali, R.; Cangro, C.B.; et al. Clinical course of polyoma virus nephropathy in 67 renal transplant patients. *J. Am. Soc. Nephrol.* **2002**, *13*, 2145–2151. [CrossRef]

10. Disease, K. Improving global outcomes (KDIGO) transplant work group. KDIGO clinical practice guideline for the care of kidney transplant recipients. *Am. J. Transplant.* **2009**, *3*, S1–S155.

11. Almeras, C.; Vetromile, F.; Garrigue, V.; Szwarc, I.; Foulongne, V.; Mourad, G. Monthly screening for BK viremia is an effective strategy to prevent BK virus nephropathy in renal transplant recipients. *Transpl. Infect. Dis.* **2011**, *13*, 101–108. [CrossRef]

12. Sawinski, D.; Goral, S. BK virus infection: An update on diagnosis and treatment. *Nephrol. Dial. Transplant.* **2015**, *30*, 209–217. [CrossRef] [PubMed]

13. Smith, J.M.; McDonald, R.A.; Finn, L.S.; Healey, P.J.; Davis, C.L.; Limaye, A.P. Polyomavirus nephropathy in pediatric kidney transplant recipients. *Am. J. Transplant.* **2004**, *4*, 2109–2117. [CrossRef]

14. Drachenberg, R.C.; Drachenberg, C.B.; Papadimitriou, J.C.; Ramos, E.; Fink, J.C.; Wali, R.; Weir, M.R.; Cangro, C.B.; Klassen, D.K.; Khaled, A. Morphological spectrum of polyoma virus disease in renal allografts: Diagnostic accuracy of urine cytology. *Am. J. Transplant.* **2001**, *1*, 373–381. [CrossRef]

15. Gabardi, S.; Waikar, S.S.; Martin, S.; Roberts, K.; Chen, J.; Borgi, L.; Sheashaa, H.; Dyer, C.; Malek, S.K.; Tullius, S.G. Evaluation of fluoroquinolones for the prevention of BK viremia after renal transplantation. *Clin. J. Am. Soc. Nephrol.* **2010**, *5*, 1298–1304. [CrossRef] [PubMed]

16. Ginevri, F.; Azzi, A.; Hirsch, H.H.; Basso, S.; Fontana, I.; Cioni, M.; Bodaghi, S.; Salotti, V.; Rinieri, A.; Botti, G. Prospective monitoring of polyomavirus BK replication and impact of pre-emptive intervention in pediatric kidney recipients. *Am. J. Transplant.* **2007**, *7*, 2727–2735. [CrossRef] [PubMed]

17. Hirsch, H.H. BK virus: Opportunity makes a pathogen. *Clin. Infect. Dis.* **2005**, *41*, 354–360. [CrossRef] [PubMed]

18. Ginevri, F.; De Santis, R.; Comoli, P.; Pastorino, N.; Rossi, C.; Botti, G.; Fontana, I.; Nocera, A.; Cardillo, M.; Ciardi, M.R. Polyomavirus BK infection in pediatric kidney-allograft recipients: A single-center analysis of incidence, risk factors, and novel therapeutic approaches. *Transplantation* **2003**, *75*, 1266–1270. [CrossRef] [PubMed]

19. Kruegel, J.; Rubel, D.; Gross, O. Alport syndrome—insights from basic and clinical research. *Nat. Rev. Nephrol.* **2013**, *9*, 170–178. [CrossRef]

20. Mallett, A.; Tang, W.; Clayton, P.A.; Stevenson, S.; McDonald, S.P.; Hawley, C.M.; Badve, S.V.; Boudville, N.; Brown, F.G.; Campbell, S.B. End-stage kidney disease due to Alport syndrome: Outcomes in 296 consecutive Australia and New Zealand Dialysis and Transplant Registry cases. *Nephrol. Dial. Transplant.* **2014**, *29*, 2277–2786. [CrossRef] [PubMed]

21. Heidet, L.; Gubler, M.C. The renal lesions of Alport syndrome. *J. Am. Soc. Nephrol.* **2009**, *20*, 1210–1215. [CrossRef]

22. Lagaaij, E.L.; Cramer-Knijnenburg, G.F.; van Kemenade, F.J.; van Es, L.A.; Bruijn, J.A.; van Krieken, J.H. Endothelial cell chimerism after renal transplantation and vascular rejection. *Lancet* **2001**, *357*, 33–37. [CrossRef]

23. Almeras, C.; Foulongne, V.; Garrigue, V.; Szwarc, I.; Vetromile, F.; Segondy, M.; Mourad, G. Does reduction in immunosuppression in viremic patients prevent BK virus nephropathy in de novo renal transplant recipients? A prospective study. *Transplantation* **2008**, *85*, 1099–1104. [CrossRef]

24. Saad, E.R.; Bresnahan, B.A.; Cohen, E.P.; Lu, N.; Orentas, R.J.; Vasudev, B.; Hariharan, S. Successful treatment of BK viremia using reduction in immunosuppression without antiviral therapy. *Transplantation* **2008**, *85*, 850–854. [CrossRef]

25. Sood, P.; Senanayake, S.; Sujeet, K.; Medipalli, R.; Zhu, Y.R.; Johnson, C.P.; Hariharan, S. Management and outcome of BK viremia in renal transplant recipients: A prospective single-center study. *Transplantation* **2012**, *94*, 814–821. [CrossRef]

26. Wali, R.K.; Drachenberg, C.; Hirsch, H.H.; Papadimitriou, J.; Nahar, A.; Mohanlal, V.; Brisco, M.A.; Bartlett, S.T.; Weir, M.R.; Ramos, E. BK virus-associated nephropathy in renal allograft recipients: Rescue therapy by sirolimus-based immunosuppression. *Transplantation* **2004**, *78*, 1069–1073. [CrossRef]

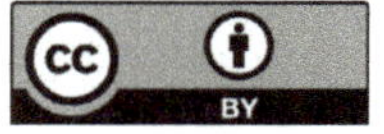

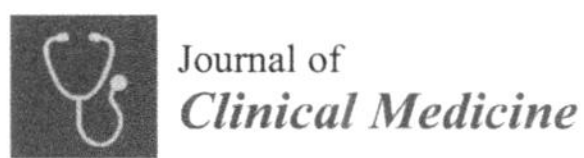 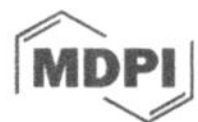

Journal of
Clinical Medicine

Article

Plasma Malondialdehyde and Risk of New-Onset Diabetes after Transplantation in Renal Transplant Recipients: A Prospective Cohort Study

Manuela Yepes-Calderón [1], Camilo G. Sotomayor [1,*], António W. Gomes-Neto [1], Rijk O.B. Gans [2], Stefan P. Berger [1], Gerald Rimbach [3], Tuba Esatbeyoglu [4], Ramón Rodrigo [5], Johanna M. Geleijnse [6], Gerjan J. Navis [1] and Stephan J.L. Bakker [1]

[1] Division of Nephrology, Department of Internal Medicine, University Medical Center Groningen, University of Groningen, 9713 GZ Groningen, The Netherlands; manueyepes@gmail.com (M.Y.-C.); a.w.gomes.neto@umcg.nl (A.W.G.-N.); s.p.berger@umcg.nl (S.P.B.); g.j.navis@umcg.nl (G.J.N.); s.j.l.bakker@umcg.nl (S.J.L.B.)

[2] Department of Internal Medicine, University Medical Center Groningen, University of Groningen, 9713 GZ Groningen, The Netherlands; r.o.b.gans@umcg.nl

[3] Institute of Human Nutrition and Food Science, Christian-Albrechts-University of Kiel, Herrmann Rodewaldstrasse 6, D-24118 Kiel, Germany; rimbach@foodsci.uni-kiel.de

[4] Institute of Food Science and Human Nutrition, Department Food Development and Food Quality, Gottfried Wilhelm Leibniz University Hannover, Am Kleinen Felde 30, D-30167 Hannover, Germany; esatbeyoglu@lw.uni-hannover.de

[5] Molecular and Clinical Pharmacology Program, Institute of Biomedical Sciences, Faculty of Medicine, University of Chile, Av. Independencia 1027, CP 8380453 Santiago, Chile; rrodrigo@med.uchile.cl

[6] Division of Human Nutrition and Health, Wageningen University and Research, P.O. Box 47, 6700 AA Wageningen, The Netherlands; Marianne.geleijnse@wur.nl

* Correspondence: c.g.sotomayor.campos@umcg.nl; Tel.: +31-061-921-08-81

Received: 17 February 2019; Accepted: 30 March 2019; Published: 4 April 2019

Abstract: New-onset diabetes after transplantation (NODAT) is a frequent complication in renal transplant recipients (RTR). Although oxidative stress has been associated with diabetes mellitus, data regarding NODAT are limited. We aimed to prospectively investigate the long-term association between the oxidative stress biomarker malondialdehyde (measured by high-performance liquid chromatography) and NODAT in an extensively phenotyped cohort of non-diabetic RTR with a functioning graft $\geq$1 year. We included 516 RTR (51 $\pm$ 13 years-old, 57% male). Median plasma malondialdehyde (MDA) was 2.55 (IQR, 1.92–3.66) μmol/L. During a median follow-up of 5.3 (IQR, 4.6–6.0) years, 56 (11%) RTR developed NODAT. In Cox proportional-hazards regression analyses, MDA was inversely associated with NODAT, independent of immunosuppressive therapy, transplant-specific covariates, lifestyle, inflammation, and metabolism parameters (HR, 0.55; 95% CI, 0.36–0.83 per 1-SD increase; $p < 0.01$). Dietary antioxidants intake (e.g., vitamin E, α-lipoic acid, and linoleic acid) were effect-modifiers of the association between MDA and NODAT, with particularly strong inverse associations within the subgroup of RTR with relatively higher dietary antioxidants intake. In conclusion, plasma MDA concentration is inversely and independently associated with long-term risk of NODAT in RTR. Our findings support a potential underrecognized role of oxidative stress in post-transplantation glucose homeostasis.

Keywords: malondialdehyde; oxidative stress; new-onset diabetes; renal transplantation

---

1. Introduction

New-onset diabetes after transplantation (NODAT) is a major metabolic complication of solid organ transplantation, with a reported incidence of up to 50% [1]. Consequences of NODAT are detrimental for renal transplant recipients (RTR) as it is associated with reduced recipient survival, increased rate of cardiovascular events, and impaired graft survival in the long term [2,3]. In the era of high-dose steroid regimens, twelve-months cumulative incidence of NODAT was significantly higher, and the main risk factor identified for the occurrence of NODAT was immunosuppressant therapy [3]. However, with new cyclosporine-based and tacrolimus-based regimens [1,4], it is well-documented that the largest number of incident cases of NODAT occurred, indeed, after the first year of transplantation [4,5], and other agents potentially involved in the long-term pathogenesis of the disease remain to be elucidated. In order to improve the outcomes of RTR, it is of great interest to know which factors contribute to this long-term NODAT development and maintenance [2].

Oxidative stress (OS) is a factor that in different studies has been linked with both physiological response to insulin and pathophysiological mechanisms of, e.g., diabetes mellitus; it is also known to be enhanced in RTR when compared to general population [6]. Higher levels of OS biomarkers, e.g., MDA [7], have been found in patients with established diabetes mellitus compared to healthy controls [8], and in patients with diabetes-associated complications compared to patients with noncomplicated diabetes [9]. However, a developing body of evidence has linked oxidative species with insulin signaling [10–13], and it has been postulated that diabetes mellitus is—to a considerable extent—caused by a failure of the organism to create enough oxidative redox potential [14]. There is, nevertheless, only limited data relating OS with insulin resistance in prediabetes states [15]. Furthermore, to the extent of our knowledge, no longitudinal studies have aimed to study the association between OS biomarkers and long-term incidence of diabetes, which makes it difficult to foresee whether OS biomarkers may prospectively be associated with positive or negative outcomes regarding glucose metabolism outcomes.

In post-transplantation setting, less evidence is available regarding the role of OS on glucose homeostasis. Indeed, the long-term prospective association of systemic OS and the development of NODAT has not been explored. The primary objective of the present study was set to test the hypothesis that post-transplantation OS is associated with the development of NODAT. Furthermore, by considering evidence reporting an effect of dietary antioxidant intake on the development of type 2 diabetes and NODAT [16,17], we aimed to assess whether the potential association of MDA with NODAT may be modified by regular dietary antioxidant fatty acids intake. Finally, we investigated whether OS is associated with the secondary end-points of long-term all-cause mortality, cardiovascular mortality, and graft failure.

2. Materials and Methods

2.1. Study Design and Patient Population

In this prospective cohort study, all adult RTR with a functioning graft for at least one year who visited the outpatient clinic at the University Medical Center of Groningen (The Netherlands) between November 2008 and May 2011 were considered eligible to participate. Baseline data was obtained at least one year after transplantation with a median of five years. We excluded RTR with diabetes mellitus at baseline or before transplant (defined as fasting plasma glucose $\geq$126 mg/dL (7.0 mmol/L) and/or use of glucose lowering drugs) (n = 173); also patients who underwent combined pancreas-kidney transplantation (n = 5) or whose plasma MDA concentration measurement at baseline was missing (n = 12), resulting in 516 RTR eligible for statistical analyses. The patients were followed-up until 1 April 2014. Collection of these data was ensured by the continuous surveillance system of the outpatient clinic of our university hospital and close collaboration with affiliated hospitals. Follow-up was performed according to the guidelines of the American Society of Transplantation [18].

The primary end-point of the current study was the long-term development of NODAT. Secondary end points were all cause-mortality, cardiovascular mortality, and graft failure. No participants were lost due to follow-up. The current study was approved by the institutional review board (METc 2008/186) and adhered to the Declarations of Helsinki and Istanbul.

2.2. Data Collection

Baseline data was collected during a visit to the outpatient clinic, following a detailed protocol described elsewhere [19]. Anthropometric measurements were taken while participants wore indoor clothing without shoes. Systolic blood pressure (SBP) and diastolic blood pressure (DBP) were measured using a semiautomatic device (Dinamap1846; Critikon, Tampa, FL, USA) every minute for 15 min, following a strict protocol as described before [20].

Three questionnaires were administered to patients: first, the Short QUestionnaire to ASsess Health-enhancing physical activity (SQUASH) score for information about the daily physical activity [21]. Second, a questionnaire regarding smoking behavior to classify patients as current, previous or never smokers. Third, a semiquantitative self-administered food frequency questionnaire (FFQ) of 177 items to collect information on dietary intake during the past month. The FFQ was developed at Wageningen university, previously validated for our population, and it has been updated several times [22]. Number of servings was recorded in natural units (e.g., slice of bread) or household measures (e.g., a teaspoon). Subsequently, all dietary data were converted into total energy and nutrient intake per day, using the Dutch Food Composition Table 2006 [23]. Specific nutrient intakes were adjusted for total energy intake according to the residual method [24].

Of note, except for discouraging excess sodium intake and encouraging weight loss in overweight individuals, no specific dietary counseling was included, nor was dietary recommendation regarding antioxidant fatty acids intake or supplementation advised to the study subjects. Other relevant recipient and transplant information was extracted from the Groningen Renal Transplant Database, as described in detail before [25].

2.3. Measurements and Definitions

Fasting blood samples and complete 24-hour urine collection were taken at baseline. Serum creatinine was determined by using the Jaffe reaction (MEGA AU510; Merck Diagnostica, Darmstadt, Germany); plasma glucose by the glucose oxidase method (YSI 2300 Stat Plus; Yellow Springs Instruments, Yellow Springs, OH, USA); total cholesterol by the cholesterol oxidase-phenol aminophenazone method (MEGA AU510); HDL cholesterol by the cholesterol oxidase-phenol aminophenazone method on a Technicon RA-1000 (Bayer Diagnostics, Mijdrecht, the Netherlands); and plasma triglycerides by the glycerol-3-phosphate oxidase-oxidase method (YSI 2300 Stat Plus). LDL cholesterol was calculated by using the Friedewald equation; estimated glomerular filtration rate (eGFR) by the serum creatinine based Chronic Kidney Disease EPIdemiology collaboration equation (CKD-EPI) [26]; and the cumulative dose of prednisolone as the sum of the maintenance dose of prednisolone from transplantation until baseline. Plasma MDA concentration was chosen as the biomarker of OS because it has been used before in studies regarding pathologies of the glucose metabolism [8,9]; it was measured by high-performance liquid chromatography with a photodiode array detector as described by Faizan et al. to improve the sensitivity offered by spectrophotometrically methods [27].

NODAT was defined according to the International Expert Panel recommendations based on the 2003 American Diabetes Association criteria [28] and the HbA1c criterion proposed by the International Expert Panel of the international consensus meeting on post transplantation diabetes mellitus [29]. The diagnosis was made with the fulfillment of one or more of the following: symptoms of diabetes (classic symptoms, including polyuria, polydipsia, and unexplained weight loss) plus random plasma glucose concentration $\geq$200 mg/dL (11.1 mmol/L); fasting plasma glucose $\geq$126 mg/dL (7.0 mmol/L); plasma HbA1c $\geq$ 6.5%; or use of glucose-lowering medication. If fasting plasma glucose was elevated, a confirmatory laboratory test was performed, after which the diagnosis of NODAT was made.

Cardiovascular death was defined as the principal cause of death being cardiovascular in nature (International Classification of Diseases (ICD)-9 codes 410–447). The cause of death was obtained by linking the number of the death certificate to the primary cause of death as coded by a physician from the Central Bureau of Statistics according to the ICD-9 [30]. Graft failure was defined as restart of dialysis or retransplantation.

2.4. Statistical Analyses

Data analyses, computations, and graphs were performed with SPSS 22.0 software (IBM Corporation, Chicago, IL, USA), R version 3.2.3 software (The R-Foundation for Statistical Computing, Vienna, Austria), and GraphPad Prism version 7 software (GraphPad Software, San Diego, CA, USA). For descriptive statistics data are presented as mean ± standard deviation (SD) for normally distributed data, and as median (interquartile range (IQR)) for variables with a non-normal distribution. Categorical data are expressed as number (percentage). Crude and age, sex, and eGFR-adjusted linear regression analyses were performed to examine the association of baseline characteristics with circulating MDA. Residuals were checked for normality and natural log-transformed when appropriate. In order to study in an integrated manner which baseline variables were independently associated with and were determinants of circulating MDA, we performed stepwise backwards multivariable linear regression analyses. For inclusion and exclusion in these analyses, p-values were set at 0.2 and 0.05, respectively.

NODAT development was visualized by Kaplan–Meier curves according to tertiles of plasma MDA concentration, with statistical significance among curves tested by log-rank (Mantel–Cox) test. The prospective association of plasma MDA concentration with the different outcomes was assessed through Cox regression analyses. We first performed crude analyses followed by additive adjustments for demographic and anthropometric factors (age, sex, and BMI) in model 1; metabolism-related variables (glucose, HbA1c, and HDL cholesterol) in model 2; lifestyle characteristics (current smoking, alcohol intake, and SQUASH score) in model 3; transplantation-related data (transplant vintage and eGFR) in model 4; immunosuppressive therapy (prednisolone dose and use of calcineurin inhibitors) in model 5; and inflammation (high sensitivity C-reactive protein (hs-CRP)) in model 6. NODAT and graft failure were censored at the date of last follow-up or death. Models were checked for the fulfillment of the assumptions of Cox regression analysis. The assumptions were met.

Furthermore, we performed prespecified analyses in which we tested for potential effect-modification by dietary intake of antioxidant fatty acids using multiplicative interaction terms over the fully adjusted model. In case of significant effect-modification, we proceeded with stratified prospective analyses for the concerned variable. Cut-off points of originally continuous variables used in the stratified analyses were determined so they would allow for an as much as possible similar number of events in each subgroup, and thus allow for similar statistical power for the assessment of the primary association under study (MDA concentration and NODAT) in each subgroup after stratification of the overall population. Since the number of events was reduced in each subgroup these analyses were adjusted analogous to model 3 of the overall prospective analyses to avoid overfitting. Also, since the dietary intake of antioxidant fatty acids could also be a potential confounder, we investigated if adjusting for this variable changed the association between MDA and NODAT.

For all statistical analyses, a statistical significance level of $p \leq 0.05$ (two-tailed) was used, except for the effect-modification analyses where the significance level was $p \leq 0.1$ (two-tailed) [31].

3. Results

3.1. Baseline Characteristics

In total 516 RTR (57% men) were included in the analyses with a mean ± SD age of 51 ± 13 years. Patients were included at a median of 5.2 (IQR 2.0–12.2) years after transplantation. The median plasma MDA concentration was 2.55 (IQR 1.92–3.66) μmol/L. Baseline characteristics of the overall RTR population are shown in Table 1. In crude linear regression analyses, glucose concentration had a significant direct association with plasma MDA concentration ($\beta = 0.10$, $p = 0.02$), which was not modified after adjustment for age, sex, and eGFR. Other variables with significant associations with plasma MDA concentration after adjustment were eGFR ($\beta = 0.10$, $p = 0.03$) and leucocytes concentration ($\beta = 0.10$, $p = 0.03$). A final reduced model of baseline variables obtained through backwards linear regression analyses ($\alpha = 0.05$) included glucose concentration ($\beta = 0.11$, $p = 0.02$), eGFR (β = 0.08, p = 0.09) leucocytes concentration (β = 0.10, p = 0.03), HDL concentration (β = 0.10, p = 0.04), and alcohol intake (β = −0.09, p = 0.07) (Table 1).

Table 1. Baseline characteristics of the study population and its association with circulating malondialdehyde (MDA) (n = 516).

Baseline Characteristics		Plasma MDA, Ln		
		Linear Regression [¥] Std. β	Adjusted Linear Regression [†] Std. β	Backwards Linear Regression [§] Std. β
Plasma MDA, µmol/L	2.55 (1.92–3.66)	–	–	–
Demographic and anthropometric				
Age, years	52 ± 13	0.01	0.02	
Male sex, n (%)	292 (57)	−0.06 *	−0.07 *	~
Weight, kg	79.0 ± 15.4	−0.04	−0.01	
Height, cm	174 ± 10	−0.04	0.02	
BMI, kg/m^2	26.0 ± 4.4	−0.03	−0.02	
Waist, cm [a]	96.4 ± 13.7	−0.07 *	−0.05	
Glucose and lipids metabolism				
Glucose, mmol/L(mg/dL) [b]	5.16 (93) ± 0.64 (11)	0.10 **	0.11 **	0.12 **
HbA1c, % [c]	5.67 ± 0.36	0.05	0.05	
Impaired fasting glucose, n (%)	122 (24)	0.06 *	0.07 *	~
Total cholesterol, mmol/L	5.12 ± 1.11	0.05	0.05	
HDL cholesterol, mmol/L [d]	1.3 (1.1–1.7)	0.09 **	0.06 *	0.09 **
LDL cholesterol, mmol/L [d]	3.0 ± 0.9	−0.04	−0.04	
Triglycerides, mmol/L [e]	1.62 (1.21–2.16)	0.03	0.05	
Transplantation-related data				
Time after transplant, years	5.2 (2.0–12.2)	0.03	0.02	
Living donor, n (%)	187 (36)	0.07 *	0.07 *	~
Pre-emptive, n (%)	92 (18)	0.03	0.02	
Immunosuppressive therapy				
Acute rejection treatment, n (%)	124 (24)	0.06 *	0.08 *	~
Use of calcineurin inhibitors				
Tacrolimus, n (%)	89 (17)	−0.01	0.02	
Cyclosporine, n (%)	194 (38)	−0.02	−0.01	
Use of proliferation inhibitors				
Azathriopine, n (%)	95 (18)	0.01	0.01	
Mycophenolic acid, n (%)	340 (66)	0.03	0.03	
Prednisolone cumulative dose, g	16.9 (5.8–36.3)	0.02	0.02	
Cardiovascular history				
History of CV disease, n (%) [f]	204 (40)	0.01	0.01	
SBP, mmHg [e]	135 ± 17	−0.03	−0.01	
DBP, mmHg [e]	83 ± 11	0.05	0.08 *	~
Use of antihypertensive medication, n (%)	448 (87)	−0.05	−0.02	
Graft function and inflammation				
Serum creatinine, µmol/L [d]	123 (100–159)	−0.07 *	0.12 *	~
eGFR (CKD-EPI), mL/mind [d]	53 ± 20	0.10 **	0.10 **	~
Protein excretion, g/day	0.18 (0.02–0.32)	0.01	0.04	
hs-CRP, mg/L [g]	1.4 (0.6–3.8)	<0.01	<0.01	
Leucocytes, × 10^9/L [e]	7.8 (6.3–9.6)	0.10 **	0.09 **	0.12 **
Nutrition				
Plasma albumin, g/L [d]	43.3 ± 3.0	0.002	−0.003	
Kcal intake, kcal/day [h]	2189 ± 617	−0.002	0.01	
Fatty acids intake [h]				
n-6 LA, g/day [∧]	15 (13–19)	0.03	0.05	
n-6 AA, g/day [∧]	0.05 (0.04–0.06)	0.02	0.02	
n-3 ALA, g/day [∧]	1.25 (1.02–1.60)	0.01	0.03	
n-3 EPA, g/day [∧]	0.04 (0.01–0.09)	0.05	0.05	
n-3 DHA, g/day [∧]	0.06 (0.03–0.13)	0.06	0.06	
Lifestyle				
Current smokers, n (%) [i]	67 (13)	−0.01	0.002	
Alcohol intake, g/day [h]	2.92 (0.04–11.52)	−0.08 *	−0.08 *	~
SQUASH-score, intensity × hours	5555 (2640–8513)	−0.02	<0.01	

* p value < 0.20; ** p value < 0.05. [¥] Crude linear regression analysis. [†] Linear regression analysis adjusted for age, sex, and eGFR. [§] Stepwise backwards linear regression analysis; for inclusion and exclusion in this analysis, p Values were set at 0.2 and 0.05, respectively. ~ Excluded from the final model. Data available in: [a] 499, [b] 514, [c] 495, [d] 455, [e] 515, [f] 398, [g] 484, [h] 468, [i] 490 patients. MDA, malondialdehyde; Std. β, standarized B coefficient; eGFR, estimated glomerular filtration rate; CV, cardiovascular; HbA1c, glycosylated hemoglobin; hs-CRP, high-sensitive C-reactive protein; kcal, kilocalories; LA, linoleic acid; AA, arachidonic acid; ALA, α-lipoic acid; EPA, eicosapentaenoic acid; DHA, docosahexaenoic acid. [∧] Adjusted for total caloric intake according to the residual method.

3.2. Prospective Analyses on NODAT

During a median follow-up of 5.3 (IQR 4.6–6.0) years, NODAT developed in 56 (11%) RTR. Kaplan–Meier curves for NODAT development by tertiles of RTRs according to circulating MDA are shown in Figure 1. NODAT distribution was significantly different according to the log-rank test (p = 0.02). Cox regression analyses showed that plasma MDA concentration is inversely associated with the risk of NODAT (HR, 0.61; 95% CI, 0.41–0.92 per 1-SD; p = 0.02). This association was independent of adjustment for demographic and anthropometric factors, metabolism-related variables, lifestyle factors, transplantation-related data, immunosuppressive medication, and inflammation (HR, 0.55; 95% CI, 0.36–0.83 per 1-SD; $p < 0.01$) (Table 2).

Plasma MDA concentration tertiles on NODAT

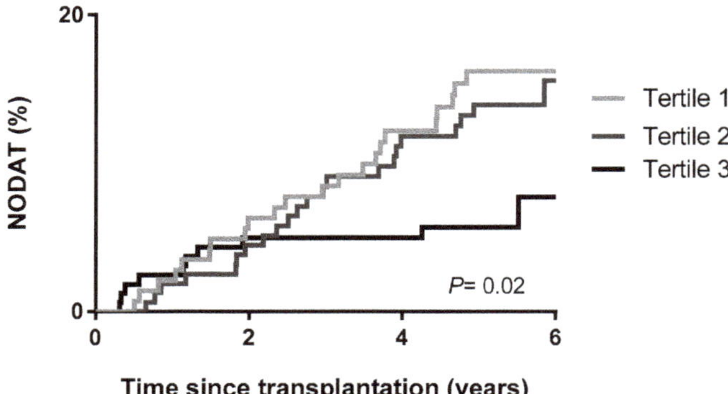

Figure 1. Kaplan–Meier curves for NODAT according to tertiles of plasma MDA concentration in RTR. Tertile 1: <2.15 μmol/L; Tertile 2: 2.15–3.09 μmol/L; Tertile 3: >3.09 μmol/L. *p* value was calculated by Log-rank (Mantel cox) test.

Table 2. Plasma MDA concentration and new-onset diabetes after transplantation (NODAT) in renal transplant recipients (RTR, n = 516).

NODAT	HR (95% CI) Per 1-SD	*p*
Crude model	0.61 (0.41–0.92)	0.02
Model 1	0.63 (0.42–0.94)	0.02
Model 2	0.54 (0.36–0.83)	<0.01
Model 3	0.54 (0.35–0.82)	<0.01
Model 4	0.56 (0.37–0.85)	<0.01
Model 5	0.55 (0.36–0.83)	<0.01
Model 6	0.55 (0.36–0.83)	<0.01

In total, 56 (11%) RTR developed NODAT. Model 1: crude model plus adjustment for demographic and anthropometric characteristics. Model 2: model 1 plus adjustment for metabolism-related variables. Model 3: model 2 plus adjustment for lifestyle characteristics. Model 4: model 3 plus adjustment for transplantation-related data. Model 5: model 4 plus adjustment for immunosuppressive therapy. Model 6: model 5 plus adjustment for inflammation.

3.3. Secondary Analysis on MDA and NODAT

In effect-modification analyses, we found that the association between MDA and the risk of NODAT was significantly modified by vitamin E, linoleic acid (LA), and α-lipoic acid (ALA) intake in regular diet ($p_{interaction}$ = 0.06, 0.02, and 0.02; respectively). Thus, we performed stratified prospective analyses by subgroups of RTR according to vitamin E intake ($\leq$ or >13.64 mg/day), LA intake ($\leq$ or >14 g/day) and ALA intake ($\leq$ or > or 1.24 g/day), in which cut-off points were determined so they would allow an as much as possible similar number of events in each subgroup. In each subgroup we assessed the association of MDA with development of NODAT and found that MDA was significantly inversely associated with the risk of NODAT in RTR with vitamin E intake >13.6 mg/day (HR, 0.52; 95% CI, 0.29–0.94 per 1-SD; p = 0.03), LA intake >14g/day (HR, 0.49; 95% CI 0.28–0.86 per 1-SD; p = 0.01), or ALA intake >1.24g/day (HR 0.42, 95% CI, 0.23–0.76 per 1-SD; $p < 0.01$), but not in the subgroups of relatively low intake (Figure 2).

Study subgroup	Subjects	Events of NODAT		Hazard ratio (95% CI)*	p-value	p_{interaction}

Study subgroup	Subjects	Events of NODAT	Hazard ratio (95% CI)*	p-value	$p_{interaction}$
Vitamin E intake					0.06
≤13.64 mg/day	193	22	0.66 (0.40–1.10)	0.11	
>13.64 mg/day	275	22	0.52 (0.29–0.94)	0.03	
LA intake					0.02
≤14 g/day	212	22	0.74 (0.45–1.20)	0.22	
>14 g/day	256	25	0.49 (0.28–0.86)	0.02	
ALA intake					0.02
≤1.24 g/day	227	21	0.80 (0.51–1.28)	0.36	
>1.24 g/day	241	26	0.42 (0.23–0.76)	0.005	

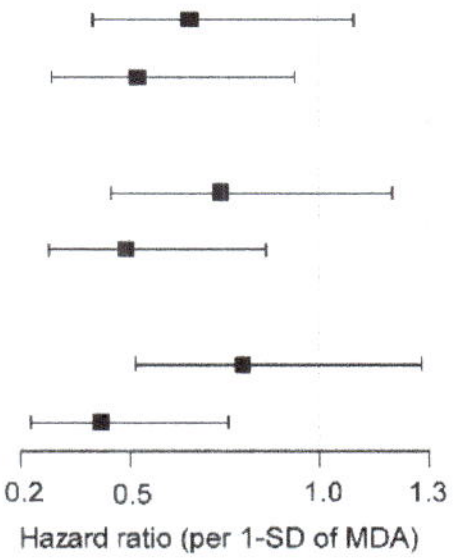

Figure 2. Stratified analysis of the association of plasma MDA concentrations with NODAT. * For the association between MDA and NODAT. HR are reported per 1-SD increase in plasma MDA concentration. Nutrient intake was adjusted for total energy intake according to the residual method. HR adjusted for age, sex, BMI, plasma glucose, HbA1c, smoking status, alcohol intake, and SQUASH score are shown.

Further, we performed Cox regression analyses with adjustment for these variables to explore if they might also be potential confounders. The association between MDA and NODAT was not significantly modified by additional adjustment for vitamin E intake (HR, 0.52; 95% CI, 0.34–0.81 per 1-SD; $p < 0.01$), ALA intake (HR, 0.55; 95% CI, 0.36–0.83 per 1-SD; $p < 0.01$), or LA intake (HR, 0.56; 95% CI, 0.37–0.84 per 1-SD; $p < 0.01$).

3.4. Prospective Analysis on All-Cause Mortality, Cardiovascular Mortality, and Graft Failure

During the same median follow up of 5.3 (IQR 4.6–5.9) years, 86 (17%) RTRs died, 29 (6%) from cardiovascular cause and 57 (11%) developed graft failure. In crude Cox regression analysis, plasma MDA concentration was not significantly associated with the risk of all-cause mortality (HR, 0.96; 95% CI, 0.73–1.25 per 1-SD; $p = 0.74$), cardiovascular mortality (HR, 0.81; 95% CI, 0.58–1.13 per 1-SD; $p = 0.21$), nor death-censored graft failure (HR, 0.89; 95% CI, 0.65–1.23 per 1-SD; $p = 0.49$). Further adjustments did not materially change these findings (Tables S1–S3).

4. Discussion

In a large cohort of stable RTR, we showed first that plasma MDA is directly associated with plasma glucose concentration. Second, plasma MDA is inversely associated with long-term risk of NODAT. This association remained present independent of potential confounders, including BMI, baseline glucose concentration and immunosuppressive therapy. Daily dietary intake of antioxidant fatty acids, e.g., vitamin E, LA and ALA were a significant effect-modifier of this association. No association was found whatsoever between MDA and all-cause mortality, cardiovascular mortality, or graft failure. These findings agree with developing evidence that proposes that oxidative status plays an important role in glucose homeostasis [10–13].

Experimental work has shown that reactive oxygen species (ROS) are part of intracellular insulin signal transmission [10,11]. ROS are upregulated in response to insulin and help to further up-regulate glucose-metabolism associated pathways related, e.g., with insulin-induced aerobic glycolysis [13]. Furthermore, ROS seem to have an effect on enzymes essential for catalytic activity, increasing glucose intake by skeletal muscle cells and glucose transport in adipocytes [11]. Also, human studies have shown that: (i) patients with severe deficiency of plasmatic antioxidants maintain supranormal insulin sensitivity, compared to healthy subjects, even if they are obese [12] and (ii) antioxidant molecules supplementation abrogates the usually generated increase in insulin sensitivity of patients on exercise interventions [32]. The current study, performed in a high-risk of new-onset diabetes population, provides for the first-time prospective evidence in line with aforementioned basic studies, and may further support the postulate of James Watson, according to which, diabetes mellitus may be caused by an incapacity of the cell to produce an oxidative redox environment [14].

Controversy may arise from data that has shown higher plasma MDA concentration in patients with diabetes mellitus than in healthy controls [8], and in patients who develop diabetes-related complications than in those without them [9]. However, it is known that ROS—as intracellular messengers—can generate opposite cellular effects. ROS can activate specific pathways whose products interfere with insulin signaling, e.g., the activation of the redox-sensitive nuclear factor-kappa beta (NF-kB) leads to the expression of cytokines such as tumoral necrosis factor α (TNF-α), and interleukins (ILs) such as IL-1β and IL-6 and all these products have a quenching effect on insulin signaling [11]. On the other hand, as mentioned before, ROS can activate signaling pathways important to fulfil insulin functions. Also, they are known to be themselves and stimuli to increase cellular antioxidant capacity [33] by the activation of specific response elements known as Nuclear factor-erythroid related factor 2- antioxidant response elements (Nrf2-ARE); this induction of endogenous antioxidant mechanisms by ROS has been specifically named mitochondrial hormesis and has gained interest in the last years [34], as it is proposed that, contrary to traditional thinking, ROS are not merely deleterious but they are necessary to reach oxidative balance inside the cell. Intensity, location, duration, and concentration of the oxidant stimulus seem to be crucial in defining whether ROS have a physiological or a pathological outcome. However, the specific thresholds that spawn the differential responses have not been determined yet [10,11]. This also might be a potential explanation of why studies regarding antioxidant supplementation have not shown to be beneficial in RTR [35], and why we did not find an association between OS and mortality, cardiovascular mortality, or graft failure.

Our data also provided evidence that LA, ALA, and vitamin E intake modify the association between MDA and NODAT. Conceivable interpretations of these findings are as follows: MDA is formed after the peroxidation of double bonds of unsaturated fatty acids such as LA [7]. Food containing important amounts of unsaturated fatty acids usually also contain substantial amounts of vitamin E, which prevents them from rancidification [36]. It is possible that in this context, high MDA concentration is a marker of a diet rich in antioxidants and unsaturated fatty acids, which has been suggested to reduce diabetes incidence [16,37]. However, when we adjusted for intake of these nutrients to evaluate them as potential confounders, the association between MDA and NODAT remained materially unaltered. An alternative explanation might be the aforementioned Nrf2-ARE pathway. This pathway has been of particular interest in the study of antioxidant molecules as therapeutic interventions, because previous authors have proposed that these interventions could show beneficial results if they were combined with unsaturated fatty acids as precursors of oxidative stress [38]. The rationale is that through Nrf2-ARE pathway activation, provision of pro-oxidant and antioxidants agents would trigger the antioxidant cellular defenses [33], thus yielding cell precondition to new oxidative challenges [39], and ultimately allowing cells to reach hormesis. This fits with our findings that high levels of MDA, although significantly inversely associated with NODAT in all our population, showed a stronger association in the patients with relatively higher intake of antioxidant in regular diet according to our subgroup analyses. Our findings might also support previous suggestions of potential protector effect of antioxidant-rich diets against NODAT [17].

The present study has several strengths. To the extent of our knowledge, it comprises the largest cohort of patients at risk of new-onset diabetes after transplantation in which the relationship between oxidative stress and NODAT has been evaluated. Moreover, our extensively phenotyped cohort allowed us to control for several potential confounders, among which anthropometric measurements, smoking status, baseline glucose metabolism markers, and immunosuppressive therapy were accounted for. Furthermore, NODAT cases were diagnosed according to International Expert Panel recommendations that were based on American Diabetes Association criteria [28], which agrees with usual clinical practice in transplant centers. Another strength of the study is that we included only stable RTRs who were 1-year post-transplantation, resulting in exclusion of transient post-transplantation hyperglycemia in NODAT diagnosis. Hyperglycemia is extremely common in the early posttransplant period and can occur as a result of rejection therapy, infections, and other critical conditions. Therefore, the formal diagnosis of NODAT in RTRs should only be based on likely maintenance of immunosuppression, stable kidney function, and absent acute infections [29]. The present study also has several limitations. It was carried out in a center with over-representation of Caucasian population, which calls prudence to extrapolation of our results to populations of other ethnicities. Another limitation of our study is that we only measured MDA concentrations in baseline samples. Most epidemiological studies use a single baseline measurement to predict outcomes, which adversely affects predictive properties of variables associated with outcomes. If intraindividual variability of predictive biomarkers is taken into account, this results in strengthening of predictive properties that, despite sometimes containing considerable intraindividual day-to-day variation, also existed for single measurements of these biomarkers [40,41]. The higher the intraindividual day-to-day variation is, the greater one would expect the benefit of repeated measurement for prediction of outcomes [40,41]. Next, although MDA has been the most commonly used OS biomarker in studies regarding glucose metabolism [9,10], further studies may want to account for other OS biomarkers to further validate our findings. Finally, the observational nature of this study makes it difficult to discern whether high levels of MDA are protective against NODAT or merely a marker of lower risk for NODAT; and, as with any observational study, residual confounding may have existed despite the substantial number of potentially confounding factors for which we adjusted, including well identified risk factors for NODAT.

In conclusion, plasma MDA concentration is inversely and independently associated with long-term risk of NODAT in stable RTR. This study provided for the first time relevant prospective data on the role of oxidative stress on glucose metabolism in a high-risk of diabetes population. This may further support already published basic studies and further promote studies to widen our knowledge on the role of oxidative stress in the pathophysiological mechanisms leading to diabetes and NODAT, which might be of relevant use in exploring novel therapeutic approaches to prevent and treat NODAT; also, it indicates that studies exploring antioxidant supplementation in RTR should explore and report metabolic outcomes in the long-term.

Supplementary Materials: The following are available online at http://www.mdpi.com/2077-0383/8/4/453/s1, Table S1: Plasma MDA concentration and all-cause mortality in RTR, Table S2: Plasma MDA concentration and cardiovascular mortality in RTR, Table S3: Plasma MDA concentration and dead-censored graft failure in RTR.

Author Contributions: Data curation, M.Y.-C., C.G.S., A.W.G.-N., and S.J.L.B.; Formal analysis, M.Y.-C., C.G.S. and A.W.G.-N.; Funding acquisition, M.Y.-C., C.G.S., and S.J.L.B.; Investigation, R.O.B.G., S.P.B., G.R., T.E., R.R., J.M.G., G.J.N. and S.J.L.B.; Methodology, G.R., T.E., J.M.G. and G.J.N.; Project administration, R.O.B.G., S.P.B., G.J.N. and S.J.L.B.; Resources, R.O.B.G. and S.P.B.; Supervision, R.R., G.J.N., and S.J.L.B.; Writing – original draft, M.Y.-C. and C.G.S.; Writing – review & editing, M.Y.-C., C.G.S., R.R. and S.J.L.B.

Funding: This study was based on the TransplantLines Food and Nutrition Biobank and Cohort Study (TxL-FN), which was funded by the Top Institute Food and Nutrition of the Netherlands (grant A-1003). The study is registered at clinicaltrials.gov under number NCT02811835.

Acknowledgments: Plasma MDA concentration was measured by Faizan et al. at the institute of Human Nutrition and Food Science, Christian Albrechts University of Kiel, Germany.

Conflicts of Interest: The authors declare no conflict of interest. The funders had no role in the design of the study; in the collection, analyses, or interpretation of data; in the writing of the manuscript, or in the decision to publish the results.

References

1. Montori, V.M.; Basu, A.; Erwin, P.J.; Velosa, J.A.; Gabriel, S.E.; Kudva, Y.C. Posttransplantation diabetes: A systematic review of the literature. *Diabetes Care* **2002**, *25*, 583–592. [CrossRef]

2. Rodrigo, E.; Fernandez-Fresnedo, G.; Valero, R.; Ruiz, J.C.; Pinera, C.; Palomar, R.; González-Cotorruelo, J.; Gómez-Alamillo, C.; Arias, M. New-Onset Diabetes after Kidney Transplantation: Risk Factors. *J. Am. Soc. Nephrol.* **2006**, *17*, S291–S295. [CrossRef]

3. Kaposztas, Z.; Gyurus, E.; Kahan, B.D. New-onset diabetes after renal transplantation: Diagnosis; incidence; risk factors; impact on outcomes; and novel implications. *Transplant. Proc.* **2011**, *43*, 1375–1394. [CrossRef]

4. Woodward, R.S.; Schnitzler, M.A.; Baty, J.; Lowell, J.A.; Lopez-Rocafort, L.; Haider, S.; Woodworth, T.G.; Brennan, D.C. Incidence and cost of new onset diabetes mellitus among U.S. wait-listed and transplanted renal allograft recipients. *Am. J. Transplant.* **2003**, *3*, 590–598. [CrossRef]

5. Cosio, F.G.; Pesavento, T.E.; Osei, K.; Henry, M.L.; Ferguson, R.M. Post-transplant diabetes mellitus: Increasing incidence in renal allograft recipients transplanted in recent years. *Kidney Int.* **2001**, *59*, 732–737. [CrossRef]

6. Pérez Fernandez, R.; Martín Mateo, M.C.; De Vega, L.; Bustamante Bustamante, J.; Herrero, M.; Bustamante Munguira, E. Antioxidant enzyme determination and a study of lipid peroxidation in renal transplantation. *Ren. Fail* **2002**, *24*, 353–359. [CrossRef]

7. Tsikas, D. Assessment of lipid peroxidation by measuring malondialdehyde (MDA) and relatives in biological samples, Analytical and biological challenges. *Anal. Biochem.* **2017**, *524*, 13–30. [CrossRef]

8. Noberasco, G.; Odetti, P.; Boeri, D.; Maiello, M.; Adezati, L. Malondialdehyde (MDA) level in diabetic subjects. Relationship with blood glucose and glycosylated hemoglobin. *Biomed. Pharmacother.* **1991**, *45*, 193–196. [CrossRef]

9. Zavar-Reza, J.; Shahmoradi, H.; Mohammadyari, A.; Mohammadbeigi, M.; Hosseini, R.; Vakili, M.; Barabadi, T.; DaneshPouya, F.; Tajik-kord, M.; Shahmoradi, E. Evaluation of Malondialdehyde (MDA) in type 2 diabetic Patients with Coronary Artery Disease (CAD). *J. Biol. Today's World* **2014**, *3*, 129–132. [CrossRef]

10. Zhang, Z.; Zhou, S.; Jiang, X.; Wang, Y.H.; Li, F.; Wang, Y.G.; Zheng, Y.; Cai, L. The role of the Nrf2/Keap1 pathway in obesity and metabolic syndrome. *Rev. Endocr. Metab. Disord.* **2015**, *16*, 35–45. [CrossRef]

11. Sottero, B.; Gargiulo, S.; Russo, I.; Barale, C.; Poli, G.; Cavalot, F. Postprandial Dysmetabolism and Oxidative Stress in Type 2 Diabetes: Pathogenetic Mechanisms and Therapeutic Strategies. *Med. Res. Rev.* **2015**, *35*, 968–1031. [CrossRef] [PubMed]

12. Schoenmakers, E.; Agostini, M.; Mitchell, C.; Schoenmakers, N.; Papp, L.; Rajanayagam, O.; Padidela, R.; Ceron-Gutierrez, L.; Doffinger, R.; Prevosto, C.; et al. Mutations in the selenocysteine insertion sequence-binding protein 2 gene lead to a multisystem selenoprotein deficiency disorder in humans. *J. Clin. Investig.* **2010**, *120*, 4220–4235. [CrossRef] [PubMed]

13. Li, Q.; Liu, X.; Yin, Y.; Zheng, J.T.; Jiang, C.F.; Wang, J.; Shen, H.; Li, C.Y.; Wang, M.; Liu, L.Z.; et al. Insulin Regulates Glucose Consumption and Lactate Production through Reactive Oxygen Species and Pyruvate Kinase M2. *Oxid. Med. Cell. Longev.* **2014**, *2014*, 504953. [CrossRef] [PubMed]

14. Watson, J.D. Type 2 diabetes as a redox disease. *Lancet* **2014**, *383*, 841–843. [CrossRef]

15. Meigs, J.B.; Larson, M.G.; Fox, C.S.; Keaney, J.F.; Vasan, R.S.; Benjamin, E.J. Association of Oxidative Stress, Insulin Resistance, and Diabetes Risk Phenotypes: the Framingham Offspring Study. *Diabetes Care* **2007**, *30*, 2529–2535. [CrossRef] [PubMed]

16. Montonen, J.; Knekt, P.; Järvinen, R.; Reunanen, A. Dietary Antioxidant Intake and Risk of Type 2 Diabetes. *Diabetes Care* **2004**, *27*, 362–366. [CrossRef]

17. Osté, M.C.J.; Corpeleijn, E.; Navis, G.J.; Keyzer, C.A.; Soedamah-Muthu, S.S.; van den Berg, E.; Postmus, D.; de Borst, M.H.; Kromhout, D.; Bakker, S.J.L. Mediterranean style diet is associated with low risk of new-onset diabetes after renal transplantation. *BMJ Open Diabetes Res. Care* **2017**, *5*, e000283. [CrossRef]

18. Kidney Disease: Improving Global Outcomes (KDIGO) Transplant Work Group. KDIGO Clinical Practice Guideline for the Care of Kidney Transplant Recipients. *Am. J. Transplant.* **2009**, *9*, S1–S155. [CrossRef]

19. van den Berg, E.; Engberink, M.F.; Brink, E.J.; van Baak, M.A.; Gans, R.O.; Navis, G.; Bakker, S.J. Dietary protein, blood pressure and renal function in renal transplant recipients. *Br. J. Nutr.* **2013**, *109*, 1463–1470. [CrossRef]

20. van den Berg, E.; Geleijnse, J.M.; Brink, E.J.; van Baak, M.A.; Homan van der Heide, J.J.; Gans, R.O.; Navis, G.; Bakker, S.J. Sodium intake and blood pressure in renal transplant recipients. *Nephrol. Dial. Transplant.* **2012**, *27*, 3352–3359. [CrossRef]

21. Wendel-Vos, G.C.W.; Schuit, A.J.; Saris, W.H.; Kromhout, D. Reproducibility and relative validity of the short questionnaire to assess health-enhancing physical activity. *J. Clin. Epidemiol.* **2003**, *56*, 1163–1169. [CrossRef]

22. Feunekes, G.I.; Van Staveren, W.A.; De Vries, J.H.; Burema, J.; Hautvast, J.G. Relative and biomarker-based validity of a food-frequency questionnaire estimating intake of fats and cholesterol. *Am. J. Clin. Nutr.* **1993**, *58*, 489–496. [CrossRef] [PubMed]

23. Stichting, N. *Nederlands Voedingsstoffen Bestand, NEVO Tabel 2006*; Dutch Nutrient Database; Voorlichtingsbureau voor de voiding: The Hague, The Netherlands, 2006.

24. Willett, W.C.; Howe, G.R.; Kushi, L.H. Adjustment for total energy intake in epidemiologic studies. *Am. J. Clin. Nutr.* **1997**, *65*, 1220S–1228S. [CrossRef]

25. De Vries, A.P.; Bakker, S.J.; Van Son, W.J.; Van Der Heide, J.J.; Ploeg, R.J.; The, H.T.; de Jong, P.E.; Gans, R.O. Metabolic Syndrome Is Associated with Impaired Long-term Renal Allograft Function; Not All Component criteria Contribute Equally. *Am. J. Transplant.* **2004**, *4*, 1675–1683. [CrossRef] [PubMed]

26. Levey, A.S.; Stevens, L.A.; Schmid, C.H.; Zhang, Y.L.; Castro, A.F.; Feldman, H.I.; Kusek, J.W.; Eggers, P.; Van Lente, F.; Greene, T.; et al. A new equation to estimate glomerular filtration rate. *Ann. Intern. Med.* **2009**, *150*, 604–612. [CrossRef] [PubMed]

27. Faizan, M.; Esatbeyoglu, T.; Bayram, B.; Rimbach, G. A fast and validated method for the determination of malondialdehyde in fish liver using high-performance liquid chromatography with a photodiode array detector. *J. Food Sci.* **2014**, *79*, 484–488. [CrossRef] [PubMed]

28. Davidson, J.; Wilkinson, A.; Dantal, J.; Dotta, F.; Haller, H.; Hernandez, D.; Kasiske, B.L.; Kiberd, B.; Krentz, A.; Legendre, C.; et al. New-onset diabetes after transplantation: 2003 international concensus guidelines. *Transplantation* **2003**, *75*, S3–S24. [CrossRef] [PubMed]

29. Sharif, A.; Hecking, M.; De Vries, A.P.J.; Porrini, E.; Hornum, M.; Rasoul-Rockenschaub, S.; Berlakovich, G.; Krebs, M.; Kautzky-Willer, A.; Schernthaner, G.; et al. Proceedings From an International Consensus Meeting on Posttransplantation Diabetes Mellitus, Recommendations and Future Directions. *Am. J. Transpl.* **2014**, *14*, 1992–2000. [CrossRef]

30. Zelle, D.M.; Corpeleijn, E.; Stolk, R.P.; de Greef, M.H.; Gans, R.O.; van der Heide, J.J.; Navis, G.; Bakker, S.J. Low Physical Activity and Risk of Cardiovascular and All-Cause Mortality in Renal Transplant Recipients. *Clin. J. Am. Soc. Nephrol.* **2011**, *6*, 898–905. [CrossRef]

31. Selvin, S. *Statistical Analysis of Epidemiologic Data*, 3rd ed.; Oxford University Press: New York, NY, USA, 2004.

32. Ristow, M.; Zarse, K.; Oberbach, A.; Klöting, N.; Birringer, M.; Kiehntopf, M.; Stumvoll, M.; Kahn, C.R.; Blüher, M. Antioxidants prevent health-promoting effects of physical exercise in humans. *Proc. Natl. Acad. Sci. USA* **2009**, *106*, 8665–8670. [CrossRef]

33. Rodrigo, R.; Prieto, J.C.; Castillo, R. Cardioprotection against ischaemia/reperfusion by vitamins C and E plus n-3 fatty acids: molecular mechanisms and potential clinical applications. *Clin. Sci. (Lond)* **2013**, *124*, 1–15. [CrossRef]

34. Ristow, M.; Schmeisser, S. Extending life span by increasing oxidative stress. *Free Radic. Biol. Med.* **2011**, *51*, 327–336. [CrossRef]

35. Blackhall, M.L.; Coombes, J.S.; Fassett, R. The Relationship between Antioxidant Supplements and Oxidative Stress in Renal Transplant Recipients: A Review. *ASAIO J.* **2004**, *50*, 451–457. [CrossRef]

36. Wood, J.D.; Enser, M. Factors influencing fatty acids in meat and the role of antioxidants in improving meat quality. *Br J. Nutr* **1997**, *78*, S49–S60. [CrossRef]

37. Risérus, U.; Willett, W.C.; Hu, F.B. Dietary fats and prevention of type 2 diabetes. *Prog. Lipid Res.* **2009**, *48*, 44–51. [CrossRef]

38. Sotomayor, C.G.; Cortés, I.A.; Gormaz, J.G.; Vera, S.; Libuy, M.; Valls, N.; Rodrigo, R. Role of Oxidative Stress in Renal TransplantationBases for an n-3 PUFA Strategy Against Delayed Graft Function. *Curr. Med. Chem.* **2017**, *24*, 1469–1485. [CrossRef]

39. Rodrigo, R.; Korantzopoulos, P.; Cereceda, M.; Asenjo, R.; Zamorano, J.; Villalabeitia, E.; Baeza, C.; Aguayo, R.; Castillo, R.; Carrasco, R.; et al. A Randomized Controlled Trial to Prevent Post-Operative Atrial Fibrillation by Antioxidant Reinforcement. *J. Am. Coll. Cardiol.* **2013**, *62*, 1457–1465. [CrossRef]

40. Koenig, W.; Sund, M.; Frohlich, M.; Lowel, H.; Hutchinson, W.L.; Pepys, M.B. Refinement of the Association of Serum C-Reactive Protein Concentration and Coronary Heart Disease Risk by Correction for within-Subject Variation Over Time: The MONICA Augsburg Studies, 1984 and 1987. *Am. J. Epidemiol.* **2003**, *158*, 357–364. [CrossRef]

41. Danesh, J.; Wheeler, J.G.; Hirschfield, G.M.; Eda, S.; Eiriksdottir, G.; Rumley, A.; Lowe, G.D.; Pepys, M.B.; Gudnason, V. C-Reactive Protein and Other Circulating Markers of Inflammation in the Prediction of Coronary Heart Disease. *N. Engl. J. Med.* **2004**, *350*, 1387–1397. [CrossRef]

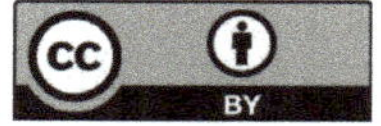

MDPI

St. Alban-Anlage 66

4052 Basel

Switzerland

Tel. +41 61 683 77 34

Fax +41 61 302 89 18

www.mdpi.com

Journal of Clinical Medicine Editorial Office

E-mail: jcm@mdpi.com

www.mdpi.com/journal/jcm